atlas of

general
surgical
technique

atlas of

general surgical technique

editors:

Francis E. Rosato, M.D.
Donna J. Barbot, M.D.

Department of Surgery
Jefferson Medical College of
Thomas Jefferson University Hospital
Philadelphia, Pennsylvania

consultant:

L. Brian Katz, M.D.

Mount Sinai Hospital
New York, New York

GOWER MEDICAL PUBLISHING
New York • London

Distributed in the USA and Canada by:
Raven Press
1185 Avenue of the Americas
New York, NY 10036
USA

Distributed in Japan by:
Nankodo Company Ltd.
42-6, Hongo 3-Chome
Bunkyo-Ku
Tokyo 113
Japan

Distributed in the rest of the world by:
Gower Medical Publishing
Middlesex House
34-42 Cleveland Street
London W1P 5FB
UK

Library of Congress Cataloging-in-Publication Data
Atlas of general surgical technique / editors: Francis E. Rosato,
        Donna J. Barbot.
                p.   cm.
        Includes bibliographical references and index.
        ISBN 0-397-44596-2
        1. Surgery, Operative—Atlases.   I. Rosato, Francis E.
II. Barbot, Donna J.
        [DNLM: 1. Surgery, Operative—methods—atlases.   WO 517 A8796]
        RD41.A78   1992
        617'.0022'2—dc20
        DNLM/DLC
        for Library of Congress   91-35429
                                                                         CIP

British Library Cataloguing in Publication Data
A catalogue record for this book is available from the British Library.

                Editors: Tim Condon, William Gabello
                Copyeditor: Joy Noel Travalino
        Illustration Supervisor: Carol Kalafatic
                Illustrators: Carol Kalafatic, Sharon T. Cavanaugh,
                        Angela DeLaura, Ruth Soffer (inking)
                Art Director: Jill Ruscoll
                Designer: Nava Anav

Printed in Singapore by Imago Productions (FE) Pte Ltd.

10 9 8 7 6 5 4 3 2 1

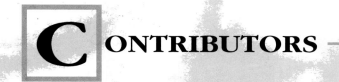

CONTRIBUTORS

Donna J. Barbot, M.D.

R. Anthony Carabasi, M.D.

Thomas L. Carter, Jr., M.D.

W. Bradford Carter, M.D.

Maryalice Cheney, M.D.

Herbert E. Cohn, M.D.

James E. Colberg, M.D.

Richard N. Edie, M.D.

John W. Francfort, M.D.

Diane R. Gillum, M.D.

Scott D. Goldstein, M.D.

Bruce E. Jarrell, M.D.

John D. Mannion, M.D.

Michael J. Moritz, M.D.

John S. Radomski, M.D.

Francis E. Rosato, M.D.

Anne L. Rosenberg, M.D.

John J. Shannon, M.D.

Stanton N. Smullens, M.D.

Robert W. Solit, M.D.

Jerome J. Vernick, M.D.

David A. Zwillenberg, M.D.

DEPARTMENT OF SURGERY
JEFFERSON MEDICAL COLLEGE OF THOMAS JEFFERSON
UNIVERSITY HOSPITAL
PHILADELPHIA, PENNSYLVANIA

PREFACE

This atlas of surgical technique was developed by members of the surgical department at Jefferson College of Thomas Jefferson University. We have asked each of the experts in our department to put down on paper the essentials needed for understanding and performing the surgical procedures in their fields of specialty. These procedures are illustrated with color diagrams and intraoperative photographs.

Although primarily geared for the surgical resident, this atlas also provides a ready basic reference on a broad range of procedures for the general surgeon. We have carefully reviewed the contents and feel that we have provided a sufficient number of individual procedures. We have also tried to offer a broad overview of each area, providing the necessary information on anatomy, exposure, and instrumentation. In this way, even if a specific procedure is not offered in detail, the reader can still attain an appreciation for concepts and technical considerations required for other or more complex operations in a particular area. No atlas can cover everything, but hopefully the material presented here is comprehensive enough to be useful to both the resident and the seasoned veteran.

We want to thank our authors for their diligent work on this large departmental project. Our special thanks go to John Novak, Jefferson's Video Production Specialist, who spent hours with our authors in the operating room to provide the intraoperative photos.

Francis E. Rosato
Donna J. Barbot
Editors

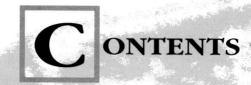ONTENTS

Chapter 1

ENDOCRINE SURGERY

Herbert E. Cohn, Thomas L. Carter, and
W. Bradford Carter

Chapter 2

HEAD AND NECK SURGERY

David A. Zwillenberg

Chapter 8

SURGERY OF THE LIVER AND BILIARY TREE

Francis E. Rosato and Donna J. Barbot

Chapter 9

SURGERY OF THE COLON, RECTUM, AND ANUS

Scott D. Goldstein and Maryalice Cheney

Chapter 10

HERNIA SURGERY

Donna J. Barbot and James E. Colberg

Chapter 11

VASCULAR SURGERY

Stanton N. Smullens and John W. Francfort

Chapter 12

RENAL AND HEPATIC TRANSPLANTATION SURGERY

Michael J. Moritz, John S. Radomski, R. Anthony Carabasi, and Bruce E. Jarrell

1

Endocrine Surgery

Herbert E. Cohn • Thomas L. Carter • W. Bradford Carter

SURGICAL ANATOMY

The thyroid gland is composed of two conical lobes joined by an isthmus that lies anterior to the second, third, and fourth tracheal rings. The superior parathyroid glands are found at the junction of the upper and middle thirds of the posterior thyroid capsule. The inferior parathyroids usually lie posteriorly or laterally on the lower thyroid poles. The thymus gland is an H-shaped organ located in the anterior mediastinum where it overlies the pericardium and great vessels (Fig. 1.1). The adrenals are small bilateral glands that sit atop the kidneys (Fig. 1.2).

THYROID GLAND SURGERY
RESECTION OF ONE LOBE AND ISTHMUS OF THE THYROID

RESECTION OF ONE LOBE AND ISTHMUS

INDICATIONS	• presence of nodule in one lobe of thyroid • if malignancy is indicated on frozen section, a total or near-total resection of opposite lobe should be performed
ANESTHESIA	• general endotracheal
POSITIONING	• patient placed in semi-sitting position with roll between shoulder blades and with neck extended (Fig. 1.3)
PREP	• patient painted with several layers of iodine solution from chin to earlobes, down neck to operating table, including shoulders to nipples • drapes placed to allow exposure of tip of chin, suprasternal notch, and both external jugular veins

PROCEDURE

After the patient is positioned, a collar incision is outlined along a skin crease, two fingerbreadths above the suprasternal notch and extending from one external jugular vein to the other (Fig. 1.4).

The skin incision is made sharply and is carried through the platysma with electrocautery (Fig. 1.5). Meticulous hemostasis is maintained throughout the procedure to ensure that vital structures are not obscured. Raising of the flaps using electrocautery minimizes blood loss and facilitates dissection.

The superior flap is elevated to the level of the thyroid notch along the avascular plane immediately subjacent to the platysma, which is just superficial to the investing layer of the deep cervical fascia. Dissection proceeds sharply with the first assistant exerting upward traction on the flap using Lahey clamps on the subcuticular tissue. The surgeon provides countertraction on the midline structures (Fig. 1.6). Occasional gentle upward force along the base of the flap, with a gauze-wrapped index finger, facilitates mobilization (Fig. 1.7).

In a similar fashion, the inferior flap is elevated to the level of the suprasternal notch. Care should be taken to avoid entering the communication arch of the anterior jugular veins at the base of the flap. A self-retaining retractor is placed to keep the flaps apart (Fig. 1.8). Sharp division of the investing fascia is performed along the midline, from the thyroid cartilage to the suprasternal notch. The dissection is carried down to the level of the thyroid (Fig. 1.9).

The entire medial edge of the strap muscles is freed from the underlying thyroid and midline fascia and is retracted laterally, exposing the lobe of the thyroid (Fig. 1.10). Alternatively, for very large glands or heavily muscled necks, the strap muscles may be divided to aid in exposure. This should be done at the junction between the upper and middle thirds of the muscles to preserve their nervous innervation. Use of a gastrointestinal stapling device allows easier reapproximation (Fig. 1.11).

The lobe of the thyroid is pulled medially, placing the middle thyroid vein in sharp relief, and the vein is divided between fine silk ligatures (Fig. 1.12). The superior pole is now retracted laterally and caudally, exposing the superior thyroid artery, which branches immediately upon entering the anterosuperior surface of the gland. These branches are divided between fine silk sutures, immediately adjacent to the thyroid tissue to avoid injury to the superior laryngeal nerve (Fig. 1.13). Occasionally, arterial branches may cross to the lateral wall of the larynx and, in such a case, must be divided to expose the avascular plane medial to the superior pole.

The entire lobe is then retracted medially and the recurrent laryngeal nerve is sought. It can often be palpated as a cordlike structure within the tracheoesophageal groove, where it is intimately associated with the inferior thyroid artery (Fig. 1.14). The latter branches anteriorly and posteriorly around the nerve to supply the inferior and lateral portions of the lobe. The nerve is exposed to its termination at the cricothyroid membrane by division of all crossing anterior arterial branches. Once the recurrent laryngeal nerve is exposed, the gland is mobilized in a cephalad direction by careful dissection of its fascial attachments to the trachea. The pretracheal fascial plane is entered just medial to the nerve, with ligation of all posterior inferior thyroid artery branches. This begins the elevation of the lobe from the underlying trachea. The recurrent laryngeal nerve is kept in constant sight during this dissection to avoid injury. The parathyroid glands are dissected from the thyroid capsule, with care taken to preserve their blood supply. If one of these glands is inadvertently devascularized, it should be diced into 1-mm sections and reimplanted into the sternocleidomastoid muscle.

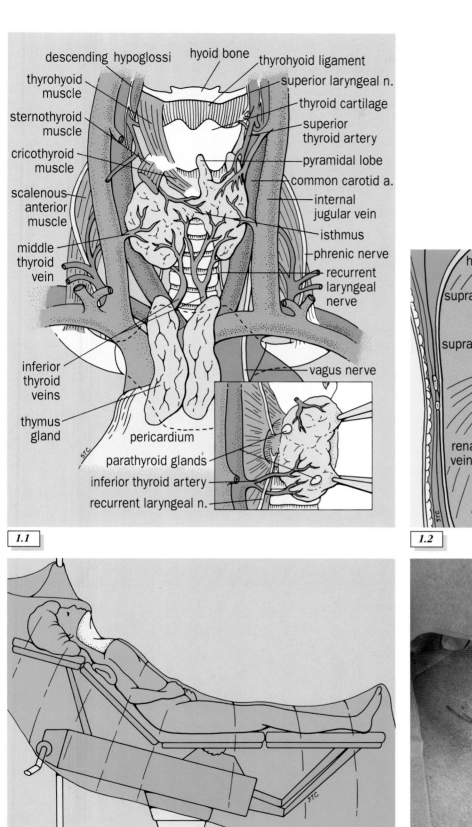

1.1

descending hypoglossi — hyoid bone — thyrohyoid ligament
thyrohyoid muscle
superior laryngeal n.
sternothyroid muscle
thyroid cartilage
superior thyroid artery
cricothyroid muscle
pyramidal lobe
common carotid a.
scalenous anterior muscle
internal jugular vein
isthmus
middle thyroid vein
phrenic nerve
recurrent laryngeal nerve
inferior thyroid veins
vagus nerve
thymus gland
pericardium
parathyroid glands
inferior thyroid artery
recurrent laryngeal n.

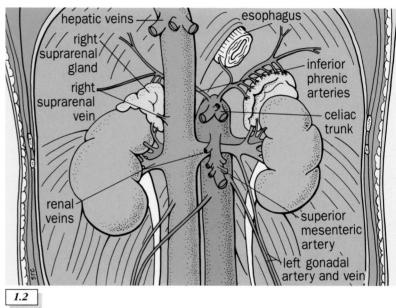

1.2

hepatic veins
esophagus
right suprarenal gland
right suprarenal vein
inferior phrenic arteries
celiac trunk
renal veins
superior mesenteric artery
left gonadal artery and vein

1.3

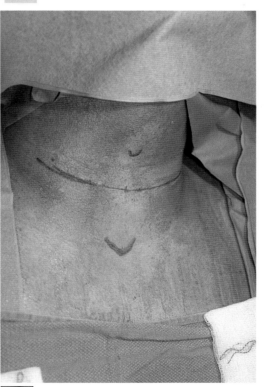

1.4

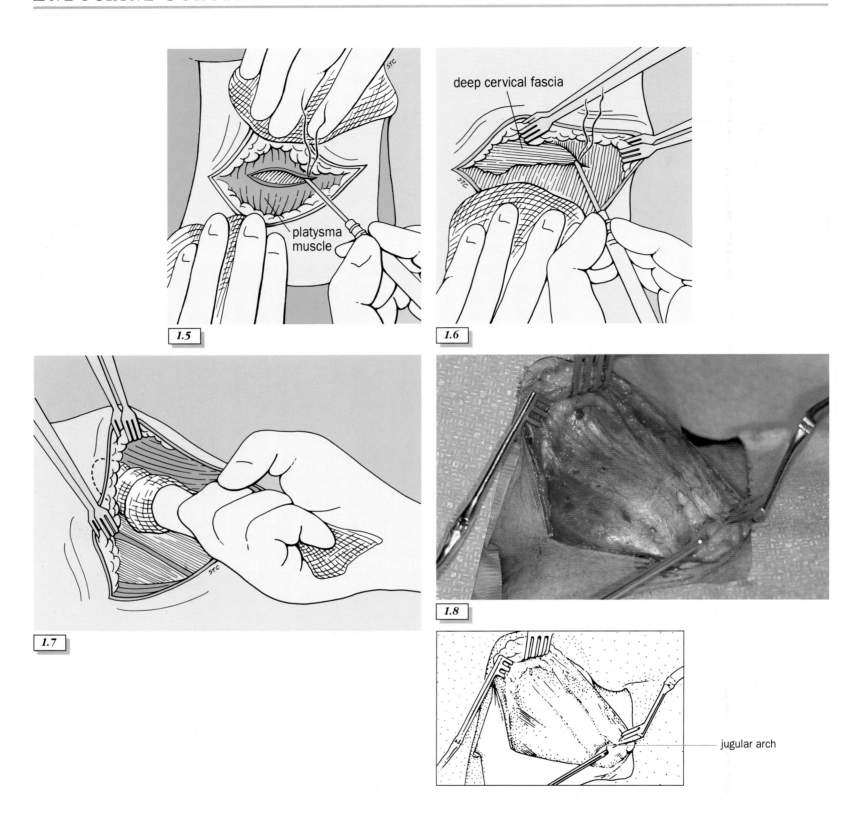

1.5

platysma
muscle

1.6

deep cervical fascia

1.7

1.8

jugular arch

1.4

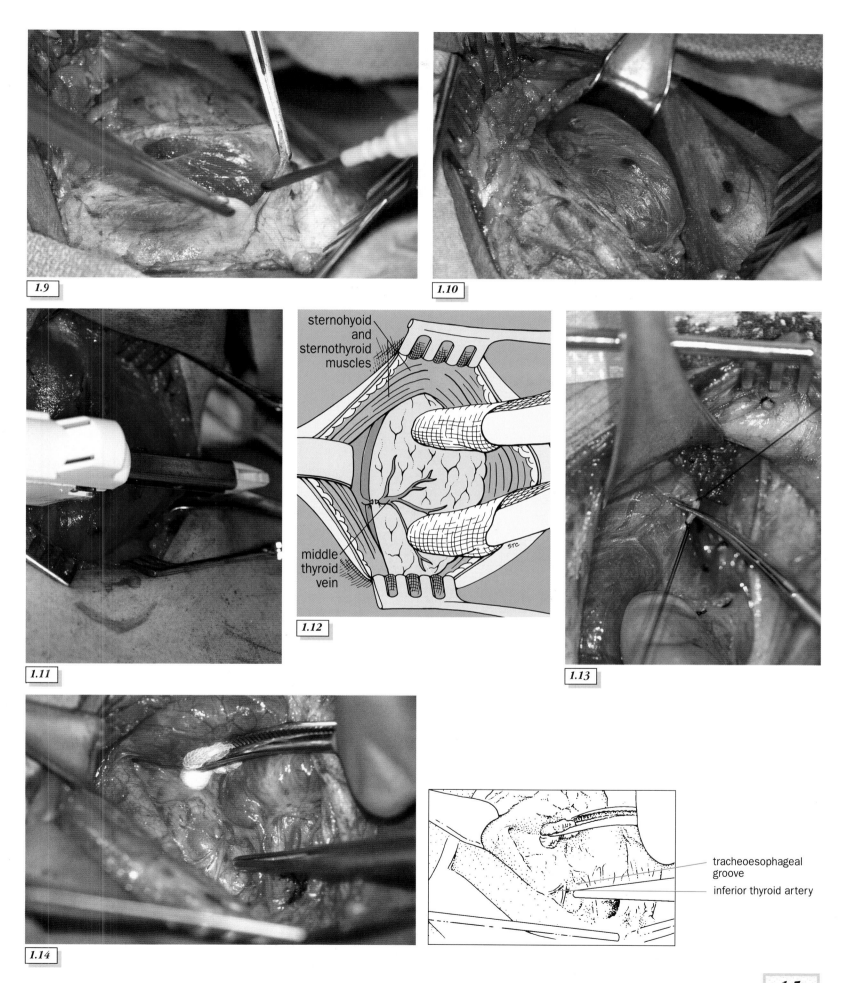

sternohyoid
and
sternothyroid
muscles

middle
thyroid
vein

1.9

1.10

1.11

1.12

1.13

1.14

tracheoesophageal
groove

inferior thyroid artery

The gland is freed medially across the trachea, with division of the inferior thyroid veins at their juncture with the lobe. Once the isthmus is mobilized, it is divided beyond its juncture with the opposite lobe (Fig. 1.15). Bleeding points are cauterized, and the capsule of the transected lobe is oversewn with absorbable sutures (Fig. 1.16). A closed drain may be placed, via a separate stab incision, along the area of dissection (Fig. 1.17). Interrupted absorbable sutures are used to reapproximate the strap muscles and platysma (Fig. 1.18). The skin is closed with a running subcuticular absorbable suture (Fig. 1.19).

SUBTOTAL RESECTION OF ONE LOBE OF THE THYROID

SUBTOTAL RESECTION OF ONE LOBE

INDICATIONS
- hyperthyroidism, in which case a bilateral subtotal thyroidectomy is performed
- malignancy confined to one lobe of the thyroid, in which case a subtotal lobectomy is performed on the contralateral lobe (and a total lobectomy performed on the ipsilateral lobe)

ANESTHESIA
- general endotracheal

POSITIONING
PREP
same as for total resection of one lobe and isthmus (see page 1.2)

PROCEDURE

The neck is opened, the flaps are raised, the strap muscles are dissected, the lobe of the thyroid gland is mobilized, and the inferior thyroid artery is identified as described for total resection of one lobe of the thyroid (see Figs. 1.4–1.14). The gland, however, is left adherent to the trachea. Branches of the inferior thyroid artery and vein that pass anterior to the recurrent laryngeal nerve are divided, whereas the posterior branches are left intact.

The amount of thyroid tissue removed is determined by the horizontal plane defined by the anterior surface of the trachea (Fig. 1.20). The surface vessels that cross this plane are clamped with hemostats (Fig. 1.21). The thyroid is then divided sharply and the glandular tissue anterior to the trachea is mobilized. The posterior thyroid tissue is left in situ. The vessels are ligated and electrocautery is used to control any intrathyroidal bleeding (Fig. 1.22). The capsule may be closed with absorbable suture. This approach leaves 3 to 5 g of thyroid tissue in situ on each side of the neck (Fig. 1.23). The wound is closed as described for total resection of one lobe of the thyroid (see Figs. 1.17–1.19).

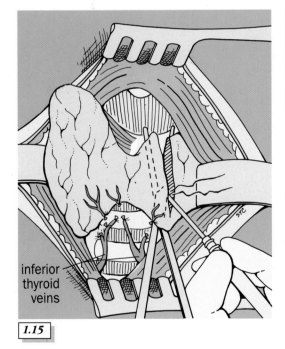

inferior thyroid veins

1.15

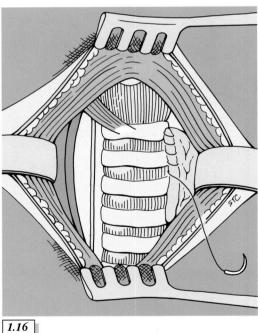

1.16

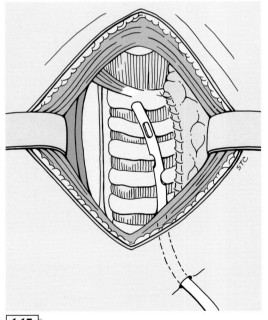

1.17

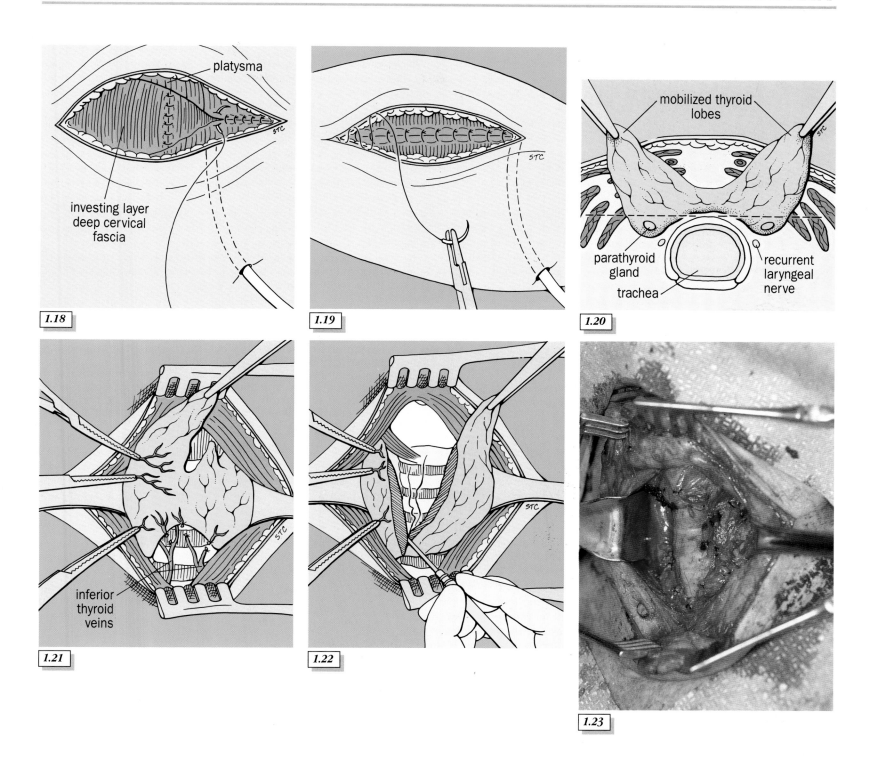

1.18 platysma / investing layer deep cervical fascia

1.19

1.20 mobilized thyroid lobes / parathyroid gland / recurrent laryngeal nerve / trachea

1.21 inferior thyroid veins

1.22

1.23

PARATHYROID GLAND SURGERY

PARATHYROID GLAND SURGERY

INDICATIONS	•primary hyperparathyroidism due to adenoma or hyperplasia •secondary hyperparathyroidism •tertiary hyperparathyroidism •parathyroid carcinoma
ANESTHESIA	•general endotracheal
POSITIONING **PREP**	same as for thyroid surgery (see page 1.2)

PROCEDURE

Exposure of the neck is performed as described for resection of one lobe of the thyroid, up to and including division of the middle thyroid vein (see Figs. 1.4–1.12). Using blunt and sharp dissection, the plane between the thyroid, trachea, and esophagus medially, and the carotid sheath laterally, is exposed to the level of the prevertebral fascia.

The recurrent laryngeal nerve is identified within the tracheoesophageal groove, as described for resection of one lobe of the thyroid (see Fig. 1.14). The inferior thyroid artery is left in situ. Normal parathyroid glands are small (approximately 4 x 6 mm), brownish-tan, and appear as flattened oval disks. They are encompassed by a thin capsule, within which they can often be moved using blunt forceps.

The superior parathyroid glands are usually located at the level of the junction of the posterior upper and middle thirds of the thyroid gland (see Fig. 1.1). Abnormal superior glands frequently follow the esophageal fascia into the posterior mediastinum (Fig. 1.24). The blood supply to the superior glands consists of branches of the inferior thyroid artery that pass posterior to the recurrent laryngeal nerve.

The inferior parathyroid glands usually are located within a 3-cm circle, the center of which is the point where the recurrent laryngeal nerve crosses the inferior thyroid artery. The glands are usually on the surface of the thyroid or are contained within the cervical thymic limb (see Fig. 1.1).

Enlarged inferior glands may descend with the thyrothymic axis into the anterior mediastinum (Fig. 1.24). The blood supply to the inferior glands consists of branches of the inferior thyroid artery that pass anterior to the recurrent laryngeal nerve. Since, regardless of their location, the blood supply to the parathyroids is the inferior thyroid artery, nearly all enlarged glands (superior and inferior) that have descended into the mediastinum can be removed via a cervical approach.

With the exception of a parathyroid carcinoma, the glands are removed easily by incising the thin capsule and mobilizing the gland back to its vascular pedicle, which is then ligated and divided (Fig. 1.25). In the case of a solitary adenoma, all four glands are exposed and identified and the adenoma is removed. To rule out asymmetrical hyperplasia, a biopsy is obtained of one of the normal parathyroids (usually the ipsilateral gland), leaving its pedicle intact. This is accomplished by placing a clip on the distal third of the gland and dividing the tissue distal to the clip (Fig. 1.26).

If all four glands are enlarged, one-half of one gland is removed, leaving 100 mg of tissue in adults and 150 mg in children. The other three glands are then removed in their entirety. Alternatively, particularly in cases of secondary and tertiary hyperparathyroidism, all four glands may be removed. One of the glands is then minced into 1-mm sections, with 150 mg of the tissue implanted into the forearm. This location allows for easy access, under local anesthesia, to the implanted tissue should hyperparathyroidism recur.

If a superior gland is not identified and careful exposure of the paraesophageal tissues and carotid sheath fails to disclose the gland, the superior pole of the ipsilateral thyroid lobe should be mobilized and the surrounding tissue examined carefully. Since, in about 10% of cases, the superior parathyroid receives its blood supply from the superior thyroid artery, it may be located more superiorly and/or medially than expected. If the gland is still not identified, the ipsilateral lobe of the thyroid gland should be removed and serially sectioned.

If an inferior gland is not identified, the thymus gland should be teased into the neck and inspected. The ipsilateral limb of the thymus should be resected if it is found to contain the parathyroid. If a thorough neck exploration fails to reveal the pathology, the procedure should be terminated and localization studies performed before proceeding with mediastinal exploration. (Note that occasionally, although the pathologic gland may not be identified, its blood supply may be destroyed during neck exploration. Consequently, calcium levels should be checked postoperatively, as the patient may have been rendered eucalcemic.)

Carcinoma of the parathyroid gland should be suspected if the gland is adherent to its capsule and surrounding tissue. In such a case, excision of all adherent tissue (eg, thyroid, thymus, nodes) should be performed. Closure of the neck is accomplished as described for resection of one lobe of the thyroid (see Figs. 1.17-1.19).

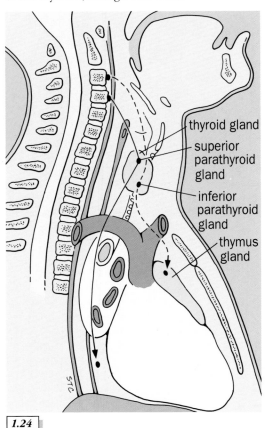

thyroid gland

superior parathyroid gland

inferior parathyroid gland

thymus gland

1.24

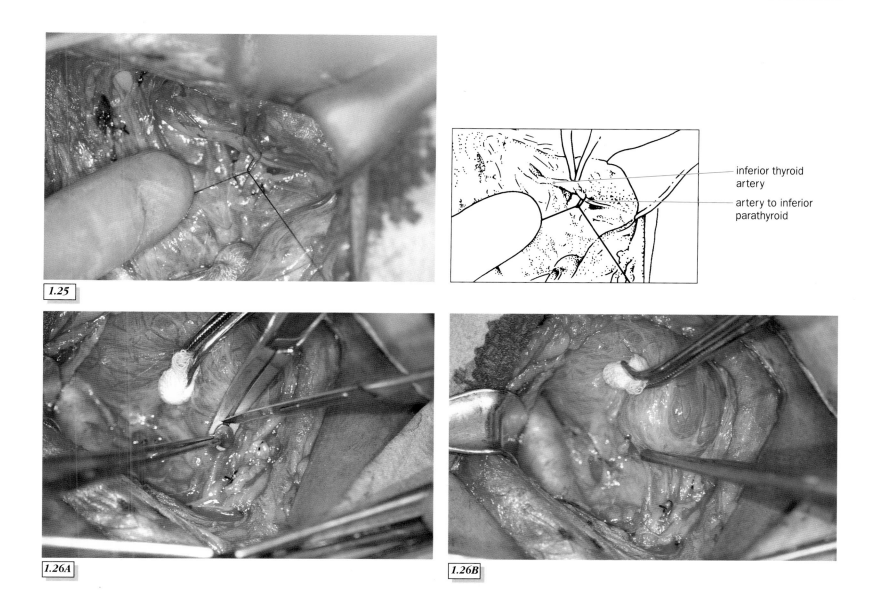

inferior thyroid
artery

artery to inferior
parathyroid

1.25

1.26A

1.26B

THYMUS GLAND RESECTION

THYMUS GLAND RESECTION

INDICATIONS	•thymoma •myasthenia gravis
ANESTHESIA	•general endotracheal
POSITIONING	•supine
PREP	•patient painted with several layers of iodine solution from chin to abdomen, with extension laterally to level of operating table •drapes placed superior to suprasternal notch, inferior to xiphoid process, and laterally, at level of nipples

PROCEDURE

For resection of a thymoma, a complete median sternotomy is performed (see Chapter 3). For those patients undergoing thymectomy for the treatment of myasthenia gravis in whom no thymoma is present, a partial median sternotomy may be performed. It is done in the same fashion as a complete sternotomy except that division of the sternum is carried down only to the fourth or fifth intercostal space and is then transected laterally (Fig. 1.27A). A sternal retractor is placed for exposure (Fig. 1.27B).

The thymus gland is now inspected to determine whether the tumor is benign or malignant. Such determination must be made in the operating room as it is usually difficult to make the distinction by histopathologic examination. The distinguishing characteristic of malignancy is invasion of surrounding structures. If such is found, resection of the invaded structures (eg, pleura, pericardium) should be performed, if feasible, with the thymectomy. (Note that the phrenic nerves are rarely invaded. Hence, though they may appear to be involved, they can usually be spared by careful dissection.)

When no thymic tumor is present, the pleura is mobilized off of all mediastinal structures, beginning posteriorly behind the sternum and chest wall and continuing laterally until the phrenic nerves are reached. Using sharp and blunt dissection, all thymic tissue, lymphatic tissue, and mediastinal fat between the phrenic nerves is removed from the level of the diaphragm to the neck. Vessels are divided between clips (see Fig. 1.28).

The final step of the dissection is division of the thymic vein where it communicates with the left innominate vein (Fig. 1.29). If a thymoma is present, both pleural spaces are entered and examined for tumor implants. The pleura can then be reapproximated over a red rubber catheter. Air is expelled by hyperinflation of the lungs prior to closure and the catheter is removed. Conversely, an anterior chest tube may be placed. Hemostasis is obtained and the sternum is reapproximated with wires. The pectoral fascia is approximated with running absorbable suture, and the skin is closed with a running subcuticular absorbable suture (see Closure of Sternotomy in Chapter 3).

ADRENAL GLAND SURGERY
RESECTION OF THE RIGHT ADRENAL GLAND: ABDOMINAL APPROACH

RESECTION OF THE RIGHT ADRENAL GLAND: ABDOMINAL APPROACH

INDICATIONS	•nonfunctioning tumors of adrenal gland that are 3 cm or more in greatest diameter or have documented evidence of growth •functioning tumors of the adrenal gland of any size; the abdominal approach is particularly applicable to situations in which both glands and/or the abdomen need to be explored, as in pheochromocytoma
ANESTHESIA	•general endotracheal
POSITIONING	•supine
PREP	•patient painted with several layers of iodine solution from nipples to pubis •abdomen draped out

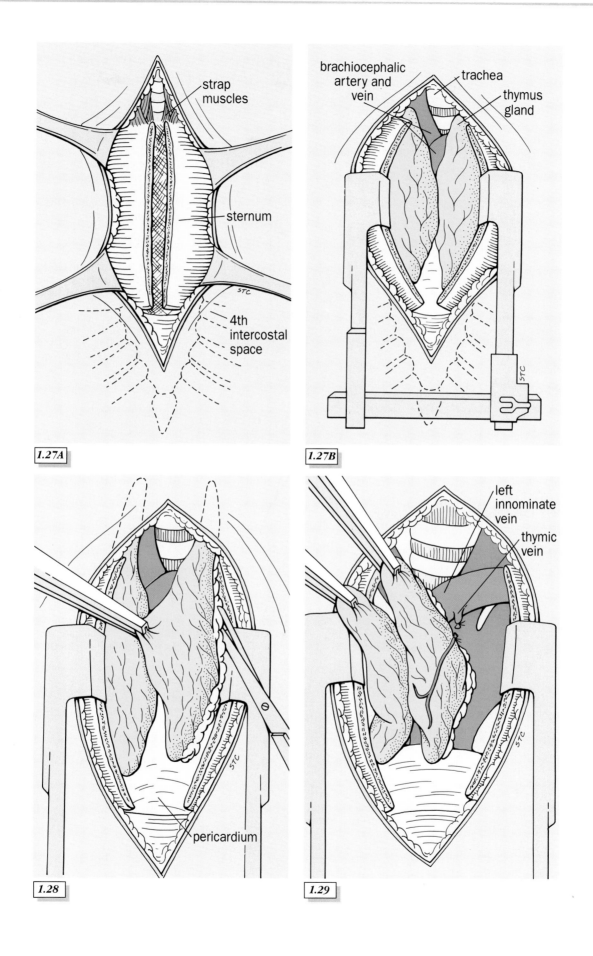

1.27A

strap muscles

sternum

4th intercostal space

1.27B

brachiocephalic artery and vein

trachea

thymus gland

1.28

pericardium

1.29

left innominate vein

thymic vein

PROCEDURE

A bilateral subcostal incision is made (Fig. 1.30) and carried down to the anterior rectus fascia, with hemostasis obtained by electrocautery. The anterior rectus sheath is incised. Each rectus muscle is elevated using a Kelly clamp and is then divided using electrocautery (Fig. 1.31). The posterior rectus sheath is incised sharply and the abdomen is entered. The falciform (round) ligament is transected between ligatures.

The hepatic flexure of the colon is mobilized and retracted caudally. The right lobe of the liver is retracted upward. A Kocher maneuver is initiated by incision of the lateral duodenoperitoneal attachments (Fig. 1.32; see also Fig. 8.41). The adrenal gland, the kidney, and the vena cava are exposed by medial retraction of the duodenum while dissecting in the plane beneath the head of the pancreas.

The kidney is retracted downward and the right adrenal vein is identified by dissection along the lateral surface of the vena cava. The vein is divided between ligatures or clips (Fig. 1.33). If the adrenal vein is obscured by tumor, ligation of minor inferior hepatic veins can be performed to provide more exposure. Dissection of the gland proceeds along its medial, superior, and lateral edges. Vessels are ligated between silk ligatures or clips.

In some cases, the tumor may extend behind the inferior vena cava. Dissection can then be accomplished by medial retraction of the vena cava. Occasionally, however, the medial border of the tumor must be freed by approach from the vena cava's left side, which may require mobilization of the left renal vein.

The remaining inferior fascial attachments between the adrenal gland and the kidney are divided, completely freeing the gland (Fig. 1.34). A closed suction drain is placed along the area of dissection via a separate stab incision, and the wound is closed in layers.

RESECTION OF THE LEFT ADRENAL GLAND: ABDOMINAL APPROACH

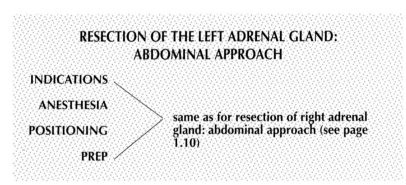

RESECTION OF THE LEFT ADRENAL GLAND: ABDOMINAL APPROACH

INDICATIONS
ANESTHESIA
POSITIONING
PREP
} same as for resection of right adrenal gland: abdominal approach (see page 1.10)

PROCEDURE

The abdomen is opened as described for the transabdominal approach to the right adrenal gland (see Figs. 1.31, 1.32). The lesser sac is entered by division of the gastrocolic ligament along the avascular plane between the omentum and the transverse pericolic fat. Larger vessels are divided between clips or ligatures. The pancreas is exposed by gentle upward traction of the stomach and downward traction on the colon (Fig. 1.35).

Mobilization of the pancreas is accomplished by division of the peritoneum along its inferior border (Fig. 1.36). Gentle blunt dissection is used to elevate the pancreas superiorly, thereby revealing the left kidney and adrenal gland. Care must be taken to avoid injury to venous communications between the pancreas and the splenic vein.

The left adrenal vein is isolated and divided as it enters the left renal vein (Fig. 1.37). The adrenal gland is dissected free, leaving the renal attachments until last. Vessels are divided between clips or ligatures. A closed suction drain is placed via a separate stab wound along the area of dissection. The wound is closed in layers.

RESECTION OF THE RIGHT ADRENAL GLAND: POSTERIOR APPROACH

RESECTION OF THE RIGHT ADRENAL GLAND: POSTERIOR APPROACH

INDICATIONS	•a single functioning cortical adenoma lateralized by preoperative anatomic and biochemical studies •if adrenocortical hyperplasia is present, a bilateral approach with two operating teams is used
ANESTHESIA	•general endotracheal
POSITIONING	•prone, with rolls placed under hips and shoulders (rolls must be large enough to allow abdomen to "hang freely," allowing abdominal contents to "fall away" from retroperitoneum) (Fig. 1.38)
PREP	•patient painted with several layers of iodine solution extending from shoulders to thighs •back draped out from midscapula to coccyx

PROCEDURE

A curved incision is made beginning at the level of the tenth rib, approximately 3 cm lateral to the midvertebral body, and extending inferiorly to the iliac crest, about 4 cm from the midline (Fig. 1.39). The incision is carried down to the level of the posterior lamella of the lumbodorsal fascia.

After hemostasis is obtained, the posterior lamella of the lumbodorsal fascia is incised, thereby exposing the sacrospinalis muscle (Fig. 1.40). The muscle is retracted medially against the spine (Fig. 1.41), and the twelfth rib is identified and resected. Care should be taken to avoid incising the underlying pleura. If the pleural space is entered inadvertently, the wound should be closed around a small catheter, allowing aspiration of air. The catheter can then be removed just prior to skin closure.

Incision of the medial and anterior layers of the lumbodorsal fascia along the lateral border of the quadratus lumborum muscle reveals Gerota's fascia and surrounding fat (Fig. 1.42). The subcostal vessels, which can be seen within the wound, are divided between ligatures or clips. The subcostal nerve is retracted superiorly or inferiorly and is preserved.

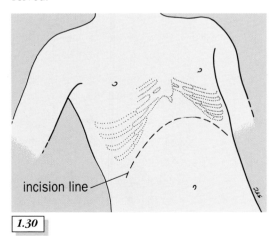

incision line

1.30

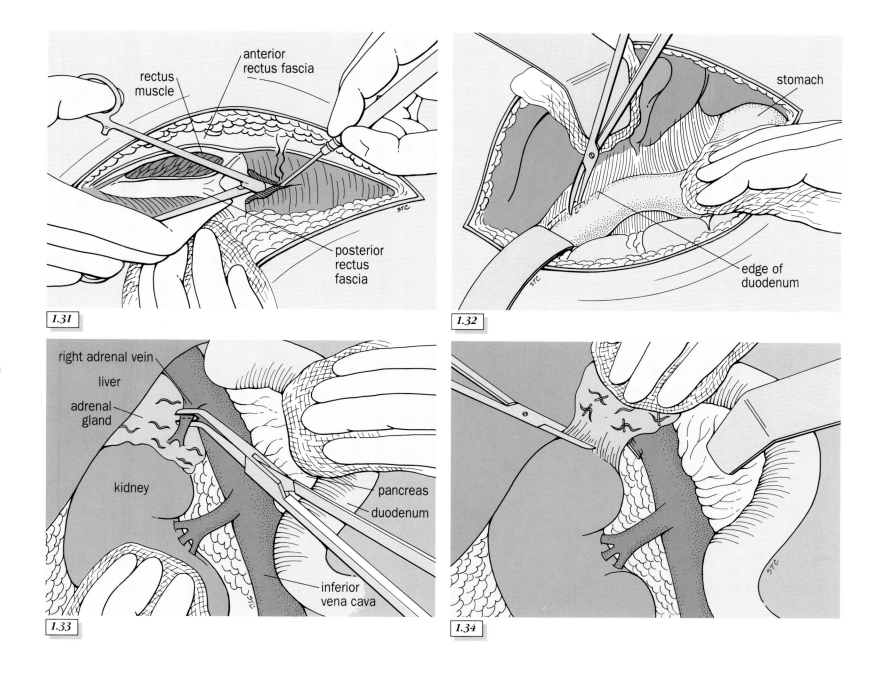

1.31

rectus muscle

anterior rectus fascia

posterior rectus fascia

1.32

stomach

edge of duodenum

1.33

right adrenal vein

liver

adrenal gland

kidney

pancreas

duodenum

inferior vena cava

1.34

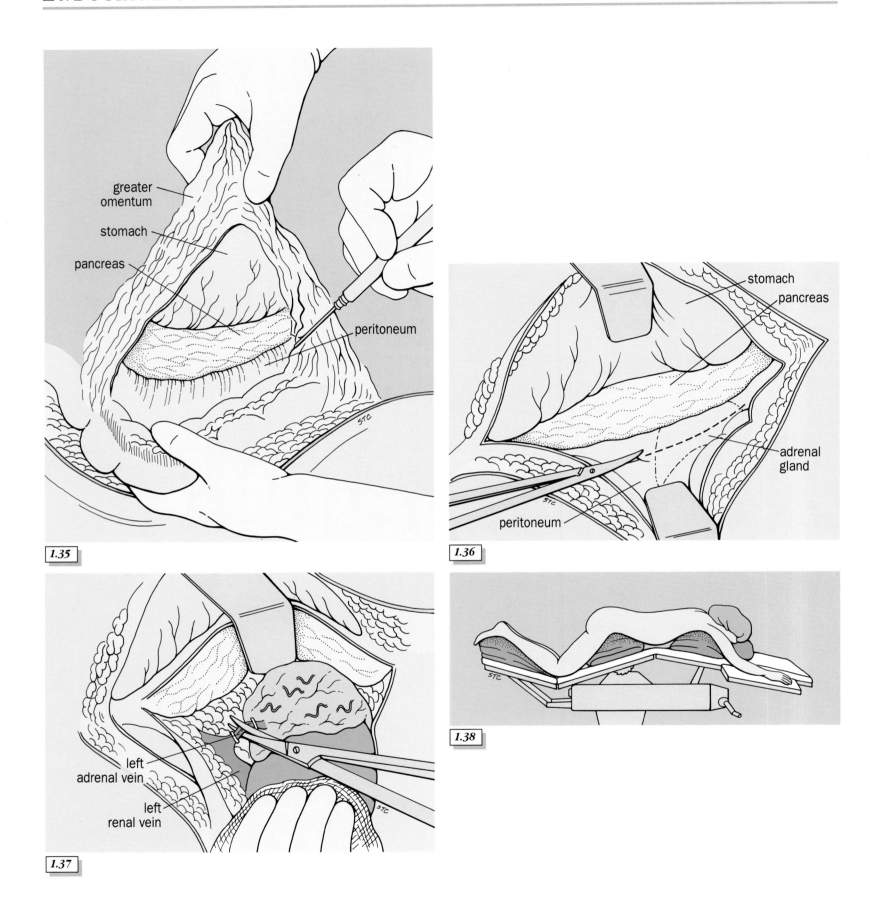

greater
omentum

stomach

pancreas

peritoneum

1.35

stomach
pancreas

adrenal
gland

peritoneum

1.36

left
adrenal vein

left
renal vein

1.37

1.38

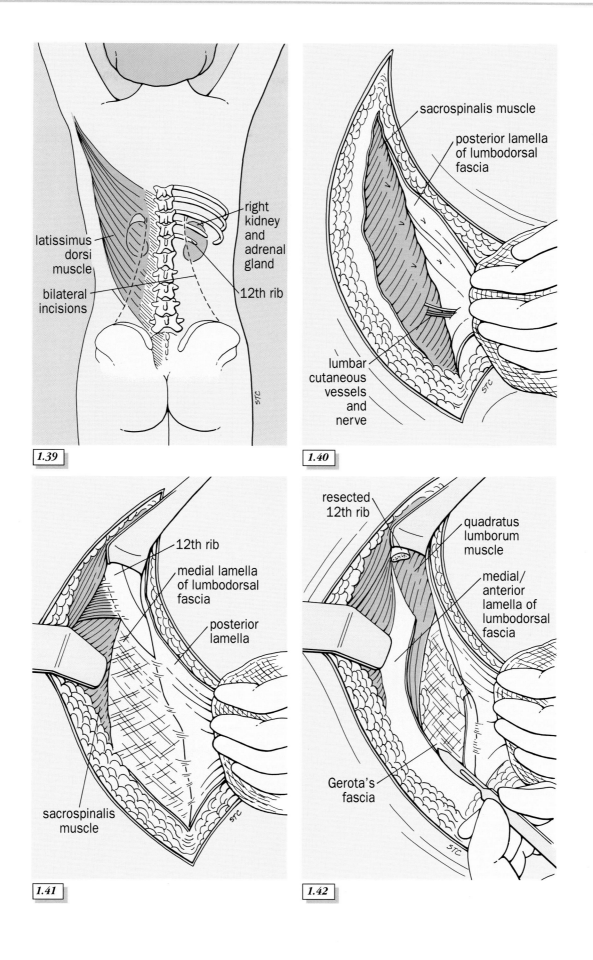

1.39

1.40

1.41

1.42

1.15

Using blunt dissection, the tissues beneath the diaphragm are dissected free and the pleura is pushed off the diaphragm's lower surface (Fig. 1.43). A self-retaining retractor is placed in the wound. If necessary for further exposure, the diaphragm can be divided between large clips (Fig. 1.44). Gerota's fascia is incised. If the surgeon is right-handed, the left hand grasps the adrenal gland exerting downward retraction, thereby aiding exposure. The left fingers gently dissect the periglandular tissue while the right hand is used to clip any potential bleeding points. Dissection continues around the gland, leaving until last the attachments to the superior pole of the kidney. Once the gland has been completely mobilized, the adrenal vein is divided between clips at its attachment to the renal vein (Fig. 1.45). Note that the left adrenal vein communicates with the left renal vein, not with the vena cava.

Closure of the wound involves approximation of the belly of the sacrospinalis muscle to the fused anterior and medial lamellae of the lumbodorsal fascia (Fig. 1.46). The edges of the posterior lamella of the lumbodorsal fascia are reapproximated as the next layer (Fig. 1.47). The skin is then closed.

RESECTION OF THE RIGHT ADRENAL GLAND: THORACOABDOMINAL APPROACH

	RESECTION OF THE RIGHT ADRENAL GLAND: THORACOABDOMINAL APPROACH
INDICATIONS	• large adrenocortical tumor or anticipated kidney removal
ANESTHESIA	• general endotracheal
POSITIONING	• supine on operating table, with small pillow or folded sheet placed beneath scapula of operative side to elevate shoulder, and ipsilateral arm suspended above chest (Fig. 1.48)
PREP	• patient painted with several layers of iodine solution from shoulder and upper portion of anterior arm to hip, and laterally to level of operating table • drapes placed superior to nipples, inferiorly above pubis, and laterally beyond umbilicus and along midaxillary line

PROCEDURE

The skin incision, begun in the tenth intercostal space at the midaxillary line, is carried medially along the rib and extended across the costal margin. It is continued vertically along the lateral edge of the rectus sheath to a point below the umbilicus (Fig. 1.48).

The intercostal muscles, the costal margin, and the muscles of the lateral abdominal wall are divided. With care taken to avoid the phrenic nerve, the diaphragm is incised circumferentially, leaving a 2-cm rim to facilitate closure. The triangular ligament of the liver is incised, and the organ is retracted into the chest (Fig. 1.49).

A Kocher manuever is performed to expose the adrenal gland (see Fig. 8.41), the adrenal vein is identified and ligated where it joins the vena cava, and the vena cava is retracted medially to allow dissection of the medial edge of the gland as described previously for abdominal approach

to resection of the right adrenal gland. Vascular communications are divided between clips or ligatures. Dissection is continued along the superior and lateral edges of the gland. Palpable nodes (periaortic or pericaval) are removed en bloc with the specimen.

The inferior portion of the tumor is inspected. If renal invasion is present, the kidney is removed en bloc. To do so, the ureter is divided first, followed by division of the renal vein where it enters the vena cava (Fig. 1.50A). The renal artery is then doubly ligated and divided (Fig. 1.50B). Sharp and blunt dissection frees the remainder of the specimen, allowing it to be removed. Hemostasis is obtained and a closed suction drain is placed along the area of dissection via a separate stab incision. A chest tube is placed via a separate stab incision and is directed anteriorly. The diaphragm is reapproximated using nonabsorbable suture in an interrupted figure-of-eight fashion and the wound is closed in layers.

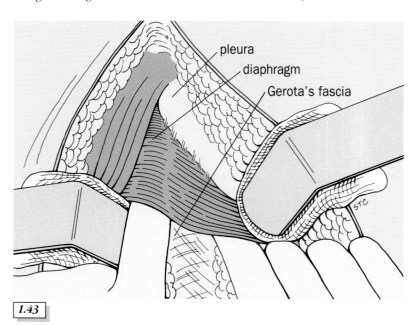

pleura
diaphragm
Gerota's fascia

1.43

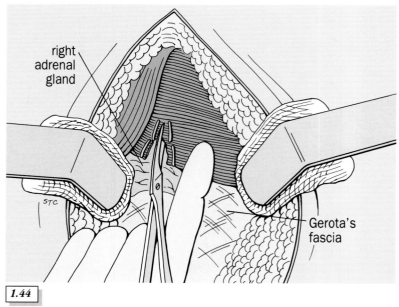

right adrenal gland

Gerota's fascia

1.44

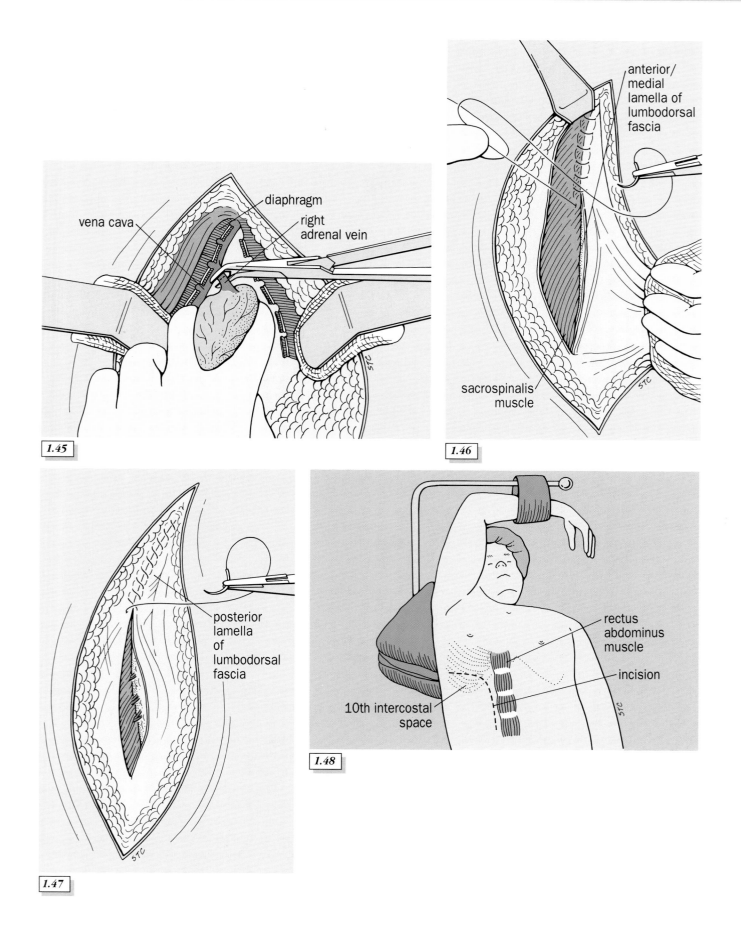

vena cava

diaphragm

right adrenal vein

1.45

anterior/ medial lamella of lumbodorsal fascia

sacrospinalis muscle

1.46

posterior lamella of lumbodorsal fascia

1.47

rectus abdominus muscle

incision

10th intercostal space

1.48

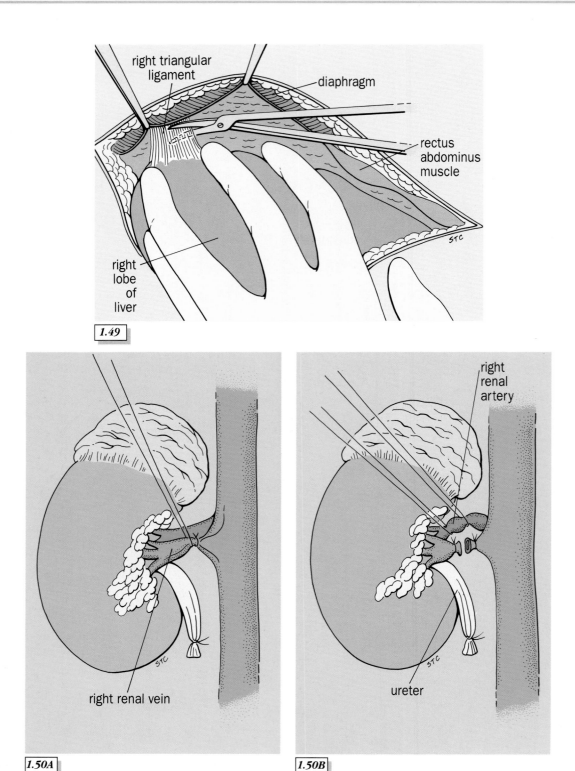

1.49

1.50A

1.50B

BIBLIOGRAPHY

Dichinson PH. *A Color Atlas of Subtotal Thyroidectomy*. Oradell, NJ: Medical Economics Books; 1983.

Edis AJ, Grant CS, Egdahl RH. *Manual of Endocrine Surgery*. New York, NY: Springer-Verlag; 1984.

Guz BV, Straffon RA, Novick AC. Operative approaches to the adrenal gland. *Urol Clin North Am*. 1989; 16(3):527–534.

Jaretzki A, Wolff M. "Maximal" thymectomy for myasthenia gravis: surgical anatomy and operative technique. *J Thorac Cardiovasc Surg*. 1988; 95(5):711–716.

2

Head and Neck Surgery

David A. Zwillenberg

RADICAL NECK DISSECTION

RADICAL NECK DISSECTION

INDICATIONS	•resection of carcinoma metastatic to the neck or directly extending into the neck from a primary malignancy in the area (may be performed prophylactically if no lymph nodes are palpable; the incidence of nodal metastases from the primary tumor is high)
ANESTHESIA	•general
POSITIONING	•neck extended by a roll beneath the shoulders and the head turned away from the involved neck
PREP	•prep from the jaw to the clavicles, from the midline anteriorly to the trapezius posteriorly •entire area should be draped out and the towels clipped, sutured, or stapled to the skin

STAGING OF NECK DISEASE

For the staging of carcinomas of the head and neck the TNM classification is employed and refers to the primary tumor. Please refer to the AJC for this information. N refers to nodal metastases and M to distant.

CERVICAL NODE CLASSIFICATION

The following regional node classification is applicable to all squamous cell carcinomas of the upper aerodigestive tract. In clinical evaluation, the actual size of the nodal mass should be measured and allowance should be made for intervening soft tissues. It is recognized that most masses over 3 cm in diameter are not single nodes, but are confluent nodes or tumors in soft tissues of the neck. There are three stages of clinically positive nodes: N1, N2, and N3. The use of subgroups a, b, and c is not required, but is recommended. Midline nodes are considered as homolateral nodes (see Table 2.1).

METASTASES

This is the classification for disease in the neck as quoted from the above-noted reference.

It is very important to identify and stage a primary tumor by laryngoscopy, bronchoscopy, and esophagoscopy. Neck nodes should never be biopsied in the adult before attempts at locating a primary source have been made. Whenever possible a single treatment plan should be developed for treating the primary and the cervical disease. Biopsying a node before neck dissection may increase mortality by as much as 20%.

PROCEDURE

Many skin incisions can be used. For the novice the Conley incision provides the easiest access to the neck and good protection to the carotid artery (Fig. 2.1). If a previous node biopsy has been carried out the incision should be designed to allow for the excision of the pre-existing wound. The skin, subcutaneous tissue, and platysma are incised; the flaps are elevated subplatysmally with the use of a knife or scissors; and the skin is retracted with heavy skin hooks (Fig. 2.2).

The heads (sternal and clavicular) of the sternocleidomastoid are sharply dissected out. They should be clamped with a Kelly clamp and cut, either sharply or with the bovie. Care should be taken not to injure the underlying jugular, carotid, or vagus.

The jugular vein is then isolated inferiorly with forceps and scissors (Fig. 2.3). The vein should then be doubly clamped and divided with a knife between the clamps. Tie each end with a 2–0 silk and then suture ligate each end with a 2–0 silk closer to the cut edge. Leave the tie on the distal end of the vein long.

Open the carotid sheath with scissors and forceps, thus exposing the carotid and vagus. Avoid the thoracic duct. If chyle is seen in the wound stop and immediately suture ligate, then proceed to strip the carotid sheath from the vagus and carotid.

As you dissect lateral to the carotid the fascia over the scalene muscles is seen. It should be left intact. As the dissection proceeds the phrenic nerve can be seen below it coursing from lateral to medial (Fig. 2.4). As the specimen is bluntly dissected cephalad, the transverse scapular and transverse cervical arteries and veins, and the anterior jugular, and external jugular veins are ligated.

TABLE 2.1 TNM STAGING OF NODES IN THE NECK

NX	Nodes cannot be assessed
NO	No clinically positive node
N1	Single clinically positive homolateral node more than 3 cm but not more than 6 cm in diameter nodes, none more than 6 cm in diameter or multiple clinically positive homolateral
N2a	Single clinically positive homolateral node more than 3 cm but not more than 6 cm in diameter
N2b	Multiple clinically positive homolateral nodes, none more than 6 cm in diameter
N3	Massive homolateral node(s), bilateral nodes, or contralateral node(s)
N3a	Clinically positive homolateral node(s), one more than 6 cm in diameter
N3b	Bilateral clinically positive nodes (in this situation, each side of the neck should be staged separately; that is, N3b: right, N2a; left, N1)
N3c	Contralateral clinically positive node(s) only

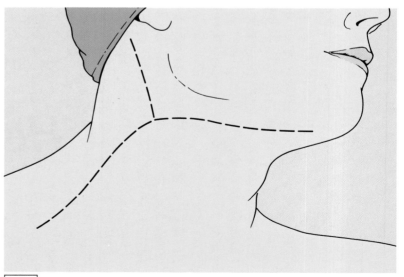

2.1

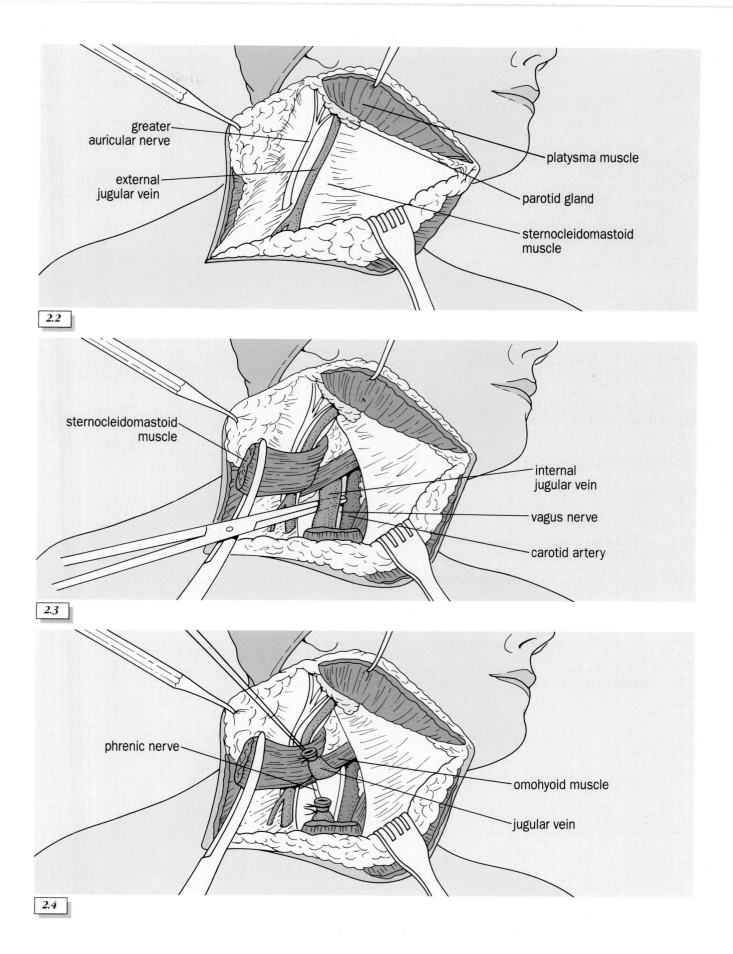

The dissection is then carried lateral to the anterior border of the trapezius. The omohyoid is transected laterally. The dissection is then carried up along the anterior border of the trapezius by serially clamping with Kelly clamps sharply dividing and ligating with 3–0 chromic.

When the superior limit of the dissection (Fig. 2.5) has been reached, place a finger between the SCM and the jugular and transect the SCM sharply or with the bovie. Suture ligate the jugular superiorly with 2–0 or 3–0 silk and divide. Retract the submandibular gland postero-interiorly after elevating the fascia superiorly to protect the marginal branch with an Allis clamp. Tie and divide the facial artery, vein, and the submandibular duct (Fig. 2.6) and remove the specimen from the field (Fig. 2.7).

Irrigate the wound and carefully and thoroughly obtain hemostasis. A drain should be placed through a separate stab incision and sutured in place. Closure should be carried out in two layers with chromic or Vicryl (3–0) and a skin closure of 3–0 nylon or staples. The wound may be dressed but since this obscures visualization postoperatively and may cause carotid compression the author prefers not to do this.

POSTOP MANAGEMENT

Keep the drain on high wall suction until drainage is below 40 cc/day, then maintain bulb suction when out of bed. Observe closely for swelling, since this may indicate a hematoma, which will require drainage. The patient should receive physical therapy to avoid the frozen shoulder that often follows the loss of CNXI.

SUBMANDIBULAR GLAND EXCISION

SUBMANDIBULAR GLAND EXCISION

INDICATIONS	•mass lesion •stone in the gland parenchyma •recurrent infection
ANESTHESIA	•may be done under local anesthesia but general anesthesia is easier on patient and surgeon alike
POSITIONING	•patient positioned with the neck extended and the head turned toward the side opposite the gland to be resected
PREP	•prepping is carried out with the drapes allowing the entire neck from the clavicle to the level of the corner of the mouth to be exposed, thus permitting the operator to note any unintentional stimulation of the marginal mandibular nerve

PROCEDURE

The whole operative technique is aimed at avoiding injury to the marginal mandibular branch of the facial nerve and other nearby structures.

The skin incision is made two fingerbreadths (4 cm) below the mandibular border from the lateral end of the hyoid almost to the level of the angle of the mandible (Fig. 2.8). The incision is carried through platysma, exposing the fascia. Retractors are placed (Fig. 2.9).

The fascia overlying the submandibular gland is exposed. It is incised on the inferior edge of the gland and elevated up off the gland (Fig. 2.10). The marginal mandibular nerve will be running horizontally in this fascia; injury to the nerve will be avoided by elevating from below up.

Once the nerve has been protected, careful dissection will permit elevation of the gland from the mylohyoid muscle which underlies it. It may be necessary to divide and ligate the anterior facial vein and the anterior branches of the facial artery.

As the mylohyoid is retracted anteriorly and the gland posteroinferiorly the lingual nerve will be exposed (Fig. 2.11). The submandibular ganglion and its vein are divided and tied. The nerve will pull up out of the field. Wharton's duct will be found immediately below the lingual nerve and should be divided and ligated (Fig. 2.12).

The specimen is then removed from the field. Hemostasis should be assured and the wound irrigated as needed. A passive or suction drain is generally left in place for a day and the wound closed with 3–0 chromic or a similar absorbable suture in the platysma (Fig. 2.13). It may be necessary to put an additional layer subcutaneously. The wound is then closed with the 4–0 to 6–0 nonabsorbable suture of the surgeon's preference.

Complications and their prevention:

1. Avoid injury to the lingual and VII nerves as described above.
2. Assure hemostasis.
3. Use antibiotics as necessary. Infections postop are not uncommon, particularly in those with chronic sialadenitis.

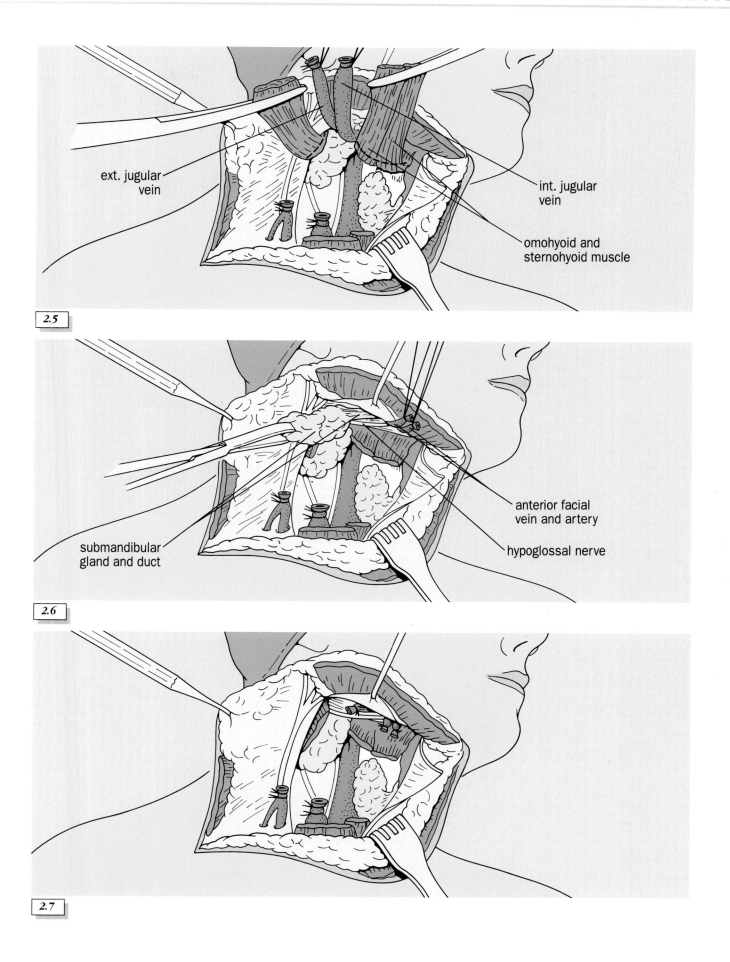

2.5

ext. jugular vein

int. jugular vein

omohyoid and sternohyoid muscle

2.6

submandibular gland and duct

anterior facial vein and artery

hypoglossal nerve

2.7

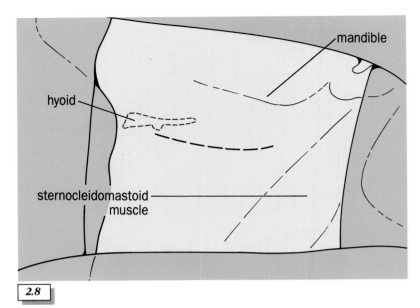

2.8

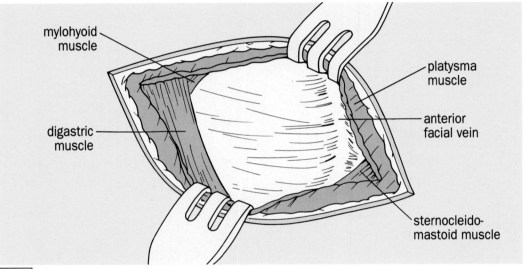

2.9

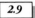

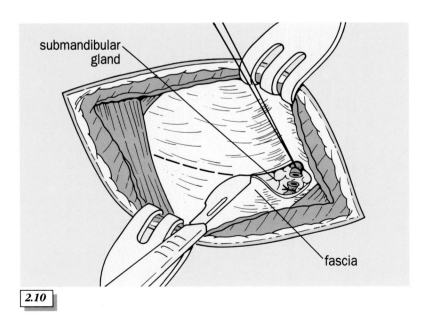

2.10

GLAND

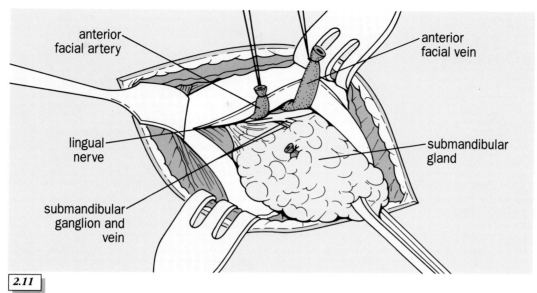

anterior
facial artery

anterior
facial vein

lingual
nerve

submandibular
gland

submandibular
ganglion and
vein

2.11

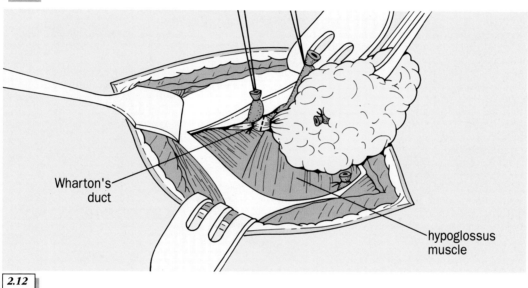

Wharton's
duct

hypoglossus
muscle

2.12

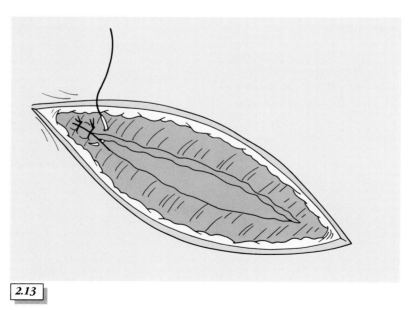

2.13

TRACHEOSTOMY

Airway obstruction can occur from many causes. Trauma to the face can result in mandibular or maxillary (LeFort II and III) fractures that permit the facial and masticatory structures to fall back and obstruct the airway. Foreign bodies can be aspirated into the larynx. Steam, irritant gases, lye, and so forth, can produce tremendous upper airway edema. Croup, epiglottitis, Ludwig's angina, and various parapharyngeal abscesses can result in airway compromise. Such congenital anomalies as choanal atresia (the newborn is an obligate nose-breather), Pierre Robin syndrome (microstomia, macroglossia, micrognathia), laryngeal webs, severe laryngo- or tracheomalacia may necessitate prolonged airway management. Hypersensitivity reactions and angioneurotic edema can result in acute airway obstruction. The inability of the vocal cords to lateralize as in bilateral cord paralysis or cricoarytenoid fixation will result in stridor and often in airway decompensation. Laryngeal, pharyngeal, or tracheobronchial tumors or cysts can also lead to respiratory compromise on an obstructive basis. Sleep apnea patients may require a tracheostomy. The inability of patients to adequately clear secretions from the lung may also require a tracheostomy. This problem is usually multifactorial in origin and includes inability to cough, swallowing dysfunction with aspiration, and poor pharyngeal function with resultant inability to expectorate.

Respiratory insufficiency may be due to a chronic or acute pulmonary process. Generally, endotracheal intubation is preferred for early management. The tracheal cartilages receive their blood supply from the mucosa. The trauma to and pressure on this mucosa due to prolonged intubation will cause necrosis of the tracheal cartilage and, consequently, a loss of support to a portion of the airway and stenosis. Subglottic stenosis is an extremely difficult problem to deal with and is best prevented. It is generally agreed that tracheostomies should be performed between 7 and 14 days after intubation in the adult. If it is known at the time of intubation that rapid extubation is not likely tracheostomy should be performed as soon as reasonably possible. In patients with neuromuscular impairment (high quadriplegics, patients with bulbar palsies, advanced Parkinsonism, Lou Gehrig's disease, etc.) who are therefore unable to handle their secretions, tracheostomies should be performed after a reasonable interval since it is considerably more comfortable than intubation.

Retractors are placed in the incision. The midline raphe of the strap muscles is then spread open with a Metzenbaum or hemostat and the retractors placed between them.

The trachea is then exposed. The tracheostomy tube should be placed in the third tracheal ring. A tracheal hook may be employed to stabilize the trachea and draw this ring into view. Very rarely is this impossible. If the isthmus of the thyroid gland is in the way it can generally be displaced upward or downward by blunt elevation directly against the trachea with a sponge or peanut. If the isthmus is too large to be avoided it should be clamped, split, and oversewn.

The third ring may be removed anteriorly, cut superiorly and laterally, and tied to the skin as a Bjork flap, cut in a cruciate manner or vertically incised (Fig. 2.15).

The Trousseau dilator is then used to expose the lumen more widely. If an endotracheal tube is present it should be withdrawn until the tip is just above the stoma. The tracheostomy tube is then inserted. The cuff must be checked before insertion for integrity.

Breath sounds are auscultated bilaterally before the endotracheal tube is withdrawn. If the insertion appears to have been unsuccessful the tracheostomy tube is withdrawn and the endotracheal tube slid back down to assure continued respiration while the tracheostomy tube is reinserted.

Complications and their prevention:

1. *Pneumothorax.* Keep the dissection in the midline. Do not close the incision tightly.
2. *Tube misplacement.* Make sure tracheal fenestra is visible as the tube is inserted. Do not remove retractors or endotracheal tube until the position has been assured.
3. *Tube displacement.* Make sure the tracheal ties are tight. Only one finger should be admissable under ties with the head flexed.
4. *Tracheo-inaminate fistula.* Make the tracheal fenestra in the third ring. Do not overinflate the cuff.
5. *Tracheoesophageal fistula.* Do not overinflate the cuff. If possible, remove any NG tube.

PAROTIDECTOMY

TRACHEOSTOMY	
INDICATIONS	•airway obstruction •prolonged ventilatory support •pulmonary toilet
ANESTHESIA	•general or sedation and 1% lidocaine 1/100,000 epinephrine (local should be injected subcutaneously and in the midline down to the trachea)
POSITIONING	•neck extended with a roll beneath the shoulders (Fig. 2.14)
PREP	•sterile prep from mandible to clavicles

PROCEDURE

When possible the patient should be intubated prior to tracheostomy. This will permit the use of more potent analgesic agents and assure the airway during the procedure. Obviously in many of the acutely obstructed patients this will be impossible.

A horizontal skin incision is made midway between the cricoid cartilage and the sternoid notch (Fig. 2.14). Make sure that you are palpating the cricoid and not the thyroid gland isthmus (the isthmus is softer). Alternatively, a vertical incision may be made in the midline from 1 cm below the cricoid to 1 cm above the notch (Fig. 2.14). If the horizontal incision is elected it should be at least 4 to 5 cm in length.

PAROTIDECTOMY	
INDICATIONS	•masses of the parotid gland •recurrent infection
ANESTHESIA	•general (endotracheal tube should be on the side opposite the lesion)
POSITIONING	•neck extended with the head turned to the side opposite the lesion
PREP	•prep should include the entire hemiface and neck •draping should leave exposed the forehead, the corners of the eye and mouth and neck to the clavicle; the drapes may be secured by clips, staples or sutures

PROCEDURE

The incision should extend from the zygoma to the bottom of the ear lobe. It should stay in the crease immediately in front of the ear. From the ear lobe it should continue back over the mastoid tip and thence out onto the neck two finger breadths below the mandible (FIg. 2.16). Incise the skin only.

Skin hooks should then be used to retract the anterior border of the incision straight up and the flap elevated with scalpel or scissors. Stay immediately subcutaneous but do not buttonhole the skin. The flap should be elevated to within 3 cm of the corner of the eye and mouth (Fig. 2.17).

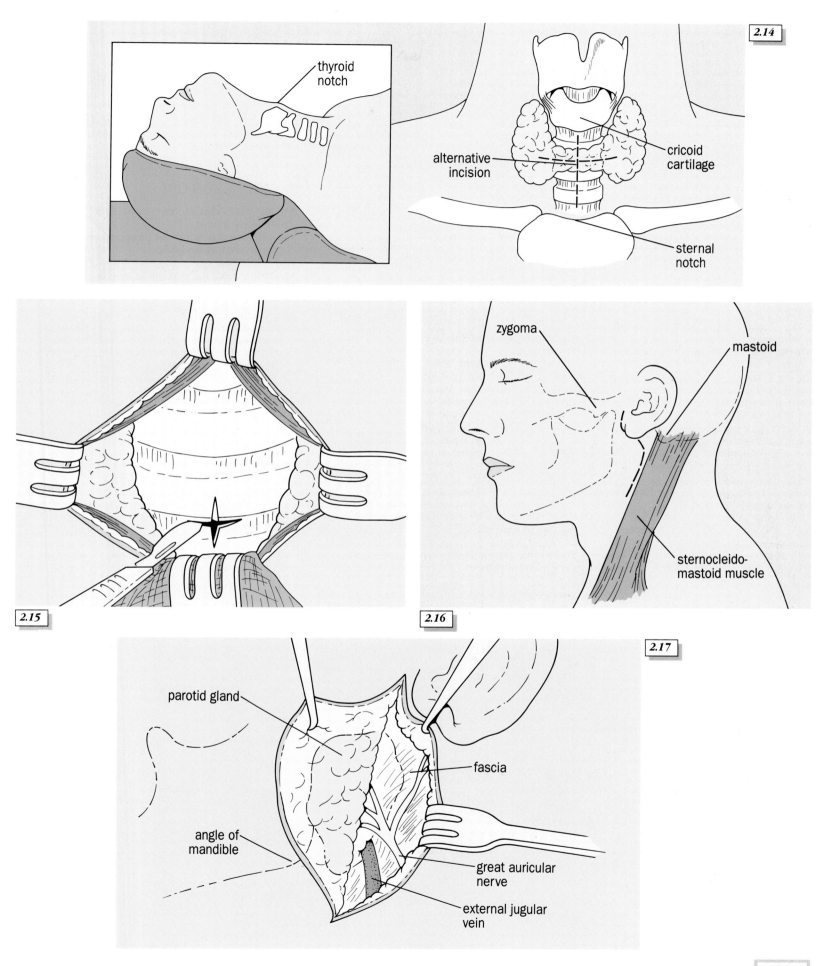

2.14

thyroid notch

cricoid cartilage

alternative incision

sternal notch

2.15

2.16

zygoma

mastoid

sternocleido-mastoid muscle

2.17

parotid gland

fascia

angle of mandible

great auricular nerve

external jugular vein

The next and most important step is to find the facial nerve. One of several different approaches may be employed:

1. The main trunk may be found by dissecting just anterior to the tragal cartilage. The main trunk will be found just caudal and medial to the inferior-most extension of the tragal cartilage (the tragal pointer) (Fig. 2.18).
2. The marginal mandibular nerve can be found overlaying the submandibular gland and dissection carried back to the main trunk (Fig. 2.19).
3. The buccal branch can be found by cannulating the parotid duct with a lacrimal probe. The nerve will run with the duct. Dissection can then be carried back to the main trunk (Fig. 2.20).
4. The nerve may be found as it exits the skull (Fig. 2.21).

A nerve stimulator should be employed to assure the inexperienced operator that he has indeed isolated the nerve. Once the main trunk has been isolated, the nerve is dissected out by bluntly spreading (a mosquito clamp is well suited to this) parallel to the main trunk and cutting the tissue above it. As the nerve branches each division must be followed and dissected out in the same manner. Do not clamp or electrocoagulate anything until you are sure that you will not injure the nerve in so doing. Use an army–navy retractor or a sponge on an assistant's finger to retract the gland as dissection continues. Tension on the retractors should be gentle and they should not directly impinge on the nerve. As the anterior edge of the gland is approached the superficial lobe is removed. Hemostasis should be obtained.

Should the mass extend deep to the nerve or lie wholly beneath the nerve, the nerve should then be bluntly elevated from the underlying tissue and the tissue medial to it removed. Prior to closure the main trunk should be stimulated. If all the branches do not work it may be necessary to perform a nerve anastomosis. A suction drain such as a Hemovac or Jackson Pratt should be inserted via a separate stab and the skin closed with a 3–0 or 4–0 absorbable suture subcutaneously and staples or a 4–0 or 5–0 nonabsorbable suture in the skin. Running suture should not be employed where the incision turns but may be employed elsewhere.

The suture anterior to the tragus should be removed in 5 to 7 days with the remainder coming out in 7 to 10 days. The drain should be removed when the drainage is below 20 cc/day.

The most common complication is facial nerve paresis. As long as the nerve was intact at the end of the procedure you can be reasonably assured that function will return.

Hematomas and seromas are also common and require evacuation. Other complications include salivary fistula, Frey's syndrome and synkinesis.

BRONCHOSCOPY

For any bronchoscopy make sure that adequate monitoring equipment (at least an EKG and/or pulse oximeter) is in use. Never perform this procedure without personnel trained in resuscitation.

BRONCHOSCOPY	
INDICATIONS	• atelectasis caused by mucous plugging or tumor, pulmonary lesions • as a staging procedure for head and neck tumors, hemoptysis, foreign body • for intubation • postaspiration, for pure sputa, and so on
ANESTHESIA	• general
INSTRUMENTS	• the flexible bronchoscope's small diameter and flexibility make it a fine diagnostic instrument (its small instrument channel is a liability that can prove frustrating in dealing with hemoptysis, foreign body or obstructing endobronchial tumor; in these cases the rigid instrument is preferred)

FLEXIBLE

Have the patient tell you which nostril is more patent by having him obstruct first one and then the other. Fill that nostril with viscous lidocaine (2 or 3 cc will do). Pass the instrument through the nose into the nasopharynx. Visualize the vocal cords and inject 2 cc of topical lidocaine onto the cords (Fig. 2.22). When the patient has stopped coughing have him inspire deeply and quickly pass the instrument through the cords. When you see the carina inject another 2 cc of topical lidocaine. Pass the instrument into each bronchus and carefully inspect for any pathology. If a lesion is seen the biopsy forceps should be passed via the instrument (suction) channel and advanced until it can just be seen.

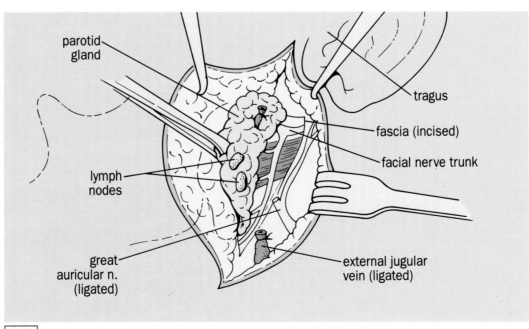

parotid gland

tragus

fascia (incised)

facial nerve trunk

lymph nodes

great auricular n. (ligated)

external jugular vein (ligated)

2.18

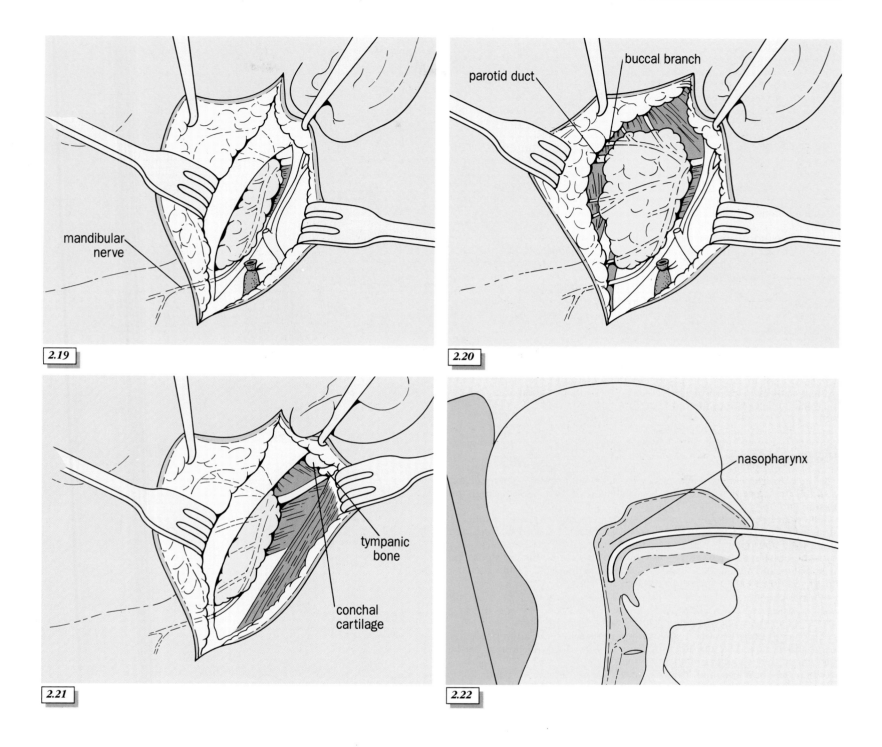

mandibular nerve

2.19

parotid duct

buccal branch

2.20

tympanic bone

conchal cartilage

2.21

nasopharynx

2.22

It should then be opened and advanced into the lesion, then closed and withdrawn. Brushings should then be taken by passing the brush down the instrument channel. The brush should be opened and passed over the lesion several times, closed, withdrawn, and immediately placed on slides and fixed. If no lesion is seen, saline should be instilled into the lobe suspected of harboring the lesion and then suctioned out into a Luken's trap which should be sent for cytology, Gram stain, and culture. Remember to have the specimen studied for TB.

In the event that the instrument is to be used to pass an endotracheal tube the operator must first make sure the tube is large enough to allow the bronchoscope to slide easily through it. The tube should be advanced enough throughout the nose and the bronchoscope then passed through it. When the cords have been visualized the bronchoscope should be rapidly advanced to the carina and the tube passed down over it. Prior to withdrawing the bronchoscope, check to make sure that you are still in the trachea then withdraw and have the anesthesiologist take over the airway.

If aspiration of gastric contents has occurred, copiously lavage out each bronchus. When performed soon after the event this helps to minimize or prevent pneumonia which is the usual sequel.

Suction and irrigation via the flexible instrument can also be used to clear mucous plugging after more conservative measures have failed. If the plugs are too thick to clear in this manner rigid bronchoscopy should be considered.

In the intubated patient, the bronchoscope may be passed via the endotracheal tube if an adapter suitable to allow respiration is employed. Remember to make sure the tube is large enough and the bronchoscope small enough to allow the patient to breath around the scope. In the patient with incipient respiratory collapse, it is often a good idea to intubate the patient prior to the bronchoscopy.

RIGID

The rigid instrument not only possesses a larger instrument channel but also has the capacity to allow for the ventilation of the patient through the instrument.

The pharynx should first be anesthetized with topical lidocaine. A straight-bladed laryngoscope is then used to visualize the vocal cords and more local anesthetic is placed directly in the cords (Figs. 2.23–2.25). The bronchoscope may then be passed through the cords, the laryngoscope withdrawn and more local instilled. The bronchoscope should then be advanced down each mainstem and lobar bronchus.

For the patient for whom a tracheostomy is necessary because of an airway obstruction, one operator should hold the bronchoscope in place above the carina while a tracheostomy is performed by others.

If a foreign body is found it should be grasped with the appropriate forceps and removed. If the foreign body is larger than the lumen of the instrument they should be withdrawn together.

When an endobronchial lesion is found, it should be biopsied. If the lesion is obstructive, the large lumen of the rigid instrument allows for the removal of large pieces of tumor, cautery or treatment with the laser. For patients with hemoptysis the larger lumen allows greater suction capacity, allowing for continued visualization, and thus maximizing attempts at localization and local control.

The procedure is terminated when the objective has been met, the instrument is withdrawn and the patient's respiratory status assured before the operator leaves the patient in the hands of other personnel.

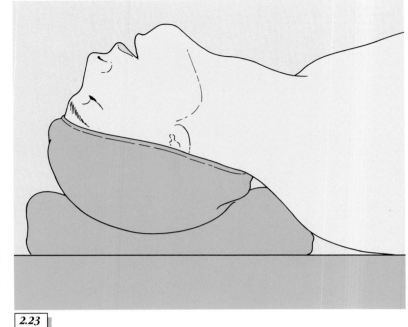

2.23

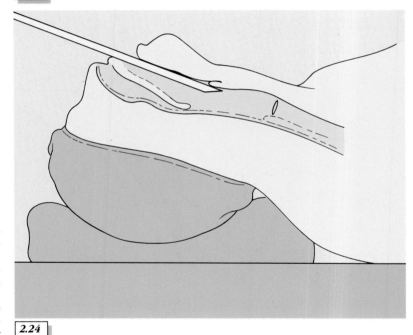

2.24

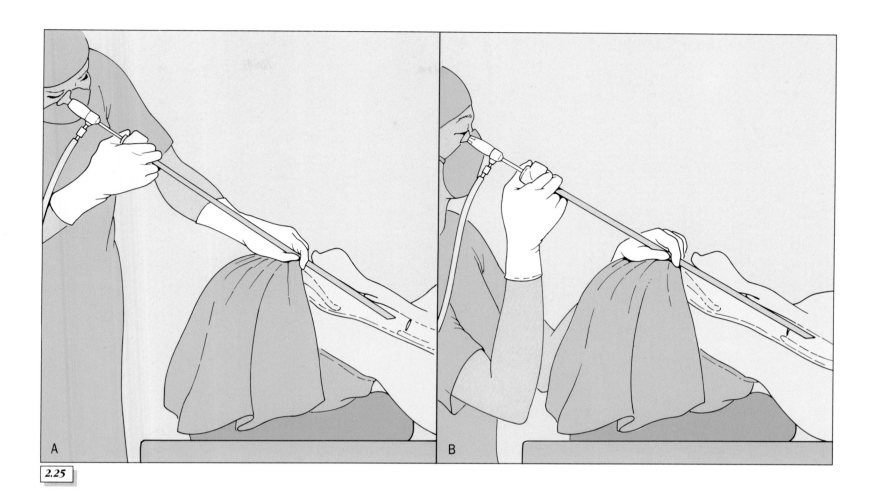

2.25

3

Thoracic Surgery

John D. Mannion • John J. Shannon • Herbert E. Cohn • Robert W. Solit • Richard N. Edie

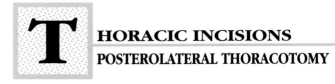

THORACIC INCISIONS
POSTEROLATERAL THORACOTOMY

The standard posterolateral thoracotomy provides excellent exposure of the anterior, middle, and posterior mediastinum, and either hemithorax. Selection of the most appropriate intercostal space for entry into the thorax depends on the procedure being performed. A fourth interspace incision is appropriate for lesions of the lung apex, or for procedures on the aortic arch or proximal descending thoracic aorta. A fifth intercostal space opening, which exposes the pulmonary hilus and the major interlobar fissures, is the preferred approach for upper lobe pulmonary resections. A lower incision in the sixth intercostal space is appropriate for a lower lobe resection and provides access to the distal intrathoracic esophagus and the esophago-gastric junction. In addition, detaching the diaphragm from its costal origin on the left side will allow exposure of the upper abdominal viscera, particularly the stomach. Further abdominal exposure with a lower posterolateral thoracotomy can be achieved with an anterior or abdominal extension of this incision. This is a thoracoabdominal incision, and is discussed subsequently.

POSTEROLATERAL THORACOTOMY

POSITIONING
- patient in full lateral position with the spinal column straight (Fig. 3.1A)
- axillary roll is placed under opposite axilla to avoid brachial plexus compression
- secure hips with broad adhesive tape to operating table
- underside leg is flexed, while the upper leg is extended
- place pillow between the legs
- upper side arm is extended on a padded armboard without fixation to allow scapula rotation and better exposure

PROCEDURE

An oblique skin incision parallels the intercostal space to be opened, is begun anteriorly. This is continued posteriorly to a point 3 cm below the tip of the scapula (Fig. 3.1B). The incision is then curved superiorly and continued between the medial border of the scapula and the thoracic spine. The extension cephalad should be carried out as medially as possible to minimize the possibility of injury to the spinal accessory nerve. Electrocautery, when placed on the cutting current, is used to incise the subcutaneous fascia and expose the muscular fascia of the chest wall. A posterior subcutaneous flap above the paraspinal musculature is elevated to a distance of 3 to 4 cm to allow for additional exposure. The auscultatory triangle, which is formed by the edges of the latissimus dorsi and trapezius muscles and the medial border of the scapula, is then opened and the fascia divided down to the level of the chest wall. Anteriorly, the latissimus dorsi muscle is then divided as well as a portion of the serratus anterior (Fig. 3.2). Posteriorly, the trapezius and a portion of the rhomboids are also divided to facilitate exposure (Fig. 3.2). A scapula retractor is used to elevate the scapula, allowing the surgeons hand to bluntly dissect and open the subscapular space. The second rib is easily identified by palpating the insertion of the serratus posterior superior muscle, as the first rib can be difficult to reach.

A rib is not resected on most thoracotomies. The thoracic cavity is generally entered through an intercostal space. A long segment of rib is resected on reoperative thoracotomies, where a wider exposure is helpful in finding the proper plane of dissection when extensive adhesions may be encountered. Also, a long section of rib is resected in thoracic exposures where it is needed for reconstruction of the thoracic spine.

The intercostal muscles of the interspace to be entered are divided using electrocautery along the upper margin of the lower rib in the interspace. Care is taken to avoid the intercostal neurovascular bundle. The parietal pleura is identified as a thin membrane where the lung can be seen moving beneath it if no adhesions are present. Positive pressure ventilation of the lungs is temporarily held while the pleural space is entered. The intercostal incision is extended anteriorly to the internal mammary vessels and posteriorly to the neck of the rib beneath the erector spinae muscles. Less force is necessary to open the ribs with a mechanical rib spreader using this longer intercostal incision. A limited intercostal incision may result in unnecessary rib fractures with a subsequent increase in postthoracotomy pain. In elderly patients, or in patients in whom a rib fracture seems likely, a subperiosteal 2-cm rib resection at the costovertebral angle of the inferior or superior ribs, or both, may prevent rib fractures. Pleural adhesions encountered within the thoracic cavity require mobilization of the lung by sharp dissection. Attempts to digitally mobilize the lung often result in tears of the fragile visceral pleura and lung which leads to multiple alveolar air leaks and excessive bleeding.

The chest can be closed in several ways. In our practice an angled, #32 posterior chest tube, and a straight, apical, #32 chest tube are then brought out through separate stab wounds at the mid-axillary line, below the incision. The apical tube evacuates air, and the posterior tube drains fluid. If an interspace incision has been used, the ribs are then approximated with #1 absorbable suture, usually four. If a rib has been resected, the intercostal muscles are approximated with interrupted 2–0 nonabsorbable dacron sutures. The latissimus and other divided muscles approximated with a #0 absorbable suture. Clips are used to approximate the skin.

MODIFICATION OF THE POSTEROLATERAL THORACOTOMY

MUSCLE-SPARING THORACOTOMIES
The standard approach for pulmonary resections has been the posterolateral incision. This incision unquestionably provides excellent exposure of the entire thoracic cavity, but requires a considerable time to open and close, and is associated with significant short- and long-term disability. Four major muscle groups can be divided—the serratus anterior, the latissimus dorsi, the trapezius, and the rhomboideus major. In selected groups of patients, ie, the elderly, in patients where bilateral thoracotomies are required, or in paraplegics or athletes where arm strength must be preserved, division of these major muscle groups can result in significant acute and chronic disability. Some surgeons tailor the posterolateral incision to the need for exposure: for instance, the serratus may be only partially divided, as well as the trapezius and rhomboids. The following adaptations of the posterolateral thoracotomy have been described formally, that minimize postoperative disability.

Muscle-sparing incisions are not ideal in heavily muscled individuals, or where the best exposure is mandatory, ie, vascular procedures or difficult pulmonary procedures. Since there is a clear-cut tradeoff of exposure for postoperative disability, the occasional thoracic surgeon should probably avoid their use. These incisions can be very useful for wedge resections or other minor thoracic procedures, and straightforward pulmonary resections.

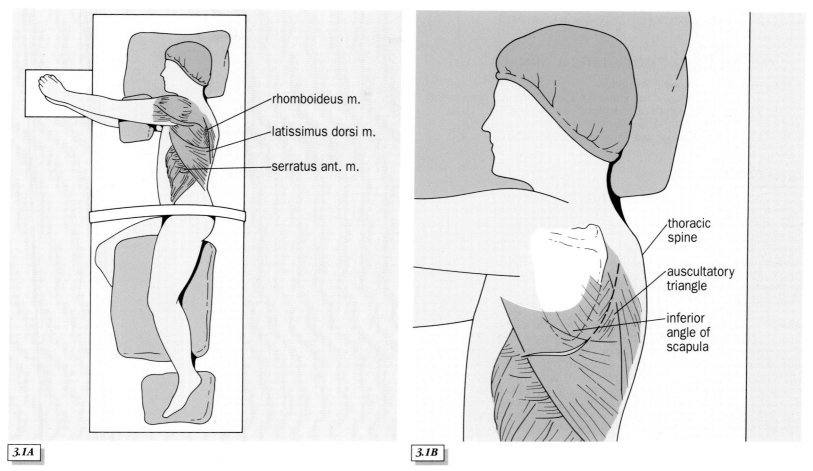

rhomboideus m.

latissimus dorsi m.

serratus ant. m.

3.1A

thoracic spine

auscultatory triangle

inferior angle of scapula

3.1B

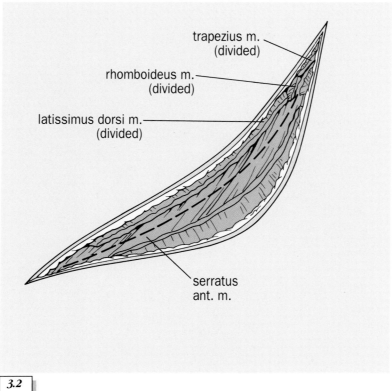

trapezius m. (divided)

rhomboideus m. (divided)

latissimus dorsi m. (divided)

serratus ant. m.

3.2

AXILLARY THORACOTOMY (LATERAL THORACOTOMY)

AXILLARY THORACOTOMY (LATERAL THORACOTOMY)

POSITIONING
- lateral decubitus
- upper arm abducted above clavicular level and stabilized on padded ether screen (Fig. 3.3) to help define the lateral borders of pectoralis major and latissimus dorsi muscles

PROCEDURE

The axillary thoracotomy was the first commonly used muscle-sparing thoracotomy. None of the extracostal muscles is divided during the exposure; thus the chest wall function is minimally impaired after this incision, and therefore this incision is often indicated in patients with poor pulmonary function. The axillary thoracotomy is commonly used to resect a ruptured apical pulmonary bleb, or a small and well-circumscribed upper lobe lung lesions. Some have advocated this technique for any pulmonary resection that does not involve operating on the diaphragm.

The second intercostal space lies along the inferior border of the axillary hair follicles, while the third intercostal space is approximately 2 cm below this margin and just above the plane with the nipple anteriorly. An oblique incision that parallels the desired interspace is made. Extension of the skin incision beyond the axillary folds over the latissimus dorsi and the pectoralis major muscles can significantly improve exposure. The latissimus dorsi muscle is retracted posteriorly and the serratus anterior is split along the direction of its fibers, with the caveat that it should not be split too far posteriorly in order to avoid injury the long thoracic nerve (Fig. 3.4). Insertion of two Tuffier retractors—one in the intercostal space, and one in the soft tissues—provides excellent exposure. Blunt finger dissection of the intercostal muscles anteriorly and posteriorly can improve exposure. Occasionally, subperiosteal resection of the third rib and incision through its subperiosteal bed is necessary.

Closure of the thoracotomy begins with placement of pleural drainage catheters, which can be brought out through the fifth intercostal space. Interrupted pericostal sutures then are used to approximate the ribs. The rib approximator is sometimes difficult to place through this incision, so a towel clip might be used. The subcutaneous tissue and skin are closed routinely. Cosmetically, the use of a subcuticular skin closure along with placement of steri-strips enhances the appearance of the wound.

SERRATUS SLING

A partial muscle-sparing incision has been described recently by Heitmiller, which is essentially a posterolateral thoracotomy, where only the latissimus dorsi muscle is divided. A standard skin incision is made, but the posterior extent stops at the anterior edge of the trapezius. The latissimus dorsi is then divided, and each edge undermined for 2 to 3 cm (Fig. 3.5). The serratus anterior is located by dissection in the auscultatory triangle, the long thoracic nerve located on the surface of the muscle, and a Kelly clamp passed from medial to the nerve around the lateral aspect of the muscle. A Penrose drain is grasped and used to retract the muscle medially (Fig. 3.6). The thoracic cavity is then entered in the chosen interspace. Closure of the incision is routine.

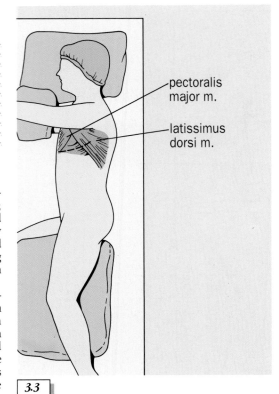

pectoralis major m.

latissimus dorsi m.

3.3

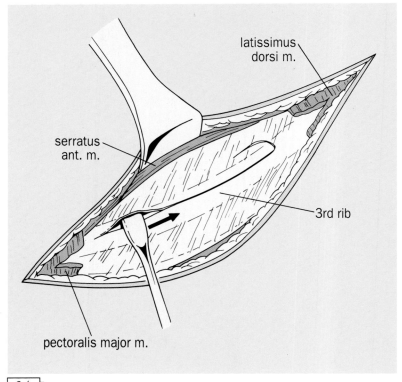

latissimus dorsi m.

serratus ant. m.

3rd rib

pectoralis major m.

3.4

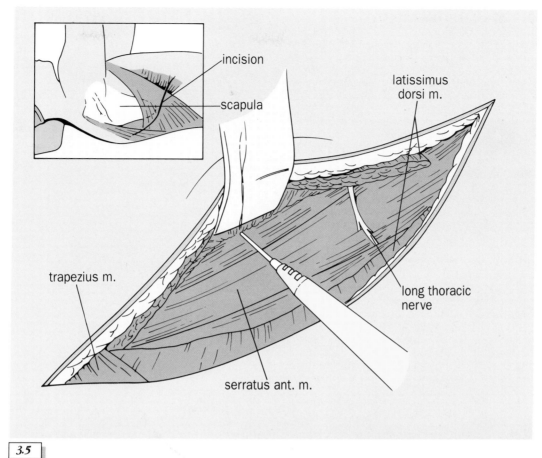

incision

scapula

latissimus dorsi m.

trapezius m.

long thoracic nerve

serratus ant. m.

3.5

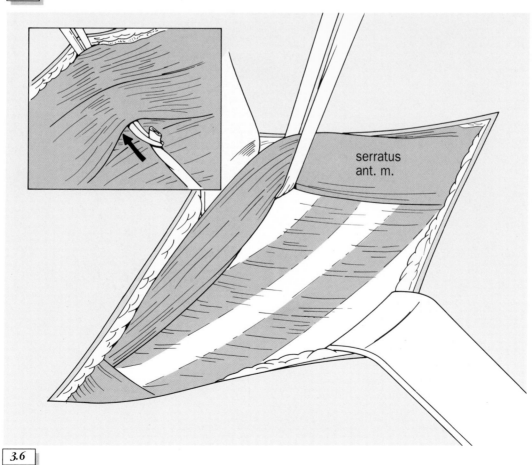

serratus ant. m.

3.6

MUSCLE-SPARING POSTEROLATERAL THORACOTOMY

Described recently by Bethencourt and Holmes, this is a posterolateral thoracotomy where no muscle groups are divided. A standard skin incision for a posterolateral thoracotomy is then made, extending from the submammary crease 2 cm anterior to the anterior axillary line, and continuing 2 cm posterior to the tip of the scapula (Fig. 3.7). The subcutaneous tissue is then dissected off the latissimus muscle, both towards the axilla and the iliac crest. The underside of the latissimus is then similarly mobilized. The lateral edge of the serratus anterior is then dissected to its insertion into the sixth rib. The thorax is entered through the chosen interspace, and two rib retractors are utilized, one to separate the ribs, and the second to separate the serratus and the latissimus (Fig. 3.8). The intercostal muscles are divided from the internal mammary vessels to the transverse processes.

Closure involves routine approximation of the ribs with pericostal sutures, and placement of a single suture on the posterior border of the serratus and the anterior border of the latissimus to anchor them to the surrounding fascia. The skin is closed over two suction drains.

THORACOTOMY THROUGH THE AUSCULTATORY TRIANGLE

This technique, described by Horowitz et al., is similar to the muscle-sparing thoracotomy depicted above, in that it preserves both the serratus and the latissimus dorsi muscles. It differs from the previously described incision, however, in that dissection and retraction of the latissimus is from a posterior direction. The usual skin incision for a posterolateral thoracotomy is made and the superficial latissimus is then dissected from the subcutaneous tissue. The fascia of the auscultatory triangle is then incised and the posterior border of the latissimus is freed both inferiorly and superiorly (Fig. 3.9). The deep aspect of the muscle is then mobilized from the chest wall, exposing the serratus anterior. The serratus and latissimus are then retracted anteriorly, and the scapula superiorly (Fig. 3.10). A greater exposure is achieved through long resection of the fifth rib. Closure is routine.

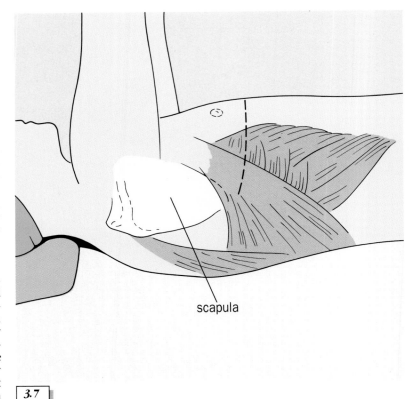

scapula

3.7

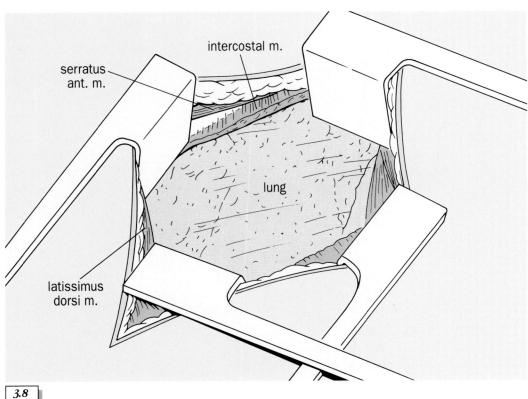

serratus ant. m.

intercostal m.

lung

latissimus dorsi m.

3.8

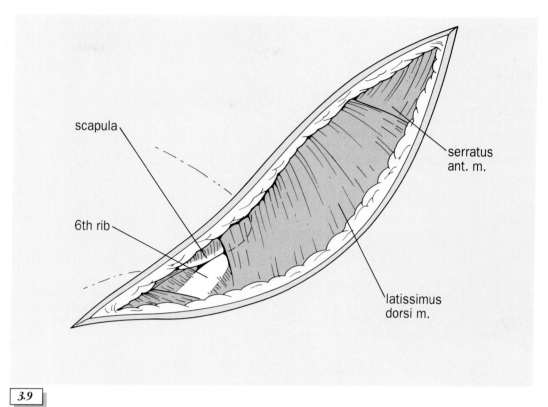

scapula

serratus
ant. m.

6th rib

latissimus
dorsi m.

3.9

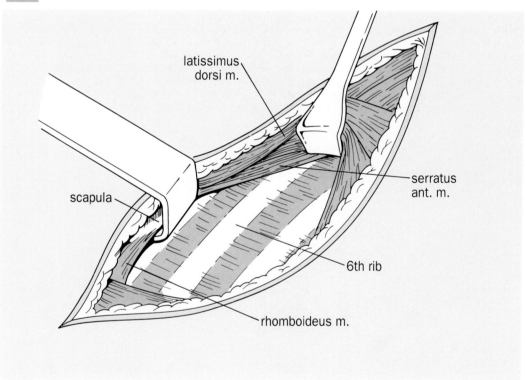

latissimus
dorsi m.

scapula

serratus
ant. m.

6th rib

rhomboideus m.

3.10

ANTEROLATERAL THORACOTOMY

ANTEROLATERAL THORACOTOMY	
POSITIONING	•supine, with a roll under the back to elevate the chest of the operative side; this maneuver allows sterile draping down to the posterior axillary line •the arm can be suspended over the patient on an ether screen, abducted outward onto an armboard, or placed along the operative side

PROCEDURE

This thoracic incision is commonly used for an open lung biopsy; on the left side it is ideal for exposure of the pericardial sac, in order to create a pericardial window or implant an epicardial pacemaker lead.

A skin incision is made just below the nipple in males (Fig. 3.11A), or within the submammary fold in females (Fig. 3.11B). It follows the curvature of the fourth rib and is extended to the midaxillary line. A common mistake is to make the incision too low in the fifth interspace. The pectoralis major muscle is divided, followed by placement of a self-retaining retractor, for exposure of the rib cage, which is covered laterally by the serratus anterior and pectoralis minor muscles (Fig. 3.12). The serratus anterior is divided along the orientation of its fibers, stopping short of the long thoracic nerve. Next the intercostal muscles and parietal pleura, in the fourth intercostal space, are transected using electrocautery, while protecting the lung. The internal mammary vessels will be found at the parasternal aspect of this intercostal incision and may require ligation and division. A wider exposure can be obtained anteriorly by obliquely transecting the adjacent costal cartilages (Fig. 3.13), and laterally, by extending the intercostal opening to the border of the latissimus dorsi muscle. A long-tipped Bovie is helpful in this maneuver.

Closure of the anterior thoracotomy is similar to the posterolateral thoracotomy, but the closure is more tenuous because of thinner overlying muscles. First, pericostal sutures of #1 absorbable are passed around the ribs, and tightened. The pectoralis major and serratus muscles are closed with continuous absorbable sutures. The superficial fascia, subcutaneous tissue and skin are then reapproximated with care taken to insure an airtight closure over the pectoralis fascia. The pleural space is usually drained with a chest tube brought out through the sixth intercostal space, at the level of the anterior axillary line.

MEDIAN STERNOTOMY

This is the standard incision employed for most cardiac surgical procedures, and provides excellent access to the anterior mediastinum, heart, ascending aorta, and great vessels. Through the median sternotomy either mediastinal pleural reflection can be opened widely. Wedge resections of bilateral pulmonary nodules can often be performed simultaneously using this approach, avoiding the need for staged thoracotomies. Some authors have even advocated the use of the median sternotomy for lobectomies, especially in patients with poor pulmonary reserve.

MEDIAN STERNOTOMY	
POSITIONING	•supine, with a roll transversely placed underneath the shoulders, which slightly hyperextends the neck and defines the suprasternal notch

PROCEDURE

A midline skin incision is made from a point beginning about 2 cm below the suprasternal notch to 3 cm below the xyphoid process. A superior extension of this incision above the manubrium at the base of the neck leaves an undesirable cosmetic result. Electrocautery is then used for hemostasis and to incise the presternal fascia and overlying midline periosteum (Fig. 3.14). However, overzealous use of electrocautery is to be avoided, as there is some evidence that it may increase the incidence of sternal infections. Retraction of the upper wound margin, followed by blunt and sharp dissection, is used to define the suprasternal notch and create a retrosternal tissue plane. Commonly a transverse vein that must be ligated is encountered during this maneuver.

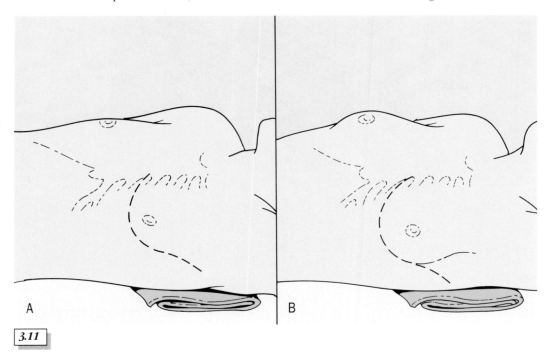

A   B

3.11

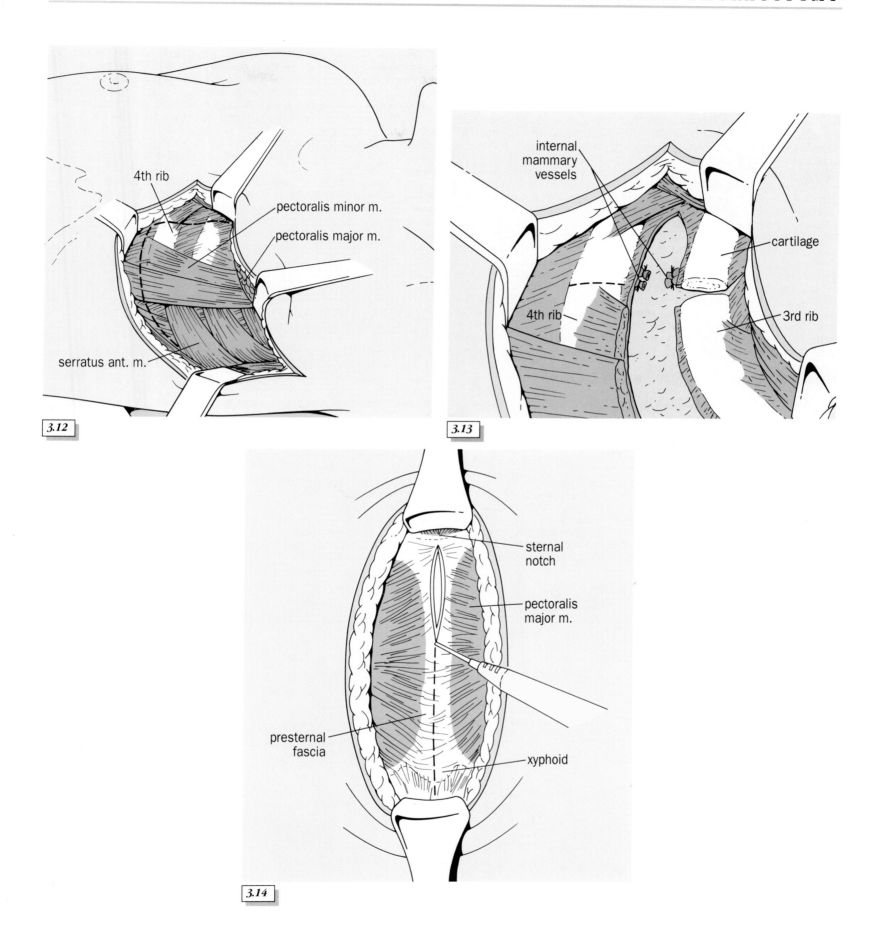

4th rib

pectoralis minor m.

pectoralis major m.

serratus ant. m.

3.12

internal mammary vessels

cartilage

4th rib

3rd rib

3.13

sternal notch

pectoralis major m.

presternal fascia

xyphoid

3.14

The xyphoid process is now exposed by dividing the linea alba, while carefully avoiding the preperitoneal tissues. The center of the sternum is then scored with the electrocautery from sternal notch to the xyphoid process. Fingertips in the edge of opposite intercostal spaces locates the center of the sternum. A powered saber saw is then hooked in the suprasternal notch, angling the blunt guide tip against the posterior sternal wall, and the sternum is divided (Fig. 3.15). Bleeding from the transected sternum can be brisk, requiring the placement of two army–navy retractors to elevate each bony half for hemostasis.

A self-retaining four-blade retractor is placed and opened gradually, in order to avoid dislocating the costal cartilage junctions or fracturing the sternum. Excessive sternal retraction may even result in a thoracic outlet neuropathy or fracture of the first rib.

Closure of the incision begins with placement of a retrosternal catheter for drainage of the anterior mediastinum. Two interrupted stainless steel wires (size 5 or 6) are placed first through the manubrium, 2 cm from the transected edge. Four or more additional wires are then placed around the sternal body, avoiding injury to the internal mammary vessels, or through the body of the sternum. The wires are twisted tight enough with a heavy needle holder to stabilize the sternum. Overtightening may result in breaking the wires. A continuous absorbable suture is used to close the abdominal and presternal pectoralis fascia in a single layer. The subcutaneous layer and skin are then approximated separately, again using a continuous suturing technique.

MEDIAN STERNOTOMY VIA SUBMAMMARY INCISION

MEDIAN STERNOTOMY VIA SUBMAMMARY INCISION

POSITIONING •supine, with shoulder roll placed, which slightly extends the neck

PROCEDURE

The bilateral inframammary skin incision is a cosmetically acceptable alternative to the midline vertical skin incision, through which the median sternotomy can be performed. This skin incision is rarely used, but is most appropriate for selected females. A symmetric butterfly incision is then made, which follows the patient's natural inframammary folds and crosses the xyphoid sternal junction at the midline (Fig. 3.16). Electro-cautery is then used to achieve hemostasis. The dissection is then carried down to the pectoralis fascia. A superior skin flap is developed to the level of the sternal notch and insertion of the cervical strap muscles. A much smaller inferior skin flap is created centrally to expose the xyphoid process completely. Subcutaneous stay sutures are placed to retract each flap, which are then covered with a moist laparotomy pad for protection. Dissection of the suprasternal notch and xyphoid process are carried out in the standard fashion.

At the completion of the procedure, the sternum is closed as described above. A closed suction system is placed under superior skin flap to obliterate the dead space and to evacuate sero-serosanguineous drainage. The subcutaneous fascia is then approximated with interrupted absorbable sutures carefully aligning the superior and inferior flaps into a midline position. The subcutaneous layer and skin are reapproximated with a running continuous suture, followed by placement of steri-strips over the wound.

BILATERAL ANTERIOR THORACOTOMY (EMERGENCY THORACOTOMY)

This approach is indicated in certain instances for penetrating thoracic trauma, which results in cardiac tamponade, or exsanguinating hemorrhage from the pulmonary hilus, heart, or great vessels. A left anterolateral thoracotomy in the fourth interspace (see Fig. 3.16), as previously described, provides access to initiate open cardiac massage. Extension of this thoracotomy, across the mid-line, into a bilateral submammary incision, enters the contralateral fourth interspace. A transverse sternotomy is then performed to interconnect these interspaces and provide extensive exposure to the heart and entire mediastinum. The use of the Gigli saw for sternal transection is depicted in Fig. 3.17. Bleeding encountered from the internal mammary vessels is temporarily controlled with a hemostat, while the major intrathoracic pathology is dealt with.

Incisional closure is begun first with sternal reapproximation, using two interrupted stainless steel wires. Pericostal sutures are then placed around the fourth intercostal spaces and tied securely; the muscle layers, subcutaneous fascia, and skin are then approximated with continuous sutures, similar to the anterior thoracotomy closure, as shown previously.

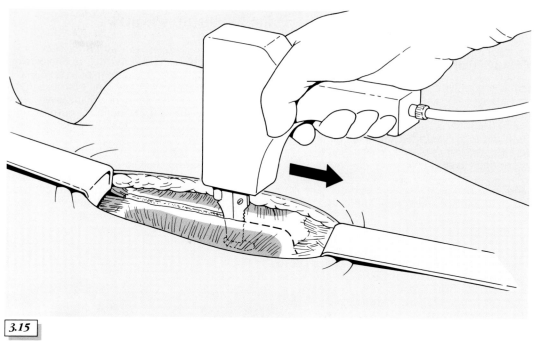

3.15

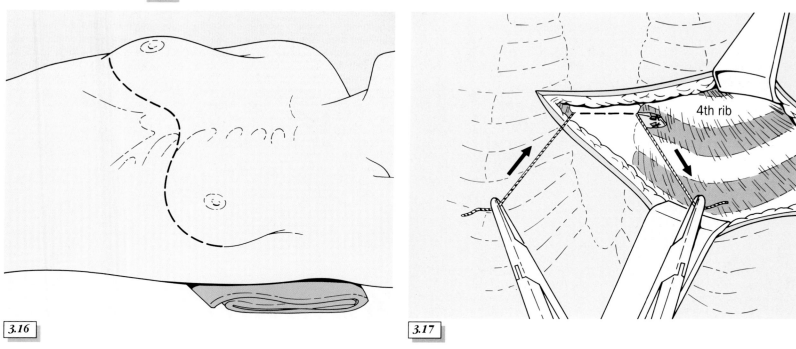

3.16

3.17

4th rib

THORACOABDOMINAL INCISION

THORACOABDOMINAL INCISION

POSITIONING • patient is placed with the hips and scapular wings forming a 45° angle to the plane of the operating table (Fig. 3.18); broad adhesive tape is placed to firmly secure the patient in the oblique position and to prevent the trunk from falling posteriorly; the arm is placed in a stockinette, and positioned as needed

PREP • the complete skin prep should extend over the lateral chest and abdomen from umbilicus

PROCEDURE

A thoracoabdominal incision provides a continuous level of exposure between the lower hemithorax and upper abdominal viscera through a single operative approach. The division of the costal margin along with its attached hemidiaphragm is the key towards developing this extended field of exposure; however, increased post-thoracotomy pain is known to occur following this incision because of the greater respiratory motion in the lower ribs, and the difficulty in stabilizing the divided costal margin. The left thoracoabdominal incision is employed for disease involving the gastroesophageal junction or for exposure of the supraceliac aorta or the anterior vertebra of the thoracolumbar spine. Rarely is the right-sided approach used because the liver fills the upper abdomen and compromises exposure. However, when there is a need for viewing the retrohepatic caval veins the right-sided approach is helpful.

A thoracotomy incision is begun overlying the sixth or seventh intercostal space and is extended anteriorly across the costal margin. The abdominal portion of the incision continues in a transverse line across the rectus sheath until the linea alba is identified. The latissimus dorsi is divided completely, along with some of the costal insertion points of the serratus anterior along the intercostal space being entered. The intercostal muscles are divided using electrocautery against the upper margin of the lower rib through the selected interspace up towards the costal cage anteriorly. Next the abdominal oblique muscles and rectus sheath are divided to expose the underlying peritoneum and cartilaginous costal margin. A large right-angle clamp is passed around the unroofed segment of costal arch for separation of the diaphragm from its undersurface. The soft cartilage is transected sharply using a scalpel and the peritoneum is then entered.

A mechanical rib retractor is placed to gradually open up the thoracotomy, which brings into view the anterior attachments of the diaphragm. The diaphragm is divided circumferentially, anteriorly and laterally, leaving behind a 2-cm rim of diaphragmatic tissue for its reattachment during closure. Silk marking sutures are placed on each side for accurate realignment during closure. The peripheral diaphragmatic incision along the lateral chest wall preserves the phrenic neurovascular pedicle supplying this muscle, avoiding its postoperative dysfunction. The posterior segment of diaphragm is divided in the direction towards the esophageal, aortic, or spinal crural fibers, depending on the surgical procedure planned.

Closure of the incision begins with realignment of diaphragmatic muscle edges, using the previously placed silk sutures as a guide. Heavy figure-of-eight silk sutures are used to plicate the diaphragm muscle together during closure. The divided costal margin is reapproximated by placing heavy interrupted sutures directly through these cartilaginous ends. Two centimeters of costal margin are often resected, to prevent painful slippage postoperatively. The ribs are closed with interrupted pericostal sutures that are passed around them adjacent to the opened intercostal space. Chest tubes are placed for drainage of the pleural space, particularly along the paravertebral gutter in proximity to any gastroesophageal anastomosis within the chest. The thoracic and abdominal muscles are closed in a routine fashion. A nasogastric tube is essential postoperatively because of the high incidence for intestinal ileus which can create tension against the diaphragmatic closure.

SUBXYPHOID WINDOW

A subxyphoid window is a useful incision for drainage of pericardial fluid or for placement of an epicardial pacemaker or an AICD. When used for pericardial drainage, it is important to note that this procedure is incorrectly named, in that a window is not created to another body cavity. Rather, drains are placed in the pericardial space, and with the drainage of fluid, the epicardium and pericardium are approximated. This, and the drains themselves, promote adhesions, which helps to prevent reaccumulation of fluid.

A subxyphoid window, which can be performed under local anesthesia, has obvious advantages in a patient with cardiac tamponade. The use of a local anesthetic does not imply, however, that this is a simple procedure. An arterial line should be positioned in all patients, and temporary pacemaker wires and pacemaker should be available, if a reflex bradycardia develops. Also, the surgeon should be capable of performing a median sternotomy, if needed.

SUBXYPHOID WINDOW

POSITIONING • same as for median sternotomy (see page 3.8)

PROCEDURE

A 6-cm skin incision is made over the lower sternum, xyphoid process, and linea alba. The upper linea alba is divided, and the xyphoid process is grasped with a Kocher clamp (Fig. 3.19). Electrocautery is then used to dissect the xyphoid and a rib shears is used to separate the xyphoid from the sternum. The attachments of the diaphragm to the underside of the xyphoid process are divided, and the preperitoneal space underneath the left rectus is bluntly dissected. An army–navy retractor is then used to elevate the lower sternum and the diaphragm is reflected inferiorly with a sponge on a stick. A finger can then be placed over the heart. The lower aspect of the anterior pericardium is covered with a layer of adipose tissue, which should be cleaned off the pericardium. Care is taken to avoid entering the right pleural cavity. The pericardium is then grasped and opened, and a biopsy taken. Considerable additional exposure can be obtained when the pericardium has been opened by placing a malleable retractor inside the pericardial cavity and retracting caudally. Also, a sponge on a stick can be used to push the inferior surface of the heart superiorly. A soft drain is placed through a separate incision and the incision is closed routinely.

MAJOR PULMONARY RESECTIONS
CONTROLLING THE PULMONARY VASCULATURE

VASCULAR DISSECTION

The primary goal during the dissection of any pulmonary vessel is to obtain enough length to allow a safe ligation. Direct clamping of the pulmonary artery with a hemostat or grasping of these fragile, low pressure vessels with forceps during their exposure can result in a crush injury or tear. As well, excessive traction applied to any branch vessel may avulse its orifice off the main vessel causing a major tangential laceration with significant hemorrhage.

Initially, sharp dissection is used while the adjacent areolar tissues are retracted off the vessel in order to incise its perivascular sheath. The potential plane between adventitial wall and perivascular sheath is an avascular layer which is developed using a blunt "peanut" dissector to separate the tissues (Fig. 3.20). Caution is used when this layer is found to be fused together as it may indicate direct vascular wall invasion from a tumor.

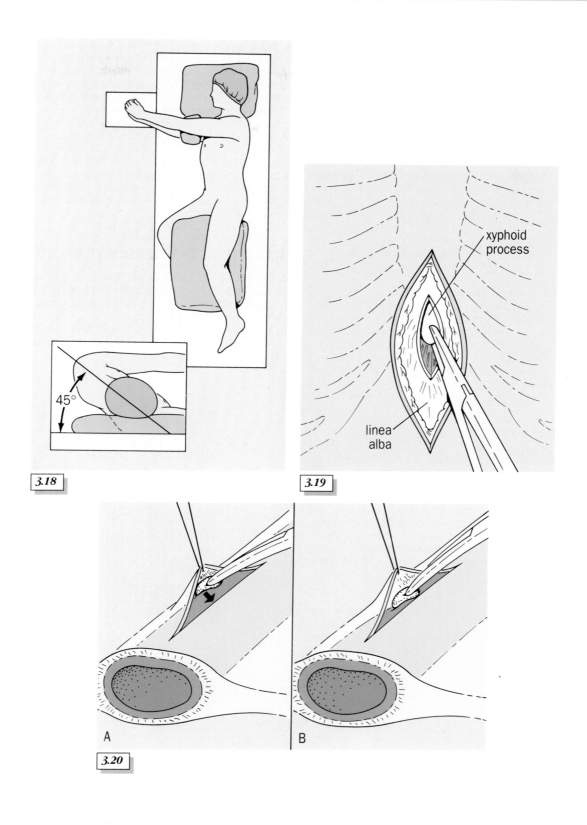

xyphoid
process

linea
alba

45°

3.18

3.19

A   B

3.20

Sharply extending an incision atop a free perivascular space is carried out to further unroof the vessel and expose a length distally. Ligating distal branches or dividing the inflammatory scar of a thickened perivascular sheath are two other methods used to obtain additional length. The vessel is freed on three sides before passing a blunt right-angle beneath the posterior wall to encircle it.

VASCULAR LIGATION

Ligation techniques vary depending on the size of the vessel and the length developed after a completed dissection. One method of proximal control involves the placement of a free ligature and a second suture or transfixion ligature separated by a small sausage of vascular tissue (Fig. 3.21). Distally, a single free ligature is tied or a temporary hemoclip is placed to prevent back-bleeding once the vessel is divided. The point of transection should always be at the expense of the distal tie as this leaves a large enough proximal "cauliflower" cuff to control ligature slippage (Fig. 3.22A). If the artery to be ligated is near a bifurcation, it might be preferable to transect the artery just distal to the bifurcation. In this way the distal cuff is enlarged, and this helps to prevent slippage.

Occasionally the vessel is transected before the distal ligature is placed. Sequestered pulmonary blood escaping from an unligated distal vascular cuff is temporarily controlled with digital pressure, followed by open placement of a hemostatic stitch. Tumor encroachment or a dense inflammatory reaction restricting adequate length are the common reasons to apply this open ligation technique of a distal cuff.

Lobar or segmental vessels are usually ligated with 2–0 silk. The main pulmonary artery can be treated with #1 or #0 silk or with one of the methods discussed below. Ligation is considered by Hood to be the least safe method.

TRANSECTION AND OVERSEWING

Another technique of control of the pulmonary artery is to transiently occlude the vessel in a noncrushing vascular clamp. The artery is then transected, leaving a long enough stump distal to the clamp to oversew the vessel. A vascular suture, usually a 4–0 monofilament Prolene, is used. Great care is taken to follow the curve of the needle when passing it through the pulmonary artery to prevent tearing of the end of the vessel. Two layers are used: the first layer is a running horizontal mattress, followed with a continuous over-and-over suture. The two ends of the suture are then tied together (Fig. 3.22B). The vascular clamp is gradually released to slowly pressurize the suture line, especially when the main pulmonary artery trunk is closed using this method.

VASCULAR STAPLING

The vascular stapling instrument is used for ligation of the bulkier pulmonary vessels such as the main pulmonary artery and veins. It has the advantage of plicating these larger vascular trunks into a single staple line rapidly to allow scalpel transection distally. The "V" staples are designed to apply a hemostatic staple closure in this situation. We prefer the instrument for the pulmonary venous trunks, controlling the artery with one of the two methods above.

CLOSURE OF THE BRONCHUS

Bronchial closure has been greatly simplified with the introduction of the mechanical stapler. There are several principles which must be adhered to with the use of this technique. Dissection of the bronchus should be performed as gently as possible. It is important that the bronchial vessels not be ligated too proximal to the intended closure site, since this will compromise the blood supply to the bronchial stump. Also, the stapler should be applied so that the anterior wall of the bronchus is apposed to the posterior wall (Fig. 3.23). For bronchial closure 4.8-mm staples are usually used.

Although the stapler is the preferred method of bronchial closure, there are circumstances when the bronchus must be closed with sutures (Fig. 3.24A). Generally, 4–0 nonabsorbable dacron sutures, on an atraumatic needle, are used. The tissues should be handled as gently as possible, and the curve of the needle should be followed, to prevent any tearing of the

bronchial walls. Simple sutures, 2 to 3 mm apart, are recommended; they are tied firmly (Fig. 3.24B), but not too tightly, to avoid strangulation of the bronchial stump. Hood recommends approximately six sutures for the main bronchus (Fig. 3.24C), and three to four for a lobar bronchus.

After the bronchial closure, the stump should be checked with 40 cm of positive pressure to ensure that there are no leaks. With a hand-sewn closure, additional sutures are occasionally required. Also, on occasion, a small leak may be noted from a stapled suture line. Additional sutures may be necessary. Coverage of a bronchial stump can be done with a pleural flap, or a flap of vascularized tissue. Probably the most beneficial flap to use is the intercostal muscle bundle. When a coverage of a bronchial stump can be anticipated, such as in a completion pneumonectomy, the muscle bundle should be harvested during entrance into the pleural cavity, to prevent compression by a retractor.

MEDIASTINAL LYMPH NODE DISSECTION

Mediastinal lymph node dissection is performed to assist in pathologic staging of pulmonary neoplasms. The precise anatomic location of the dissected region should be noted to differentiate between N1 and N2 nodes at the time of resection.

The regional stations for lymph node involvement in lung cancer as adopted by the International Joint Committee for Cancer Staging and End Results Reporting, in November 1981, are shown in Fig. 3.25.

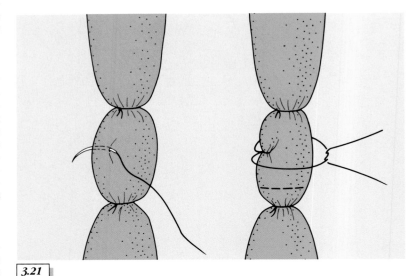

3.21

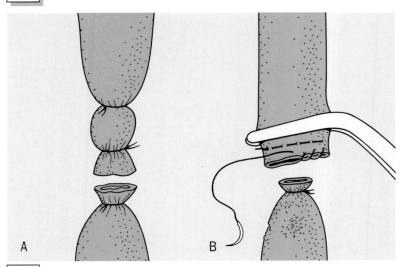

A   B

3.22

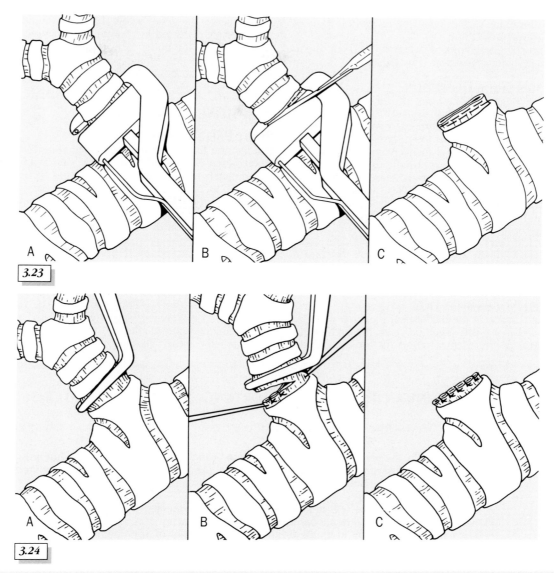

3.23

3.24

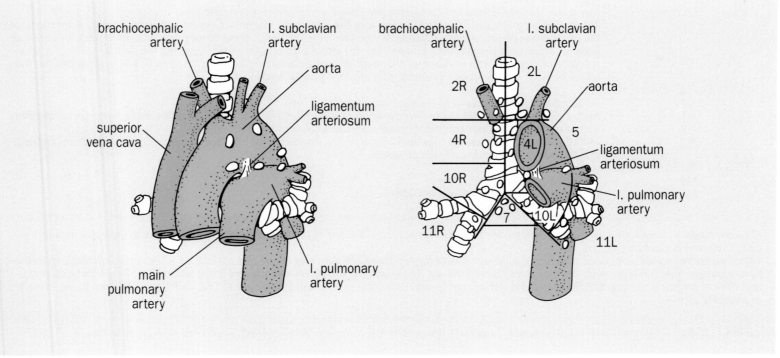

3.25

This system designates the locations of the lymph nodes on the basis of readily identifiable adjacent structures (Table 3.1).

The technique for dissection at thoracotomy differs right from left due to the asymmetry of the thoracic cavities, as reported by Cahan.

RIGHT MEDIASTINAL LYMPH NODE DISSECTION

On the right, the dissection begins at the apex of the thoracic cavity (Fig. 3.26). The vagus nerve is identified near the subclavian artery, just distal to the takeoff of the right recurrent laryngeal nerve. An incision is then made in the pleura, from this point to the azygous vein, immediately anterior to the vagus. A pleural flap is then created anteriorly by pulling the superior vena cava and phrenic nerve anteriorly. Starting at the apex, the mediastinal tissue between the trachea and superior vena cava, is then swept towards the azygous vein (Fig. 3.27). This can be divided or left intact, but there is usually a large lymph node beneath the azygous.

The subcarinal nodes are then dissected by incising the parietal pleura anterior to the esophagus, immediately beneath the right mainstem bronchus. Usually three or four large nodes are encountered. The nodes from the inferior pulmonary ligament are taken when that structure is divided. Care should be taken to avoid injury to the esophagus, which is located adjacent to the node-bearing tissue.

LEFT MEDIASTINAL LYMPH NODE DISSECTION

On the left side, an incision is made in the mediastinal pleura at the apex of the chest, and is extended along the vagus nerve to the arch of the aorta (Fig. 3.28). An anterior pleural flap is raised to the level of the phrenic nerve; the tissue below the subclavian vein, and above the subclavian artery is dissected inferiorly. The subaortic space, beneath the aortic arch and above the pulmonary artery, is then dissected out with the specimen. The dissection of the subcarinal space and posterior mediastinal nodes is similar to the right side.

PNEUMONECTOMY

RIGHT PNEUMONECTOMY

The incision used routinely for a pneumonectomy is a right posterolateral thoracotomy. Sharp dissection of any pleural adhesions is then performed to completely mobilize the lung.

HILAR DISSECTION

The initial step with a right pneumonectomy, as with any pulmonary resection, is division of the inferior pulmonary ligament up to the level of the inferior pulmonary vein. The mediastinal pleura over the anterior hilum is then sharply incised, from the level of the inferior pulmonary vein to the azygous vein. The lung is reflected posteriorly, and the loose areolar tissue is gently swept away onto the mediastinum using a wet sponge; this exposes the anterior hilar vessels (Fig. 3.29). The incision is then extended down the posterior surface of the hilum, just anterior to the esophagus. With the hilar dissection completed, the tissues above the right main pulmonary artery and the superior pulmonary vein are sharply dissected to expose their glistening adventitial tissue layer.

TABLE 3.1 NEW INTERNATIONAL STAGING FOR LUNG CANCER: TNM DEFINITIONS

PRIMARY TUMOR (T)	
TX	Tumor proven by the presence of malignant cells in bronchopulmonary secretions but not visualized by roentgenography or bronchoscopy, or any tumor that cannot be assessed as in a retreatment staging.
T0	No evidence of primary tumor.
TIS	Carcinoma in situ.
T1	A tumor that is 3.0 cm or less in greatest dimension, surrounded by lung or visceral pleura, and without evidence of invasion proximal to a lobar bronchus at bronchoscopy.*
T2	A tumor more than 3.0 cm in greatest dimension, or a tumor of any size that either invades the visceral pleura or has associated atelectasis or obstructive pneumonitis extending to the hilar region. At bronchoscopy, the proximal extent of demonstrable tumor must be within a lobar bronchus or at least 2.0 cm distal to the carina. Any associated atelectasis or obstructive penumonitis must involve less than an entire lung.
T3	A tumor of any size with direct extension into the chest wall (including superior sulcus tumors), diaphragm, or the mediastinal pleura or pericardium without involving the heart, great vessels, trachea, esophagus, or vertebral body, or a tumor in the main bronchus either 2.0 cm of the carina without involving the carina.
T4	A tumor of any size with invasion of the mediastinum or involving heart, great vessels, trachea, esophagus, vertebral body, or carina or with presence of malignant pleural effusion.†
NODAL INVOLVEMENT (N)	
N0	No demonstrable metastasis to regional lymph nodes.
N1	Metastasis to lymph nodes in the peribronchial or the ipsilateral hilar region, or both, including direct extension.
N2	Metastasis to ipsilateral mediastinal lymph nodes and subcarinal lymph nodes.
N3	Metastasis to contralateral mediastinal lymph nodes, contralateral hilar lymph nodes, or ipsilateral or contralateral scalene or supraclavicular lymph nodes.
DISTANT METASTASIS (M)	
M0	No (known) distance metastasis.
M1	Distant metastasis present—specify site(s).

*The uncommon superficial tumor of any size whose invasive component is limited to the bronchial wall and that may extend proximal to the main bronchus is classified as T1.

†Most pleural effusions associated with lung cancer are due to tumor. There are, however, some few patients in whom cytopathologic examination of pleural fluid (on more than one specimen) is negative for tumor and the fluid is nonbloody and is not an exudate. When these elements and clinical judgment dictate that the effusion is not related to the tumor, the cases should be staged T1, T2, or T3, with effusion being excluded as a staging element.

Mountain CF. The new international staging system. Surgical Clinics of North America, October 1987. Reprinted with permission.

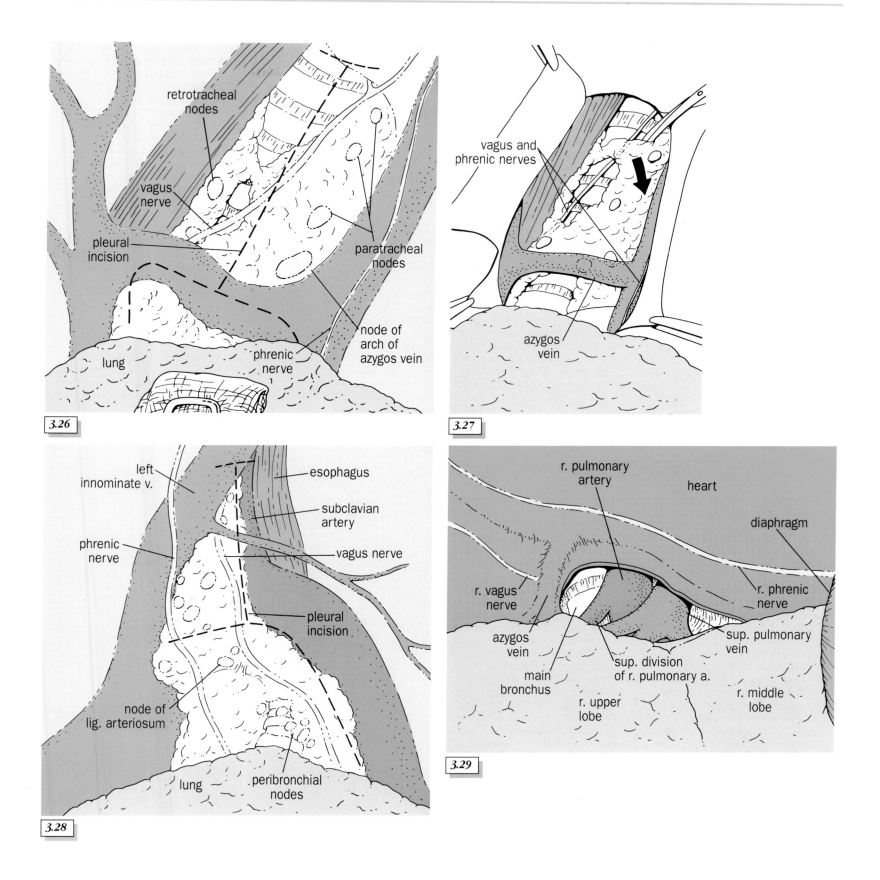

3.26

retrotracheal nodes

vagus nerve

pleural incision

paratracheal nodes

node of arch of azygos vein

phrenic nerve

lung

3.27

vagus and phrenic nerves

azygos vein

3.28

left innominate v.

phrenic nerve

esophagus

subclavian artery

vagus nerve

pleural incision

node of lig. arteriosum

lung

peribronchial nodes

3.29

r. pulmonary artery

heart

diaphragm

r. vagus nerve

r. phrenic nerve

azygos vein

sup. division of r. pulmonary a.

sup. pulmonary vein

main bronchus

r. upper lobe

r. middle lobe

ARTERIAL DISSECTION

Adequate exposure of the right main pulmonary artery is essential for the performance of a safe pneumonectomy. One technique that helps in exposing the artery is to develop a cleavage plane between the artery and the right superior pulmonary vein, which is the most anteriorly located hilar structure and overlies and partially covers the main pulmonary artery. Division of the apical anterior branch of this vein is occasionally helpful, and allows downward displacement of the superior pulmonary vein and permits better exposure of the right pulmonary artery. When necessary, a second technique that aids in exposure of the pulmonary artery is division of the azygous vein, followed by retraction of the superior vena cava medially. This exposes the anterior surface on the pulmonary artery near the mediastinum. The pulmonary artery is sharply dissected in the proper plane; often the posterior aspect of the dissection is best completed with the finger. On occasion, the truncus anterior branch of the right pulmonary artery should be divided so as to gain length and perform a safer division of the pulmonary artery. The main pulmonary artery may then be stapled, transected and oversewn, or ligated, as previously discussed (Fig. 3.30). Pictured in Fig. 3.30 is division after ligation.

VENOUS DISSECTION

Next, the lung is retracted posteriorly, and the superior pulmonary vein is exposed, and surrounded. The main trunk can be doubly ligated proximally with #0 silk, with the distal branches individually tied or clipped. Often the wider and sometimes bulky superior pulmonary vein is more easily controlled proximally using the vascular stapler. If sufficient length of the vein is freed, two rows of staples can be placed, and the vein divided between the staples.

The lung is then retracted anteriorly for exposure of the posterior hilum and inferior pulmonary vein. The pulmonary ligament has been previously divided and the mediastinal pleura has been opened, parallel to the azgous vein. The dissection around the inferior pulmonary vein is completed, followed by simple ligation distally and passage of the vascular stapler proximally. Division of this vein releases the hilum inferiorly, allowing blunt dissection of the mediastinal connective tissue up to the right mainstem bronchus. The lateral esophageal wall can sometimes be bowed outward from the mediastinum by hilar inflammation or tumor and must be protected during this phase of the dissection (Fig. 3.31). Visualization of the esophagus is also necessary during the skeletonization of the right main bronchus. Enlarged hilar lymph nodes adherent to the bronchus are dissected out and sent to pathology for staging.

BRONCHIAL DISSECTION

The lung is then picked up and reflected anteriorly. The bronchus is divided just beyond the tracheal bifurcation without leaving a long stump. Subcarinal lymph nodes, located after opening the space between the esophagus and the pericardium are dissected out to expose the carina for accurate placement of the stapling instrument. The entire lung is retracted posteriorly to draw the proximal bronchus out from the mediastinum. A TA-30 stapler using 4.8-mm staples is passed around the bronchus from an anterior approach and positioned at a right angle to the bronchus. The instrument is fired, approximating the anterior and posterior bronchial walls, 1 cm from the carina. The bronchus is transected, the specimen removed from the field, and the bronchial stump checked for leaks under positive pressure. Different methods of covering the bronchial stump have been previously described.

After a pneumonectomy, the unoperated lung must be carefully protected. No compromise of the opposite lung volume is well tolerated. Different methods can also be used to balance the mediastinum after a

pneumonectomy. Often the thoracotomy incision is closed, the patient placed in the supine position, and an 18-gauge needle inserted into the pleural space. Air is then aspirated with a glass syringe until the piston of the syringe is sucked towards the chest, indicating a negative intrapleural pressure. Alternatively, a single chest tube can be placed, which allows for fluid drainage. A postoperative chest x-ray is essential in determining the position of the mediastinum. Air can then be withdrawn or added to the pleural space as needed to equilibrate the mediastinum. A watertight closure of the thoracotomy is performed, particularly for a pneumonectomy where the hemithorax will accumulate proteinaceous fluid postoperatively that can organize into a fibrothorax. Subcutaneous emphysema is not unexpected in the postoperative period, as the hemithorax fills with fluid.

LEFT PNEUMONECTOMY

The standard incision for a left pneumonectomy is a posterolateral thoracotomy. The left hemithorax is entered through the fifth intercostal space. Pleural adhesions are divided using sharp dissection to free the lung completely, and to expose the pulmonary hilum. The thoracic cavity is then explored by inspecting the pleural and diaphragmatic surfaces for evidence of metastatic disease; the mediastinal surface is then inspected and palpated to detect evidence of mediastinal lymphadenopathy.

HILAR DISSECTION

The inferior pulmonary ligament is first taken down, followed by dissection of the anterior hilum. The lung is retracted posteriorly to expose the mediastinal pleura overlying the anterior hilum. A pleural incision is then made parallel and posterior to the phrenic nerve and pericardial reflection. The incision should extend from the inferior pulmonary vein upwards to the transverse aortic arch (Fig. 3.32), without injuring the recurrent laryngeal nerve. The superior pulmonary vein is easily identified as the most anteriorly located vascular structure in the hilum.

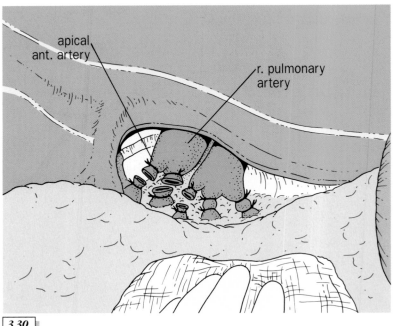

apical ant. artery

r. pulmonary artery

3.30

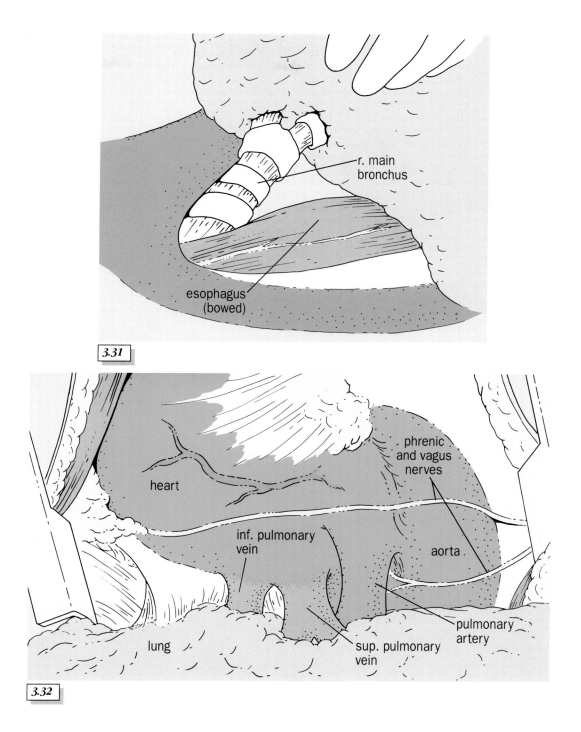

3.31

3.32

ARTERIAL DISSECTION

Located above the superior pulmonary vein is the main pulmonary artery, which is the most cephalad structure in the left hilum as it emerges from beneath the transverse aortic arch. Sharp dissection of this vessel in the perivascular plane exposes its glistening adventitial layer. Further blunt digital dissection can be used to develop a plane posteriorly and the vessel can be encircled by passing a finger between the artery and the main bronchus. If needed additional arterial length can be obtained by dividing the first branch of the pulmonary artery between silk ligatures—usually this is the apical–posterior branch. This step also helps to avoid excess tension on the artery during inferior retraction of the lung. The main artery is transected and oversewn with a 4–0 Prolene suture (Fig. 3.33). Alternatively, it can be divided between two proximal heavy silk ligatures and a single distal ligature. Leaving a generous "cauliflower" cup is essential to avoid slippage of the ligature from the proximal stump. A vascular staple can also be used.

VENOUS DISSECTION

Next, the superior pulmonary vein is dissected. A vascular stapling instrument is placed across the vein proximally, and a right-angle is used to control the vein distally. The vein is stapled proximally, clamped distally, and divided. The distal stump is then tied with a 2–0 silk. If an adequate length of vein is not obtained to permit both proximal and distal control, the vessel can be transected proximally against the stapling instrument edge, initially allowing sequestered pulmonary blood to drain. Removal of the stapler exposes the distal venous cuff which can be oversewn for hemostasis. The inferior pulmonary vein is now exposed by retracting the lung anteriorly, so that the vein can be approached from behind (Fig. 3.34). Division of the pulmonary ligament previously along with dissection of the vein allows the vascular stapler to be passed behind the vessel. The same technique used for division of the superior pulmonary vein is used for division of the inferior pulmonary vein.

BRONCHIAL DISSECTION

With the pulmonary artery and pulmonary veins divided, the bronchus can be easily approached. The areolar tissue remaining within the hilum and surrounding the bronchus is divided while carefully obtaining hemostasis of the small bronchial arteries. The lung is retracted posteriorly, exposing the bronchus, which is located beneath the ligated pulmonary artery cuff. The bronchus is divided with the stapler on the aorta. Care must be taken not to injure the arterial closure or the recurrent laryngeal nerve during application of the automatic stapler. Identifying the carina is important to accurately place the staple line across the orifice of the left main bronchus to minimize the size of the left main bronchial stump. Next, the bronchus is divided, followed by removal of the specimen and testing of the bronchial closure beneath a water level during positive pressure ventilation. Coverage of the bronchial stump and treatment of the postpneumonectomy space has been discussed in the right pneumonectomy section.

LOBECTOMY

LEFT UPPER LOBECTOMY

HILAR DISSECTION

The pleural space is entered using a fifth interspace posterolateral thoracotomy, followed by sharp dissection of pleural adhesions. The thoracic cavity is explored in a routine fashion, and the inferior pulmonary ligament is then divided up to the inferior pulmonary vein. Mobilization of the hilum is continued by retracting the lung posteriorly and incising the pleura covering the anterosuperior left hilum. This step allows a superficial dissection and inspection of the superior pulmonary vein in order to assess tumor entrapment of this vessel. The main pulmonary artery and aortopulmonary window located in the superior hilum are similarly examined as tumor from the upper lung frequently extends towards these areas.

ARTERIAL DISSECTION

If the tumor appears resectable, the dissection of the main pulmonary artery is then begun. The pleura over the main pulmonary artery is incised in the area of the aortopulmonary window. The vagus and recurrent laryngeal nerve are identified and protected. The arterial supply to the upper lobe is variable. The first branch of the pulmonary artery can be a short, fat trunk, which quickly divides into the apical and posterior arteries, or these arteries can arise separately (Fig. 3.35). Alternatively, the anterior branch to the upper lobe may be the first branch encountered. A lymph node, often calcified, is invariably found between the apical and posterior branches, and can be adherent to the upper lobe bronchus, making dissection difficult. In 20% of patients, a lingular branch arises from the proximal portion of the artery, and proceeds to the lingula anterior to the bronchus. This branch can be injured if the apical–posterior branches are dissected blindly. In 20% of patients, a superior pulmonary vein must be ligated before dissection of the pulmonary artery can be safely undertaken. It is oftentimes best to identify the proximal arteries, and then to proceed with the interlobar arterial dissection.

The major fissure is then opened and the lateral surface of the interlobar pulmonary artery is identified (Fig. 3.36). The vessel is located within the base of the main fissure towards the posterior third of its length as it curves behind the upper lobe bronchus. The major fissure is often completely developed, but may require division with the GIA stapling device.

Separation of the difficult fissure fused by apparent inflammatory adhesions is indicated to rule out tumor extension across the interlobar hilum which might require pneumonectomy for complete resection. Packing with a gauze sponge will control bleeding from capillary ooze and smaller interlobar venules. Persistent bleeding points, after several minutes of pressure, should be immediately ligated to regain a clear operative field. Densely adherent lobes may be divided along their periphery using the GIA auto-stapler for hemopneumostasis while carefully avoiding injury to the major lobar vessels. The pulmonary artery should be sufficiently exposed within the base of the major fissure by sharply dividing the perivascular fascia, and dissecting within this plane to clearly identify the segmental arteries penetrating into the upper lobe. In about 50% of patients, there is a single arterial trunk to the lingula, which quickly divides into a superior and inferior division. In 20% of patients, there are two or more separate lingular branches. Additional arterial branches to the anterior segment of the upper lobe are identified. Anomalous segmental vessels, as well as the superior segmental artery supplying the lower lobe arising opposite the lingular segmental branch are also defined. The dissection is extended superiorly along the surface of the pulmonary artery making certain that tumor invasion of the arterial wall is not present.

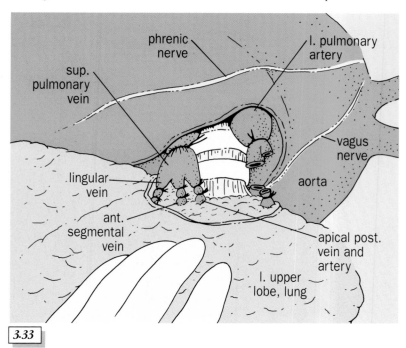

3.33

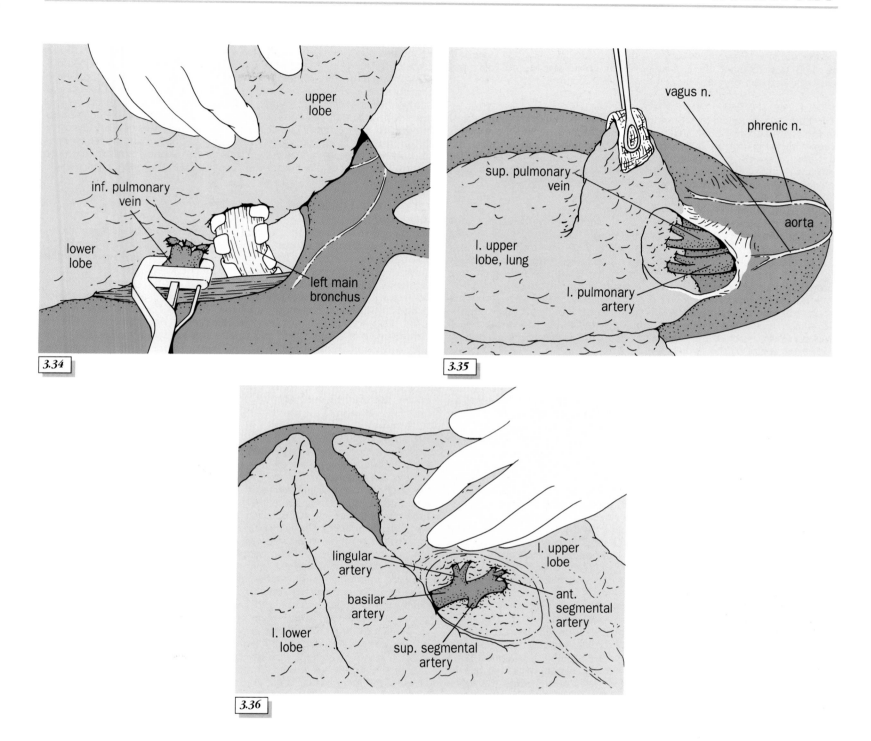

3.34

3.35

3.36

After the arterial supply is defined, the individual vessels are ligated. It is often best to ligate the apical–posterior vessel last, as this may put excessive traction on the vessel, and cause a laceration.

VENOUS DISSECTION
The lung is now retracted posteriorly to expose the superior vein located in the anterosuperior hilum. The bronchus is located behind the superior vein with separation of these structures being required to mobilize the vessel up towards the pericardial sac. A vascular staple line is placed for proximal control, followed by ligation distally when possible, with transection of the vein against the instrument edge as a scalpel guide.

BRONCHIAL DISSECTION
Complete division of the vascular supply leaves only the upper lobe bronchus remaining. The majority of the peribronchial tissues are cleared off by blunt "peanut" dissection reserving electrocautery for hemostasis of the smaller bronchial arteries. The upper lobe is again retracted anteriorly to use the interlobar approach for bronchial stapling. Adherent peribronchial lymph nodes are dissected sharply and removed until the bifurcation between upper and lower bronchus is seen clearly. The bronchus is closed without creating a stenosis of the lower lobe bronchus using the TA stapler with 4.8-mm staples. Commonly, the pulmonary trunk which arcs posteriorly around the upper lobe bronchus is gently retracted away to prevent injury by the stapler.

LEFT UPPER SLEEVE LOBECTOMY
A sleeve resection is usually indicated for the upper lobe carcinoma which has extended proximally to involve the bronchial orifice and its junction with the main bronchus. In this situation, the standard upper lobectomy would leave a bronchial stump of residual carcinoma, whereas a "sleeve" resection includes the lobar orifice and a cuff of the main bronchus allowing a complete resection. The two bronchial ends are reanastomosed together with this type of reconstruction collectively considered a "bronchoplastic" procedure (Fig. 3.37). A variety of bronchial resections has been described including the partial removal of the carina and trachea. For simplicity, only the left upper sleeve procedure is presented; however, a right upper sleeve resection is essentially a mirror-image technique. The procedure is valuable in the patient with marginal respiratory reserve as it preserves a functional lower lobe. A preoperative bronchoscopic examination is extremely important to evaluate the need and extent of bronchial resection. Postoperatively, bronchoscopy is performed to control secretion formation at the bronchial suture line during the first days after the operation.

Left upper lobe dissection with division of the vascular supply is similar for the standard upper lobectomy and should be reviewed. The upper lobe is then rotated forward with a posterior approach used for dissection to isolate the left main bronchus proximally towards the carina and distally until the superior segmental bronchus is defined. Umbilical tapes are passed around the bronchus for its retraction laterally to facilitate the exposure. The main bronchus is divided transversely while the lower lobe bronchus (bronchus intermedius on the right) is obliquely divided to compensate for the difference in their diameters. The open main

bronchus can be easily occluded with inflation of a Foley balloon catheter for temporary control of the air leak and single lung ventilation if a right-sided double-lumen tube was not inserted at induction. The bronchial ends are sent for frozen pathologic exam to check for a clear margin of resection. Guy sutures are then placed to align the bronchial ends with an open anastomosis performed for careful placement of an interrupted suture line. Four–0 sutures on a tapered needle are used for the anastomosis. The knots are tied outside the lumen, and the anastomosis is tested beneath a water level against a sustained positive pressure breath. Wrapping of the anastomosis using a pleural or intercostal pedicle flap is usually recommended.

LEFT LOWER LOBECTOMY
HILAR DISSECTION
The pleural space is entered through a fifth interspace posterolateral thoracotomy, with sharp division of any pleural adhesions, followed by inspection of the thoracic cavity. The lung is first retracted anterosuperiorly, with division of the inferior pulmonary ligament between ligatures to release the lower lobe. The mediastinal pleura overlying the posterior hilum is opened with an incision extending from the divided edge of the inferior pulmonary ligament superiorly until the left main bronchus is seen (Fig. 3.38). The perivascular fascia encircling the inferior pulmonary vein is cleared, with the vessel left undivided until verifying a resectable lobe with a completed interlobar dissection. Next, the mediastinal pleura over the superior pulmonary vein is incised, and the inferior aspect of the vein is identified. This maneuver confirms the presence of two separate veins on the left side. A single, extrapericardial vein is present in 8% of patients on the left side. Identification of the superior pulmonary vein also facilitates later division of the interlobar fissure.

ARTERIAL DISSECTION
Next the major fissure is separated by retraction of the upper lobe anteriorly. Blunt and sharp dissection is begun downward within the posterior third of the major fissure to expose the interlobar pulmonary artery. A difficult fissure fused by inflammatory adhesions requires a careful approach while attempting to remain in the true interlobar plane and avoid upper lobe parenchymal injury. Temporary gauze packing of the operative field will usually control venous oozing. Frequently the interlobar plane is incomplete posteriorly between the lingula and basilar segments of the lower lobe. It requires division peripherally using the GIA auto-stapler.

The perivascular tissues encasing the pulmonary artery are incised. Any enlarged interlobar lymph nodes are sent for pathologic study. The pulmonary artery is dissected superiorly beneath the upper lobe until its lingular branch is clearly identified. The superior segmental artery will arise opposite or proximal to the origin of the lingular branch from the posterior pulmonary arterial wall (see Fig. 3.36). In one-third of patients, there are two arterial branches to the superior segment. Individual ligation and division between fine silk ligatures of the superior segmental branch preserves the interlobar artery supplying the lingular segmental vessel. Distally, the main basilar trunk is doubly ligated as well as the individual basilar segmental branches, followed by their division to complete the arterial dissection.

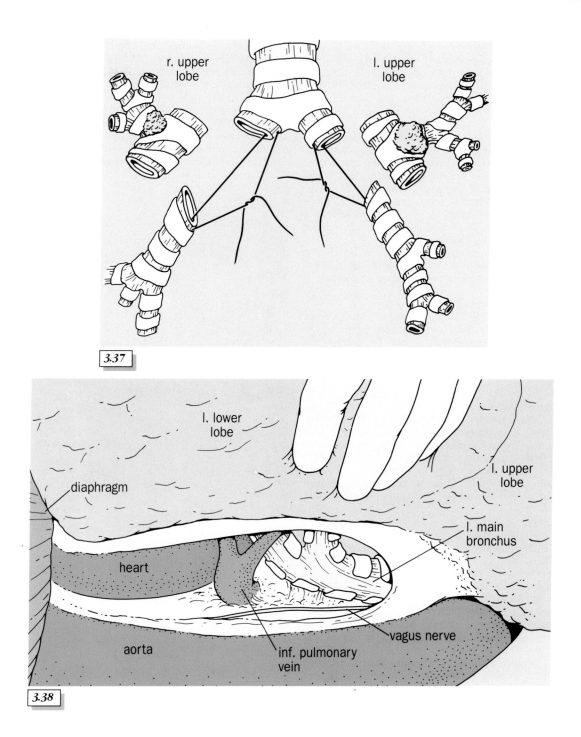

3.37

3.38

VENOUS DISSECTION

The lower lobe is retracted anteriorly for placement of the vascular stapler across the venous trunk of the inferior vein that was previously isolated. Using the instrument as a scalpel guide the vessel is transected distally, while the vessel is controlled proximally with a ligature, or a clamp.

BRONCHIAL DISSECTION

The lower lobe bronchus is located behind the proximal interlobar arterial cuff with a plane of dissection developed between these structures to expose the origin of the upper lobe bronchus. The TA stapling instrument is placed around the lower bronchus and the upper bronchus insufflated with air, to ensure against compromise of the upper lobe bronchus. The stapler is fired to close the bronchus, which is then transected (Fig. 3.39). The bronchial closure is submerged and tested for any air leaks against a sustained positive pressure breath. A viable pleural flap is rotated over the bronchial stump and sutured on top to buttress this closure.

Inspection of the interlobar dissection with control of the significant bleeding points and air leaks is carried out prior to thoracotomy closure. Two pleural drainage catheters are left in place, as described previously.

RIGHT UPPER LOBECTOMY

A posterolateral thoracotomy through the fifth interspace is used to enter the right hemithorax, followed by sharp dissection of pleural adhesions in order to mobilize the entire lung and define the fissures. Frequently, the horizontal or minor fissure between the lower and middle lobe is not easily distinguished because of its incomplete development.

HILAR DISSECTION

The initial step in a right upper lobectomy is mobilization of the hilum. The inferior pulmonary ligament is divided to the level of the inferior pulmonary vein; the anterior pleural reflection is then divided from the inferior pulmonary vein cephalad to the azygous vein. The posterior hilar reflection is also dissected, from superiorly to past the takeoff of the right upper lobe bronchus. Another preliminary step for upper lobectomy is inspection of the minor fissure. The middle lobe may occasionally require removal as part of an en bloc upper lobectomy due to neoplasm crossing the minor fissure in this area.

VASCULAR DISSECTION

As in a right pneumonectomy, arterial dissection is begun by developing a cleavage plane between the superior pulmonary vein and the right pulmonary artery. The lung is retracted caudad, exposing the right main bronchus as the most cephalad hilar structure; the pulmonary artery is anterior and inferior to the bronchus. Dissection is sharp, along the superior surface of the artery, and in the proper periarterial plane. The division of the pulmonary artery into superior and inferior divisions is noted and the superior division, with its apical and anterior branches, is ligated and divided (Fig. 3.40).

The lung is then retracted posteriorly, and the superior pulmonary vein is seen. Care must be taken in defining the venous drainage of the upper lobe, so as not to compromise the middle lobe drainage. The superior pulmonary vein has two divisions, upper and lower, and the lower division drains the middle lobe, and must be preserved. The upper division has three branches to the upper lobe—the apical, anterior, and posterior. If the tumor is close, the upper division should be ligated, realizing that the inferior division of the pulmonary artery lies beneath the vein, and can be injured with careless technique. If possible, however, the tributaries of the vein should be ligated separately because a portion of the middle lobe often drains into the anterior branch, and simple division of the upper division of the superior pulmonary vein can compromise drainage to the middle lobe (Fig. 3.41). The upper lobe tributaries are individually ligated between heavy silk ties and divided. Afterwards, the superior venous trunk is mobilized along its back wall until the inferior division of the pulmonary artery is identified. This step is indicated to avoid missing a posterior venous tributary that can be avulsed later on.

The interlobar phase of the dissection is now begun by retracting the upper lobe superiorly and sharply opening the parenchymal pleura covering the oblique fissure. Dissection is begun at the junction of the horizon-

tal and oblique fissures, and the inferior division of the pulmonary artery identified. The segmental pulmonary arteries supplying the middle lobe and superior segment of the lower lobe segment should be noted to avoid their inadvertent ligation at this juncture. An ascending posterior segmental artery to the right upper lobe is usually found about 1.5 cm cephalad to these branches, and should be carefully ligated (Fig. 3.42). In 25% of cases, there are two upper lobe branches. Control of the upper lobe arterial and venous segmental branches is now complete. The fissure between the upper and middle lobes is divided with the GIA stapling device. Similarly, the fissure between the upper and lower lobes is divided.

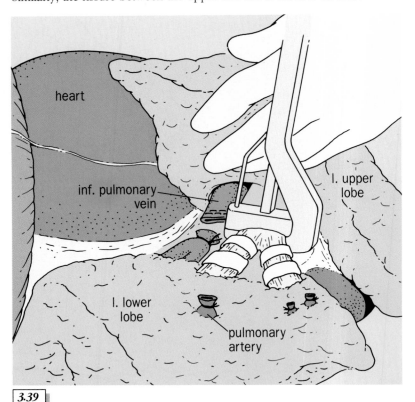

3.39

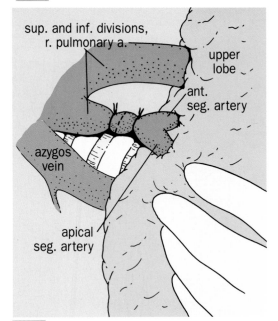

3.40

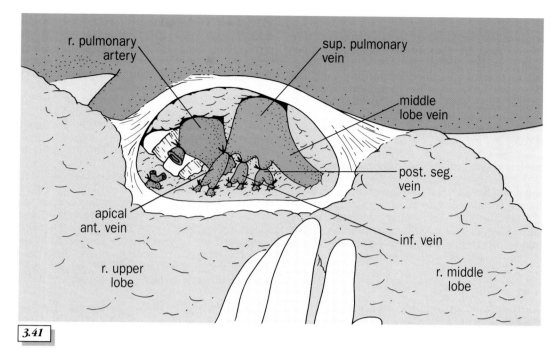

3.41

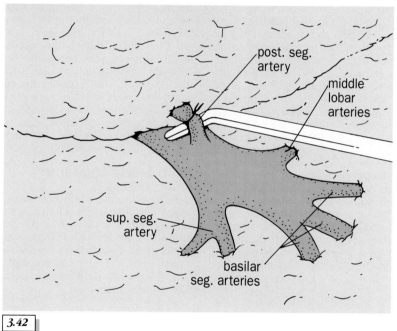

3.42

BRONCHIAL DISSECTION

The lung is again retracted posteriorly. The lateral surface of the pulmonary artery is unroofed next by sharply dissecting the upper lobe parenchyma off within a periadventitial plane working from an anterior approach. This dissection is continued posteriorly until the peribronchial tissue of the upper lobe bronchus is cleared. The lung is reflected anteriorly, and the upper lobe bronchus divided with the TA stapler (Fig. 3.43).

RIGHT MIDDLE LOBECTOMY

As the right middle lobe represents only 8% of the total lung mass, removal of the middle lobe would not ordinarily compromise lung function. However, because of the close proximity of the middle lobe bronchus to the superior segmental bronchus to the lower lobe, a middle and lower bilobectomy is often necessary to remove a middle lobe tumor. Similarly, because of the fusion of the lung parenchyma of the upper with the middle lobe, an upper and middle bilobectomy is often required for an upper or middle lobe lesion. Although the middle lobe is small, a middle lobectomy can be a more difficult procedure than any other lobectomy.

ARTERIAL DISSECTION

The safest approach in evaluating whether a middle lobectomy is possible is to open the major or oblique fissure between the middle and lower lobe. Dissection within this fissure is facilitated by the fact that it is usually well defined and completely developed, in comparison to the horizontal fissure. The upper and middle lobes are retracted anteriorly, while the lower lobe is allowed to lay in a dependent posterior position. Sharp dissection begins at the junction of the oblique and horizontal fissures in order to define the inferior division of the pulmonary artery. Frequently, a periarterial lymph node is encountered, and must be carefully removed. The periarterial plane is entered and the middle lobe, the superior segment of the lower lobe, and the posterior segment of the upper lobe arteries are identified. The artery to the superior segment of the lower lobe comes off posteriorly, opposite the middle lobe artery, while the recurrent artery to the upper lobe comes off laterally, more proximally (Figs. 3.45, 3.46). All arteries should be identified before division of the middle lobe branches. Should the pulmonary artery or its associated middle lobe arterial branches be invaded by hilar tumor, consideration should be given to a bilobectomy. Occasionally, careful sharp dissection and blunt "peanut" dissection can elevate a tumor mass from the pulmonary artery when direct arterial wall invasion is absent. Surgical judgement is used in order to avoid a major pulmonary artery laceration and hemorrhage. One or two separate middle lobe arterial branches are found to course anteriorly from the pulmonary artery onto the middle lobe base. The middle lobe arteries are then doubly ligated, and divided; if identification of the arteries is uncertain, the suspected middle lobe arteries are looped with a 2–0 silk, and divided after the venous dissection is complete.

VENOUS DISSECTION

A technique of differential inflation is employed to easily define the incomplete minor fissure. Holding positive pressure reinflates the upper lobe, while the middle lobe remains atelectatic due to its bronchial disconnection. The right middle lobe is now retracted posteriorly, while continuing differential inflation to localize the middle lobe vein. A single middle lobe vein most commonly enters the inferior aspect of the superior pulmonary vein. This branch vein is ligated and divided completing the division of the middle lobe bronchovascular connections. In approximately 50% of patients, a second middle lobe vein is encountered; in 14% of these patients, the second vein drains into the upper lobe, while in 8%, the additional vein drains into the inferior pulmonary vein. These anomalies should be looked for so as not to injure the venous drainage from the other lobes.

The specimen is now retracted laterally from the pulmonary hilum with the remaining oblique fissure divided using a sequential GIA stapling technique. This avoids excessive entrapment of the upper lobe parenchyma within a single staple line. The right lung is reinflated while the lower lobe is checked for segmental atelectasis and the possibility of an iatrogenic bronchial stenosis. Hemostasis of the dissection site is obtained followed by two pleural drainage catheter placements. Thoracotomy closure proceeds in a routine fashion.

BRONCHIAL DISSECTION

The inferior pulmonary artery trunk can now be rolled posteriorly to approach the peribronchial tissues surrounding the bronchus intermedius and middle bronchus. The middle lobe bronchus represents the one instance in pulmonary surgery where the bronchus comes off anterior to the pulmonary artery. The bronchi are directly palpated and blunt dissection with a "peanut" instrument is used to sweep off the peribronchial tissue, plus any enlarged lymph nodes up towards the middle lobe parenchymal specimen. This technique brings into clear view the bifurcation between bronchus intermedius and the middle lobe bronchus (Fig. 3.45). Bleeding from any bronchial arteries disrupted during this maneuver are controlled with individual hemoclips or direct electrocautery. A circumferential segment of middle bronchus is closed using the smaller TA stapler. Bronchial transection followed by placement of a bronchus clamp distally is used to prevent spillage of any endobronchial secretions and also to provide traction during the division of the minor fissure.

RIGHT LOWER LOBECTOMY

HILAR DISSECTION

The thorax is entered through the sixth intercostal space. The dissection is begun by dividing the inferior pulmonary ligament up to the inferior pulmonary vein. The division of the pleural reflection is then extended anteriorly, above the level of the superior pulmonary vein, and posteriorly to the origin to the bronchus to the upper lobe. The inferior pulmonary vein is skeletonized and the inferior pulmonary hilum is examined. Manual palpation of the entire right hilum is performed in a circumferential fashion and aids in initial assessment.

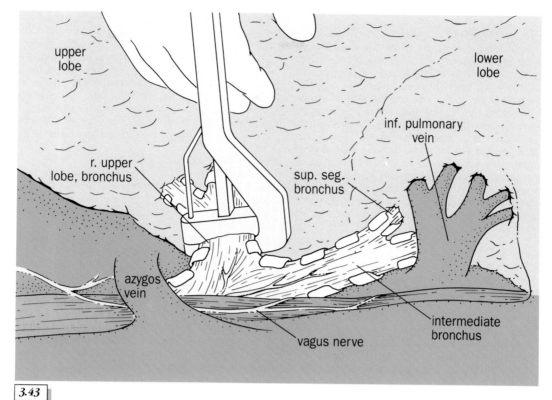

upper lobe

lower lobe

inf. pulmonary vein

r. upper lobe, bronchus

sup. seg. bronchus

azygos vein

vagus nerve

intermediate bronchus

3.43

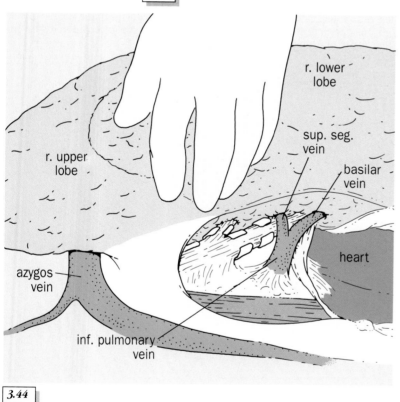

r. lower lobe

sup. seg. vein

basilar vein

r. upper lobe

azygos vein

heart

inf. pulmonary vein

3.44

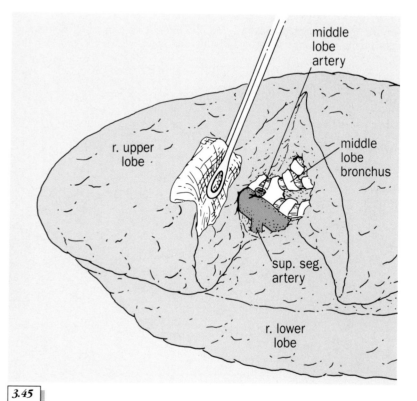

middle lobe artery

middle lobe bronchus

r. upper lobe

sup. seg. artery

r. lower lobe

3.45

ARTERIAL DISSECTION

The interlobar pulmonary artery is located by incising the pleura at the junction of the horizontal and oblique fissures. Often a lymph node is encountered and this must be carefully dissected. The perivascular tissues around the artery are opened with the dissection carried superiorly in this plane to expose the various segmental arterial vessels. Branches supplying the middle lobe, posterior segment of upper lobe, and superior segment of lower lobe all comprise the interlobar arterial anatomy in this area (Fig. 3.46). The superior segmental artery to the lower lobe begins directly opposite the middle lobe vessels, and courses posteriorly. Ligation and division of the superior segmental branch between heavy silk ligatures is carried out leaving an adequate proximal arterial cuff. In 20% of patients, two arteries to the superior segment of the lower lobe will be found. Also, in 10% of patients the recurrent posterior branch to the upper lobe comes off the superior segmental artery; the superior segmental artery should be dissected, and ligated distal to this branch. The basilar artery with its segmental branches is then dissected from within its perivascular bed to gain enough arterial length for its ligation and division. The most proximal arterial ligature should be carefully placed to avoid compromising flow through the lowest middle lobe branch. Frequently some of the lower lobe parenchyma needs to be divided to uncover a greater length of the basilar vessels to obtain an adequate proximal cuff.

If exposure of the basilar segmental arteries is difficult, then the posterior third of the major fissure can be divided before the basilar segmental arteries are ligated. Keeping the interlobar pulmonary artery under direct vision, blunt finger dissection between artery and lung parenchyma is used until the posterior mediastinal pleura is reached, followed by passage of a GIA stapler to complete the fissure. This step releases the superior segment from the interlobar hilum allowing its retraction inferiorly for good exposure of the basilar artery trunk to the remaining lower lobe.

VENOUS DISSECTION

A posterior approach is used to view the inferior venous trunk within the right pulmonary hilum by retracting the lung anteriorly (see Fig. 3.44). The TA instrument with vascular staples is passed around the vessel to occlude it proximally adjacent to the mediastinum. Distal ligatures are placed on the segmental veins before dividing the inferior venous trunk. Occasionally because of tumor encroachment the segmental veins are left unligated allowing the sequestered lower lobe blood to drain after their transection. Suture ligation of the severed distal end is easily accomplished using upward retraction on the lung after its release from the tethering inferior vein. The inferior pulmonary vein is rarely single on the right, but in 4% of patients a branch of the middle lobe vein drains to the inferior pulmonary trunk, and this must be dissected and preserved.

BRONCHIAL DISSECTION

Outward retraction on the specimen up from the mediastinum exposes the hilar connective tissues attached to the lower lobe bronchus. Sharp dissection is then used to free the bronchus superiorly until the intermediate bronchus is identified. Frequently, our preference is to divide the lower bronchus through the main fissure in order to clearly view the anteriorly located middle lobe bronchus and avoid its luminal compromise. Manual palpation is used constantly during the dissection of peribronchial tissues within the major fissure and during completion of the interlobar space anteriorly to pinpoint the origin of middle lobe bronchus. Sequential division of the incomplete interlobar space between the middle and lower lobes is performed using the GIA stapler. The anteriorly located middle lobe vein is preserved during this step as it is kept under direct view using posterior lung retraction. If the middle lobe bronchus arises opposite the superior segmental bronchus, as is often the case, it will be necessary to divide the superior segmental bronchus separately from the basilar bronchus. These bronchi are individually stapled using a TA instrument, followed by transection distally. The lower lobe specimen is removed followed by careful hemostasis of any severed bronchial arteries. Positive pressure testing of the bronchial closure is carried out beneath a pleural space fluid level to detect any air leaks. Apical and posterior chest tubes are placed followed by thoracotomy closure in the standard fashion.

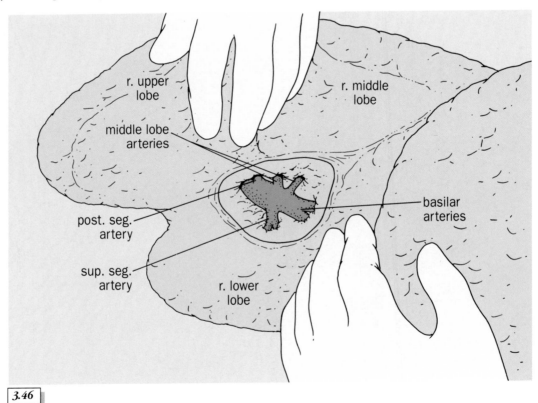

r. upper lobe

r. middle lobe

middle lobe arteries

basilar arteries

post. seg. artery

sup. seg. artery

r. lower lobe

3.46

BIBLIOGRAPHY

Edmunds LH Jr, Norwood WI, Low DW. *Atlas of Cardiothoracic Surgery.* Philadelphia, Pa: Lee & Febiger; 1990.

Hood RM. *Techniques in General Thoracic Surgery.* Philadelphia, Pa: WB Saunders; 1985.

Humphrey EW, McKeown DL. In Egdahl R (ed.), *Comprehensive Manual of Pulmonary Surgery.* New York: Springer-Verlag; 1982.

Ravitch MM, Steichen FM. *Atlas of General Thoracic Surgery.* Philadelphia, Pa: WB Saunders; 1988.

Shields TW. *General Thoracic Surgery,* 3rd ed. Philadelphia, Pa: Lea & Febiger; 1990.

4

Esophageal Surgery

Richard N. Edie • Robert W. Solit • John D. Mannion • John J. Shannon

URGERY OF CRICOPHARYNGEAL MUSCLE FOR CONDITIONS OF INCOORDINATION OF UPPER SPHINCTER

CRICOPHARYNGEAL MUSCLE MYOTOMY

CRICOPHARYNGEAL MUSCLE MYOTOMY

INDICATIONS	•Zenker's diverticulum •severe dysphagia not responding to medical therapy •aspiration with pulmonary complications secondary to cricopharyngeal muscle spasm with competent distal esophageal sphincter
ANESTHESIA	•general endotracheal
POSITIONING	•supine, with neck in moderate hyperextension turned from surgeon
PREP	•neck and upper chest prepared with Betadine and draped into a sterile field

PROCEDURE

The incision is begun along the anterior border of the sternocleidomastoid muscle approximately 2 cm above the suprasternal notch, and is carried to a point approximately 4 cm above the cricoid cartilage (Fig. 4.1). It extends deeply through the subcutaneous tissue and the platysma.

The sternocleidomastoid muscle is now retracted laterally, and the omohyoid muscle is mobilized and retracted medially or it is transected at the junction of the anterior and posterior bellies. The middle thyroid veins are ligated and divided. The carotid sheath containing the carotid artery and the internal jugular vein is retracted laterally. The thyroid, larynx, trachea, and esophagus are retracted medially (Fig. 4.2). Often the inferior thyroid artery must be divided between ties. The recurrent laryngeal nerve is located carefully to protect it from harm throughout its course.

If a Zenker's diverticulum is present, it is now located above the cricopharyngeal muscle, inferior to the inferior constrictor muscle (Fig. 4.3). If the diverticulum is small, it is generally not necessary to resect it. For the patient with achalasia, or spasm, of the cricopharyngeal muscle, complete relief of symptoms generally can be obtained with transection of the muscle fibers. The fibers of the cricopharyngeal muscle are transected in a vertical plane posteriorly, allowing the mucosa and submucosa to pout through the transected area (Fig. 4.4). If there are no constricting bands around the diverticulum and if the diverticulum is small, this completes the procedure.

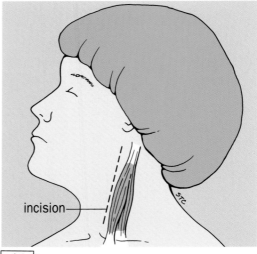

incision

4.1

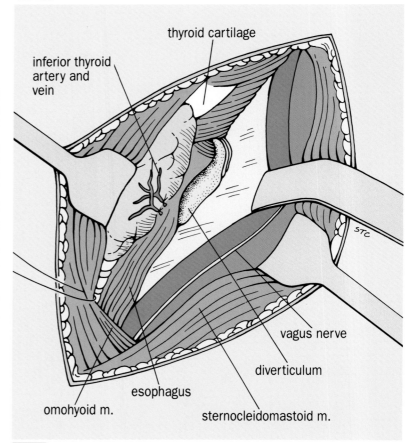

thyroid cartilage

inferior thyroid artery and vein

vagus nerve

diverticulum

omohyoid m.

esophagus

sternocleidomastoid m.

4.2

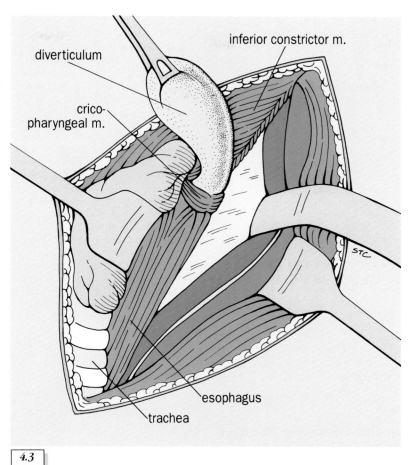

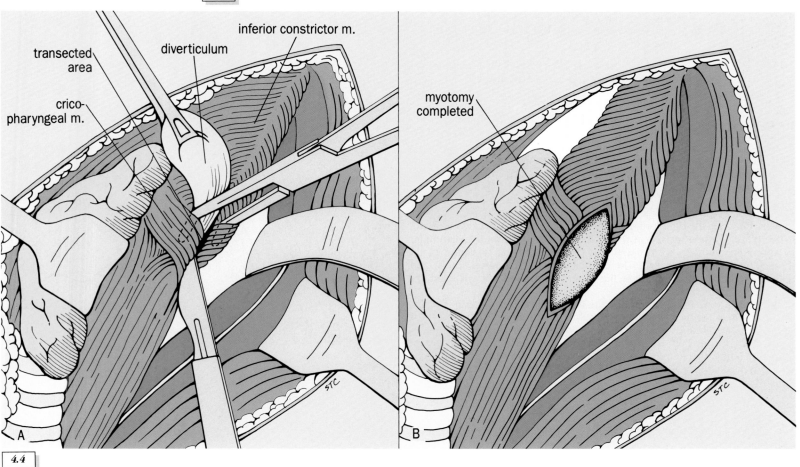

If a large Zenker's diverticulum is present, a diverticulopexy may be performed, in which the diverticulum is sutured to the anterior spinal ligament using an interrupted suture technique (Fig. 4.5). Usually, the diverticulum is then removed, following ligation of its base with a stapler or with interrupted sutures of 3–0 Vicryl (Fig. 4.6). Diverticulopexy or diverticulectomy is always combined with cricopharyngeal myotomy.

Following resection, the area is drained with a closed drainage system. If no resection has been performed, drainage is not necessary. The area is then irrigated with saline solution, following which the platysma is approximated using interrupted sutures of 3–0 Vicryl. A subcuticular suture of 5–0 Vicryl follows, and the skin is approximated using steri-strips. The patient must wait 36 to 48 hours following diverticular resection to begin oral intake of liquids. If no resection has been performed, the patient can be started on liquids that evening.

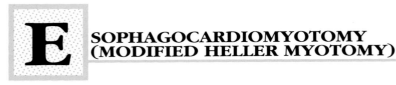

ESOPHAGOCARDIOMYOTOMY (MODIFIED HELLER MYOTOMY)

ESOPHAGOCARDIOMYOTOMY

INDICATIONS	• achalasia of the esophagus
ANESTHESIA	• general endotracheal with a double lumen endotracheal tube
POSITIONING	• after anesthesia is induced with patient placed in supine position, appropriate arteriovenous lines in place, a nasogastric tube may be inserted into the stomach before the patient is placed in the lateral position or it may be placed later in the procedure, when in the right lateral decubitus position
PREP	• left chest, front and back from neck to umbilicus is prepped and draped into a sterile field

PROCEDURE

The patient is placed in the right lateral decubitus position on a Vac-pack (bean bag). A left posterolateral thoracotomy incision is made (Fig. 4.7) and the left pleural space is entered after the latissimus dorsi muscle has been divided and the serratus anterior muscle retracted anteriorly. An incision is made through the bed of the nonresected eighth rib. The lung is mobilized by division of the pulmonary ligament. The left lung is allowed to collapse while the right lung is ventilated. The lung is retracted cephalad.

The pleura is then incised in a longitudinal fashion from the diaphragm to approximately 2 to 3 cm above the beginning of the dilatation of the thoracic esophagus (Fig. 4.8). The esophagus is then carefully mobilized, with care taken to avoid injury to the vagus nerves, and it is encircled and elevated with a Penrose drain.

The esophagogastric junction should be mobilized for a short distance into the chest, with care taken to avoid disturbance to the phreno-esophageal membrane or incision of the diaphragm. Usually there is no need to divide any of the hiatal attachments of the esophagogastric junction. Using the left (nondominant) hand to elevate the esophagus, which is kept under tension, a longitudinal myotomy is begun on the

anterolateral surface of the esophagus, just above the esophagogastric junction. It is continued caudad to a point 1 cm distal to the esophagogastric junction (Fig. 4.9) and is carried through the serosa and muscularis of the stomach to reveal the submucosal venous plexus. Proximally, the incision is deepened through the encircling muscles of the lower end of the esophagus down to mucosa. In general, the thick musculature over the narrowed area is incised first, followed by extension of the incision proximally over the dilated thick-walled portion of the esophagus. The incision is usually between 6 and 10 cm long (Fig. 4.10). The cephalad extent of the incision can be determined by preoperative manometry and by the appearance of the esophagus on an orally placed bougie. The muscular wall of the esophagus is now dissected laterally from the mucosa so that at least half of the circumference of the esophageal mucosa is free, allowing it to pout freely through the incision (Fig. 4.11).

Any perforation of the esophagus should be closed carefully with fine catgut sutures. A nasogastric tube may now be placed down beside the bougie into the stomach, if it has not been placed earlier.

Removal of the Penrose drain allows the esophagus to return to its normal position in the mediastinum, following which the esophagogastric junction usually resumes its normal intraabdominal position (Fig. 4.12). If there is a coincidental diaphragmatic hernia, the esophagogastric junction is restored below the diaphragm with interrupted sutures in the front of the esophageal membrane through the diaphragm. The mediastinal pleura is then closed longitudinally over the operative area with continuous or interrupted sutures of fine Vicryl. Large chest tubes are placed in the usual fashion and are brought out through intercostal incisions inferior to the thoracotomy incision, which is closed in the usual fashion.

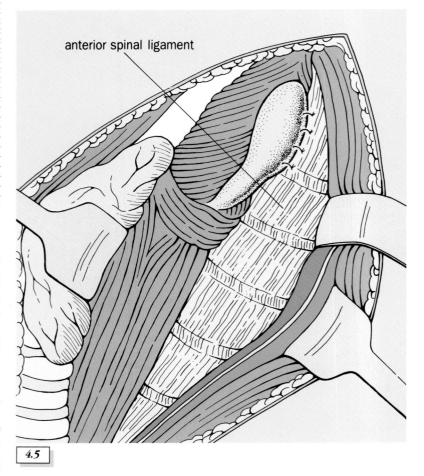

anterior spinal ligament

4.5

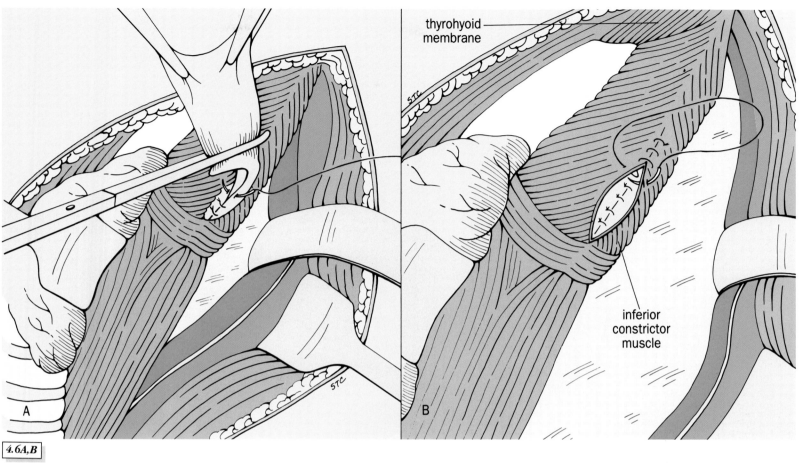

4.6A,B

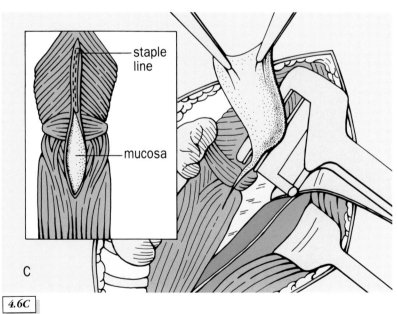

4.6C

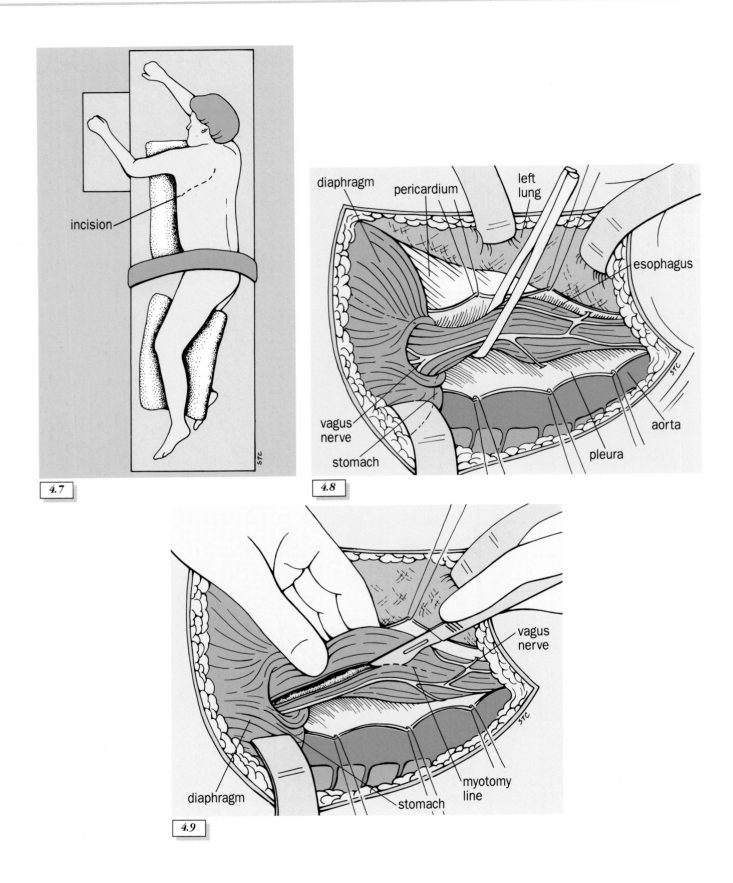

incision

4.7

diaphragm · pericardium · left lung

esophagus

vagus nerve

stomach

aorta

pleura

4.8

vagus nerve

diaphragm

stomach

myotomy line

4.9

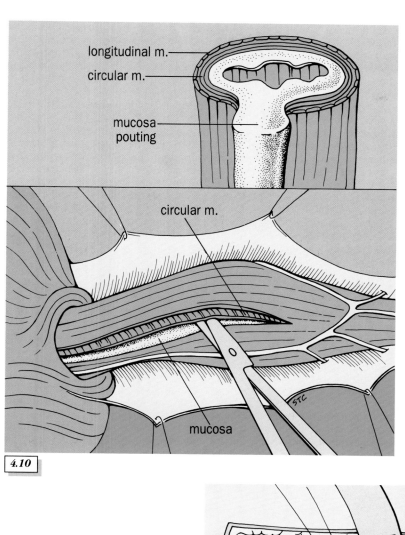

4.10

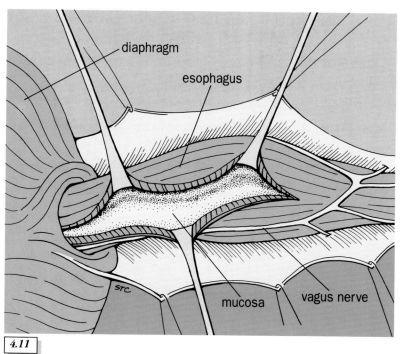

4.11

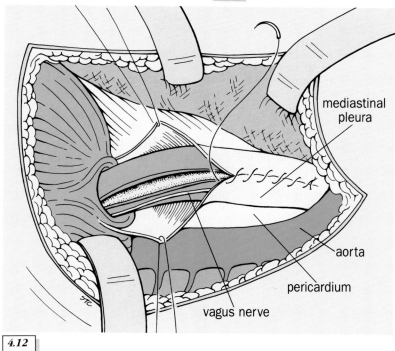

4.12

ESOPHAGOGASTRECTOMY WITH LAPAROTOMY AND RIGHT THORACOTOMY

ESOPHAGOGASTRECTOMY WITH LAPAROTOMY AND RIGHT THORACOTOMY

INDICATIONS	• carcinoma of the mid- and lower esophagus and esophagogastric junction ✓ • severe stenosis of the mid- and distal esophagus an occasional indication (eg, lye ingestion) ✓
ANESTHESIA	• general endotracheal with a double lumen endotracheal tube ✓
POSITIONING	• patient placed on operating table on a Vac-pack (bean bag), with right chest elevated approximately 45° from the horizontal and the abdomen in a general supine position slightly elevated; the right hip is raised approximately 30° from the horizontal (Fig. 4.13) • right upper extremity is carefully padded and either draped across the chest or kept secure on the transverse bar of an ether screen • patient is secured with tape so that the operating table can be rotated laterally to facilitate exposure of each operative field
PREP	• neck, chest, and abdomen prepped into the field

PROCEDURE

Two surgical teams may be used. The first team opens the abdomen through a midline upper abdominal incision (Fig. 4.14). The presence and extent of intra-abdominal metastasis, in the liver, along the celiac axis and left gastric artery, and at the esophageal hiatus, are assessed. If no metastasis is present, the patient is a suitable candidate for a curative resection.

The stomach is then assessed for its viability as a bypass organ. If it is deemed satisfactory, the second surgical team begins a long, anterolateral thoracotomy incision (Fig. 4.15) as the first team proceeds by dividing the gastrocolic omentum, with care taken to avoid injury to the right gastro-epiploic vessels. Short gastric vessels are ligated and divided. The left gastric artery is divided close to the celiac artery.

If the tumor is near the esophagogastric junction or if it is located in the fundus of the stomach, the spleen should be included in the resection specimen and the splenic attachments to the diaphragm and the splenic ligament must be divided (Fig. 4.16). If the spleen is not to be included in the resection specimen, it can be left in place by division of the short gastric vessels.

At the same time, the second surgical team proceeds with the right anterolateral thoracotomy incision (see Fig. 4.15). After division of the latissimus dorsi and serratus anterior muscles, the right chest is entered through the resected bed of the right fifth rib. The azygos vein is divided close to the highest intercostal vein, and the pleura overlying the esophagus is incised down to the diaphragm (Fig. 4.17). Using blunt and sharp dissection, the esophageal tumor and surrounding lymph nodes are resected en bloc (Fig. 4.18). Care is taken to secure all vessels entering the esophagus. This procedure can be facilitated by use of a double lumen endotracheal tube, which allows the right lung to be decompressed and removed from the operative field. The esophagus is mobilized from its bed, including the surrounding lymph nodes from just above the azygos vein to the diaphragm.

The first surgical team, working in the abdomen, uses a GIA stapler to transect the fundus of the stomach from the greater curvature proximally to the lesser curvature down to the gastric notch (Fig. 4.19). This essentially tubes the stomach (Fig. 4.20), following which a pyloromyotomy or a pyloroplasty (a one-layer Weinberg type) is performed. To increase the mobility of the stomach, the lateral peritoneal reflection is now divided along the second and third portions of the duodenum (see Kocher maneuver, Fig. 8.41), allowing the proximal duodenum to be mobilized close to the esophageal hiatus.

The distal end of the esophagus and stomach is brought through the esophageal hiatus, with division of any attachments. The esophagus is mobilized well above the azygos vein. The tubed proximal end of the stomach, which is to be used for the bypass, is brought gently through the esophageal hiatus, which occasionally must be enlarged. An esopha-gogastrostomy is performed either with sutures or using the EEA stapler (Figs. 4.21–4.23).

The stomach is fixed with sutures placed at 2- to 3-cm intervals along the lesser curvature of the stomach to the cut edge of the mediastinal pleura. Usually, the stomach lies easily in the esophageal hiatus without tension (Fig. 4.24). Occasionally, sutures must be placed along the diaphragm to the stomach to prevent any herniation of abdominal contents through the hiatus. A nasogastric tube must be placed carefully through the esopha-gogastrostomy and into the distal stomach under direct vision before the specimen is removed (Fig. 4.25).

All incisions are closed in layers in the usual fashion. If the spleen is removed, a closed-system drain is placed under the left leaf of the diaphragm and is brought out through a stab wound to the left of the abdominal incision. Two large chest tubes, one posterior to and one anterior to the hilum, are placed in the apex of the pleural space, and they are brought out through intercostal incisions inferior to the thoracotomy incision. The thoracotomy incision is then closed in layers in the usual fashion.

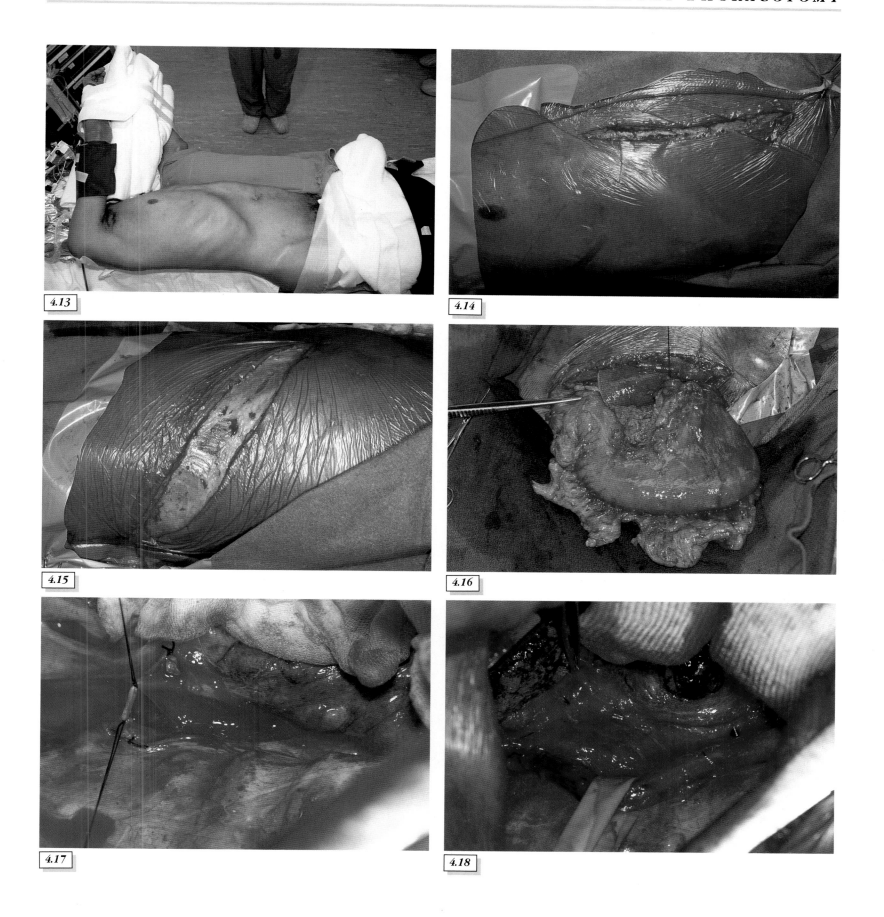

4.13

4.14

4.15

4.16

4.17

4.18

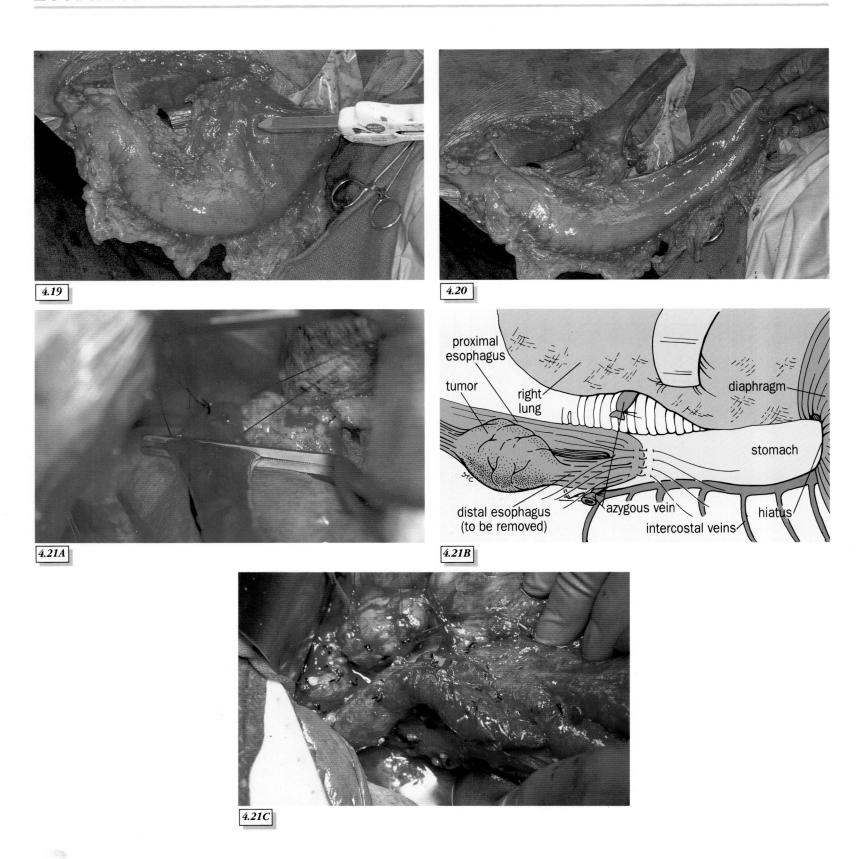

4.19

4.20

4.21A

4.21B

proximal
esophagus

tumor

right
lung

diaphragm

stomach

distal esophagus
(to be removed)

azygous vein

intercostal veins

hiatus

4.21C

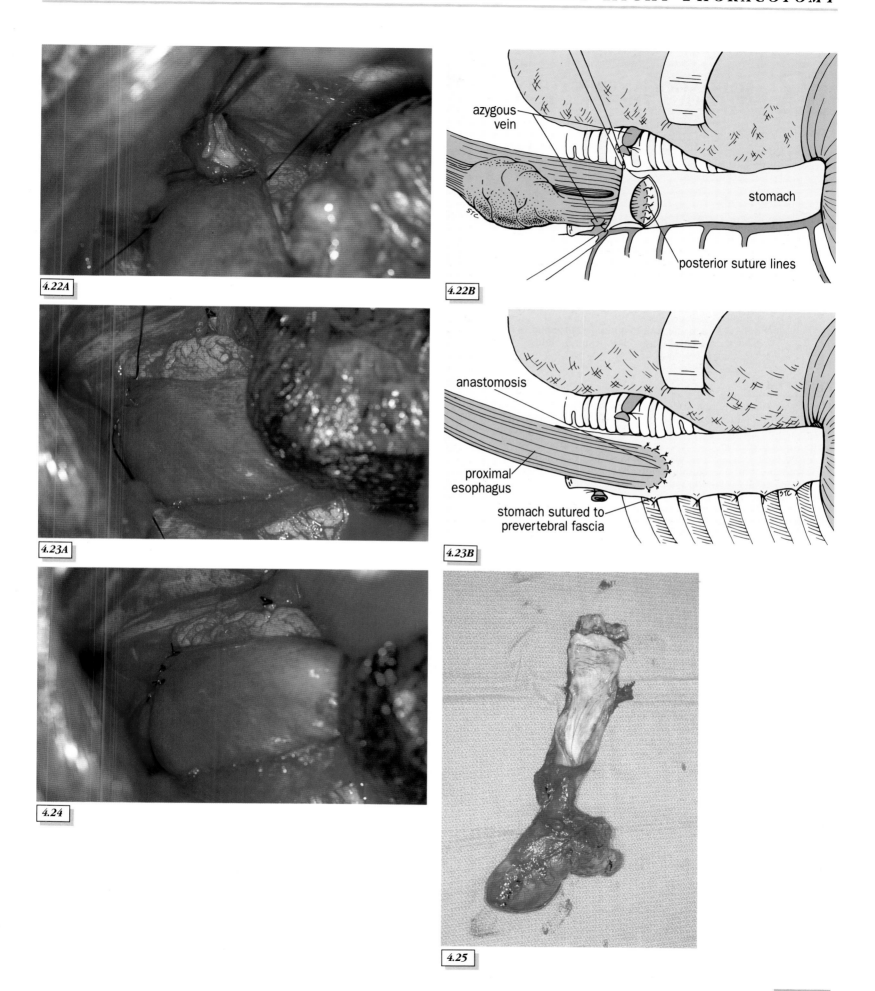

4.22A

4.22B

azygous vein

stomach

posterior suture lines

4.23A

4.23B

anastomosis

proximal esophagus

stomach sutured to prevertebral fascia

4.24

4.25

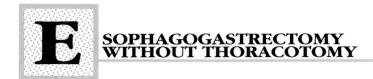

ESOPHAGOGASTRECTOMY WITHOUT THORACOTOMY

Apparent advantages of this technique over esophagogastrectomy with thoracotomy include shorter operating time, less postoperative pain, and lower morbidity and mortality.

ESOPHAGOGASTRECTOMY WITHOUT THORACOTOMY

INDICATIONS	•carcinoma of the mid- and lower esophagus •severe stricture of the esophagus
ANESTHESIA	•general endotracheal
POSITIONING	•supine, with head angled to the right
PREP	•neck, chest, and abdomen prepped to mid-thigh area and draped into a sterile field

PROCEDURE

A long, generous, midline abdominal incision is made (Fig. 4.26), following which the greater and lesser curvatures of the stomach are mobilized and the short gastric vessels are divided between ties of 3–0 silk. The left gastric artery is divided between silk ties so the operative procedure is facilitated by the use of an upper hand retractor, which helps to expose the esophageal hiatus at the esophagogastric junction (Fig. 4.27). The lower portion of the intrathoracic esophagus is freed from the surrounding tissues and any observed vessels are controlled with surgical clips. The esophagus can now be visualized through the hiatus almost to the area of the carina. The dissection is facilitated by placing a large bougie into the esophagus.

An incision is made along the anterior border of the sternocleidomastoid muscle in the neck (see Fig. 4.26), and the upper esophagus is mobilized and encircled with a Penrose drain. Working from both the top incision and the abdominal incision by way of the hiatus, the entire esophagus is now mobilized (Fig. 4.28).

If the stomach is to be used for bypass, it is tubed from the greater to the lesser curvature using the GIA stapler. Prior to mobilization of the stomach, a pyloromyotomy or a pyloroplasty must be performed. The blood supply to the stomach will be based on the right gastric and right gastroepiploic arteries. Following division of the stomach, the esophagus is delivered from the cervical incision. The upper end of the divided stomach is passed up along the esophageal bed, with care taken to ensure that no torsion occurs. An esophagogastrostomy is now performed through the cervical incision using an outer layer of silk and an inner layer of Vicryl (Fig. 4.29). The stomach can also be brought up through a substernal or a subcutaneous tunnel. All incisions are closed in the usual fashion (Fig. 4.30).

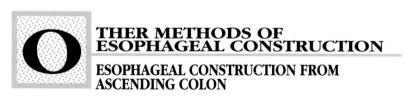

OTHER METHODS OF ESOPHAGEAL CONSTRUCTION

ESOPHAGEAL CONSTRUCTION FROM ASCENDING COLON

As seen in the above procedures, the esophagus is most commonly replaced with stomach. However, colon can also be used when stomach is not acceptable because of vascular insufficiency, or having been previously removed. Several variations have been used with success, including isoperistaltic, antiperistaltic, right colon, left colon, substernal, and subcutaneous construction. All of these variations require thorough bowel preparation prior to surgery and meticulous care throughout.

ESOPHAGEAL CONSTRUCTION FROM ASCENDING COLON

INDICATIONS	•stomach not suitable for bypass (see above)
ANESTHESIA	•general endotracheal
POSITIONING	•supine
PREP	•thorough bowel preparation; neck, anterior chest, and abdomen prepped to mid-thigh and draped into a sterile field

PROCEDURE

A long, midline, abdominal incision is made (Fig. 4.31). The ascending colon is mobilized by incision of the peritoneum lateral to the colon and by mobilization of the terminal ileum, cecum, ascending colon, and hepatic flexure toward the midline (Fig. 4.32). Injury to the duodenum must be carefully avoided. The terminal ileum is divided approximately 6 to 8 cm from the ileocecal valve using a GIA stapler. The transverse colon is then divided to the left of the midcolic artery, also using the stapler (Fig. 4.33). The ileocolic and right colic arteries are occluded with vascular clamps and the cecum is observed for evidence of vascular insufficiency. If no evidence is found, these arteries are then divided close to their origin, with care taken to leave intact the vascular arcades in the major anastomosis of the vessel supplying the ascending colon. In this way, the entire blood supply of the ascending colon and proximal transverse colon will be maintained by the midcolic artery and veins.

The length of the colonic segment can be tested for adequacy by placing it on the anterior chest wall. In most cases the colonic segment will be long enough to enable removal of the cecum. The cervical esophagus is now approached and mobilized through either a left or a right cervical incision parallel to the anterior border of the sternocleidomastoid muscle. A substernal tunnel is developed by blunt dissection, with the fingers working from above in the neck and from below through the abdomen. The exposed end of the cecum is covered with a rubber glove or dam and is secured with a heavy ligature. The end of the ligature is then placed through the previously made substernal tunnel. The esophagus is transected, with stapling of its distal portion and anastomosis of its proximal portion to the cecum or ascending colon in two layers. Sutures of 3–0 Vicryl are used for the inner layer, with 3–0 silk used for the outer layer.

An end-to-side gastrocolic anastomosis is now performed, with the proximal transverse colon anastomosed to the stomach in two layers, using interrupted 3–0 Vicryl on the inner layer and interrupted 3–0 silk on the outer layer (Fig. 4.34). There must be no tension on either suture line. Finally, an ileocolic anastomosis is performed in two layers, again, with an inner layer of 3–0 Vicryl and an outer layer of 3–0 silk, or with a stapler. All incisions are closed in layers without drainage. A chest radiograph should be obtained immediately following the procedure to ensure that the pleura was not entered and that the patient did not develop a pneumothorax. If a pneumothorax is present, appropriate chest drainage should be instituted.

A similar bypass using the left transverse colon, the splenic flexure, and the proximal descending colon also can be performed based on the middle colic artery (Fig. 4.35). Careful evaluation of the marginal artery and avoidance of injury to it must be undertaken. Some surgeons prefer to clamp the vessels along the intended lines of resection early in the procedure to assess the adequacy of both the arterial supply and the venous drainage. If any evidence of vascular insufficiency is noted, the colon segment cannot be used.

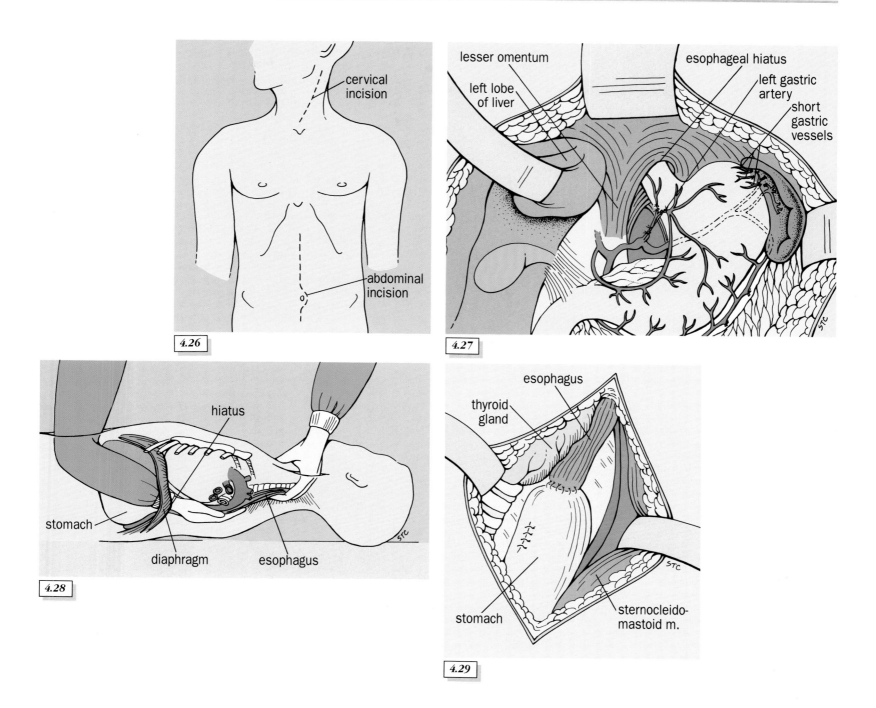

4.26

4.27

4.28

4.29

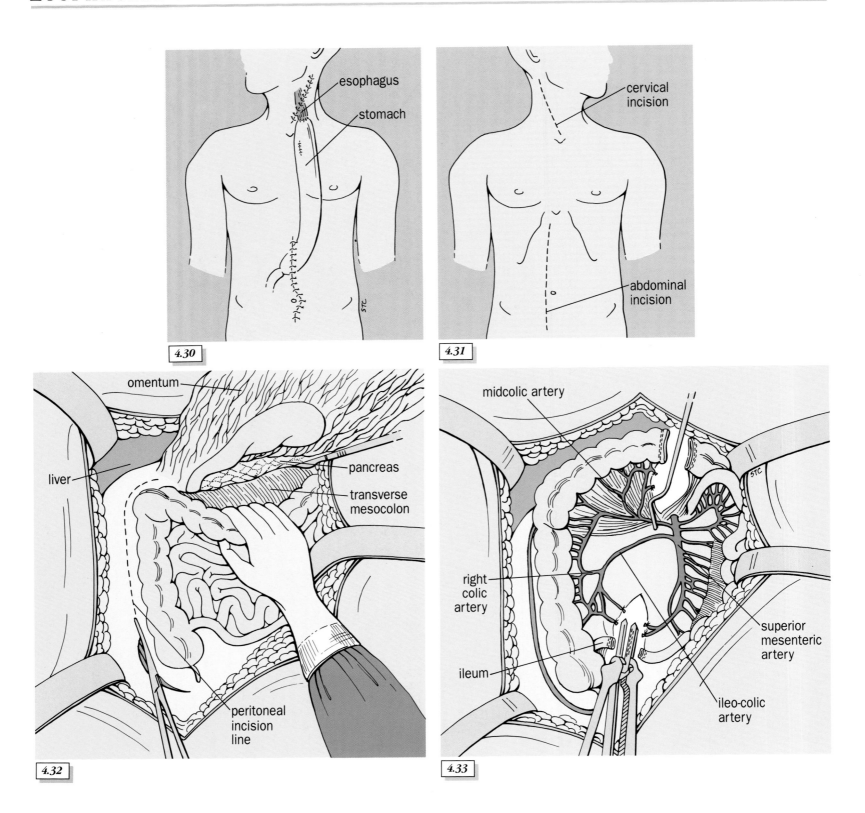

esophagus

stomach

4.30

cervical incision

abdominal incision

4.31

omentum

liver

pancreas

transverse mesocolon

peritoneal incision line

4.32

midcolic artery

right colic artery

ileum

superior mesenteric artery

ileo-colic artery

4.33

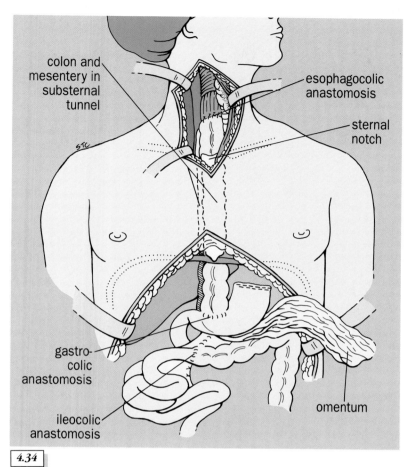

4.34

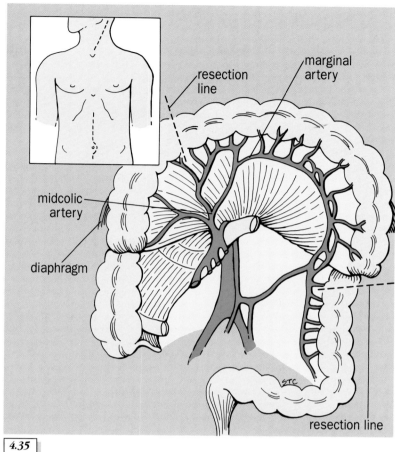

4.35

BIBLIOGRAPHY

Shackleford RT. *Surgery of the Alimentary Tract*. Philadelphia, Pa: Saunders; 1978:173–196, 152–158.

Skinner DB, Belsey RH. *Management of Esophageal Disease*. Philadelphia, Pa: Saunders; 1988:409–429, 474, 475, 753, 756.

Waldhausen JA, Pierce WS. *Johnson's Surgery of the Chest*. Chicago, Il: Yearbook; 1985:204–209, 214–219, 222–225.

5

Breast Surgery

Anne L. Rosenberg • Francis E. Rosato

The first surgeon to approach breast cancer with a therapeutic operation was Jean Louis Petit in the early 18th century. He employed wide excision, en bloc axillary dissection, and evaluation of the pectoralis fascia. Later, the Halsted-championed radical mastectomy became the standard. Most recently, an increasing number of patients are treated with breast-sparing procedures. Based on physical examination findings, the surgeon determines a preliminary diagnosis and plans the surgical approach, taking into account diagnostic and therapeutic factors. Surgical treatment options should be considered carefully, in light of additional factors such as patient history and risk, adequacy of nearby radiation facilities, and patient preference and compliance.

BREAST BIOPSY

ROUTINE BREAST BIOPSY

ROUTINE BREAST BIOPSY

INDICATIONS	• solid, dominant mass on physical examination
	• dominant lesion that cannot be successfully aspirated
	     • bloody aspirated fluid
	     • unresolved mass after aspiration
	     • recurrent mass less than 3 months after aspiration
	• excisional biopsy: lesions under 3 cm in diameter
	• incisional biopsy: malignant lesions over 3 cm in diameter

ANESTHESIA	• local, with or without intravenous sedation
POSITIONING	• patient supine, with arms abducted 90° or, for medial lesions or patient comfort, with arms at side
PREP	• Hibiclens preferable to Betadine in outpatient setting (less staining of skin and clothes) • surgical field extends from clavicle to costal margin and sternum to latissimus dorsi muscle (edge of table), including entire breast and axilla

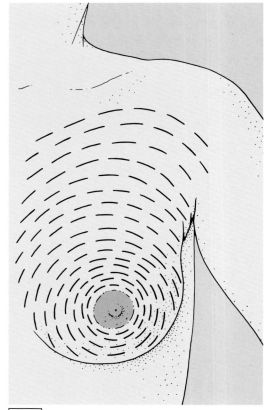

5.1

PROCEDURE

After prepping the patient, the incision is planned along Langer's lines (Fig. 5.1). The possibility of subsequent surgery must always be kept in mind in selecting an incision site. For lesions thought to be benign, a circumareolar incision is preferred (Fig. 5.2). With the use of Haagensen hooks and then appropriately sized retractors, a skin flap is developed to approach the lesion by sharp dissection (Figs. 5.3, 5.4). For lesions thought to be carcinoma, an incision directly over the lesion is preferred (Fig. 5.5). A skin flap is then developed in the same manner as that described for the circumareolar incision (Fig. 5.6).

Sharp dissection is used to cut through the breast tissue to the palpable lesion (Fig. 5.7), which is then excised from the surrounding tissue together with a small margin of normal tissue. This specimen is submitted to the pathologist for histologic evaluation.

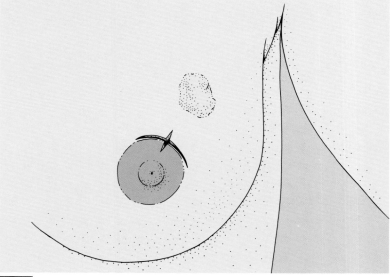

5.2

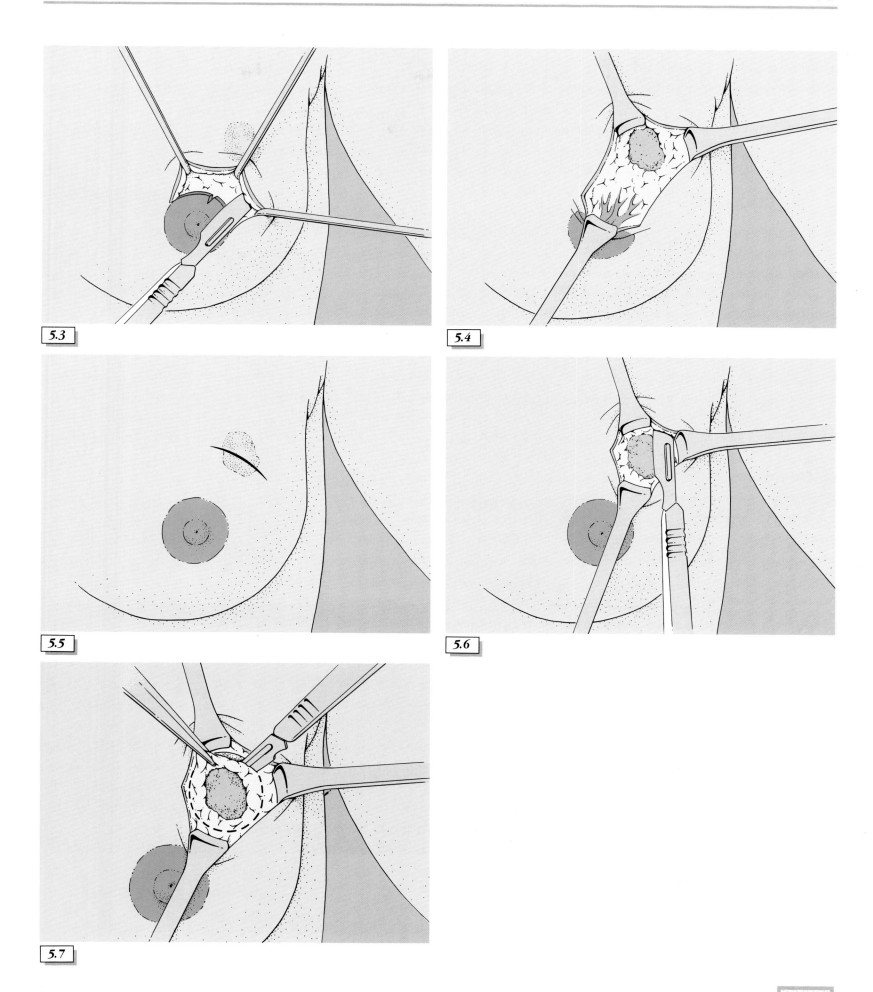

5.3

5.4

5.5

5.6

5.7

Electrocautery is not used until the lesion has been removed because heat denatures the protein measured in the estrogen- and progesterone-receptor assay, thereby altering the accuracy of the test. After hemostasis is obtained, the wound is closed. The dermis is closed using interrupted absorbable sutures (5–0 Vicryl or Dexon); the skin is then closed with interrupted 5–0 nylon sutures. If a drain is indicated, a Penrose drain is preferred (Fig. 5.8).

The wound is dressed with fluff gauze dressings, which are secured in place with two 6-inch Ace wraps around the chest wall (Fig. 5.9).

NEEDLE-GUIDED BREAST BIOPSY

NEEDLE-GUIDED BREAST BIOPSY

INDICATIONS	•nonpalpable lesion demonstrated on mammogram, which may show:
	  •calcifications
	  •mass or asymmetric density
	  •mass with calcifications
	•ultrasound to determine cystic or solid nature of lesion

ANESTHESIA	
POSITIONING	same as for routine breast biopsy (see page 5.2)
PREP	

PROCEDURE

The patient is taken to the mammography unit where needle localization of the lesion is performed (Figs. 5.10, 5.11). With the needle in place, the patient is then taken to the operating room for the biopsy procedure. Care must be taken to avoid dislodging the needle during prepping and positioning of the patient.

The biopsy is performed in a similar fashion to that of the routine biopsy (see Figs. 5.1–5.8). The dissection is carried sharply down to the area indicated by needle as the site of the abnormality. This tissue is then excised and submitted for specimen radiography (Fig. 5.12). If the radiograph confirms the presence of the lesion within the specimen, the wound is closed and the specimen is submitted for histologic evaluation. If the lesion is not present in the specimen, additional tissue from the surrounding area is taken and specimen radiography is again performed. This is repeated until the presence of the lesion within the specimen is confirmed by radiography.

ULTRASOUND-GUIDED BREAST BIOPSY

ULTRASOUND-GUIDED BREAST BIOPSY

INDICATIONS	•nonpalpable, solid lesion demonstrated by ultrasound (possibly also evident on mammogram)
ANESTHESIA	
POSITIONING	same as for routine breast biopsy (see page 5.2)
PREP	

PROCEDURE

After ultrasound examination, performed to locate and mark the lesion (Figs. 5.13, 5.14), the surgical procedure is performed using the same technique as that for routine breast biopsy (see Figs. 5.1 through 5.8). Once the lesion has been excised, ultrasound examination is repeated, with a sterile sleeve over the transducer, to confirm complete resection of the lesion (Fig. 5.15). The wound is then closed, and the specimen is submitted for histologic examination.

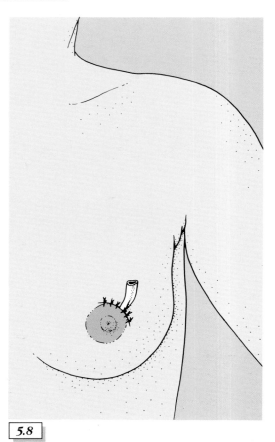

5.8

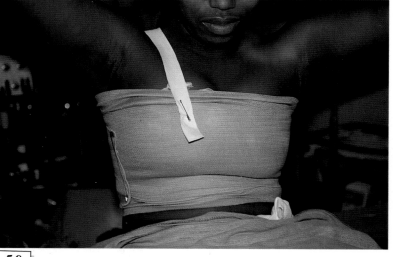

5.9

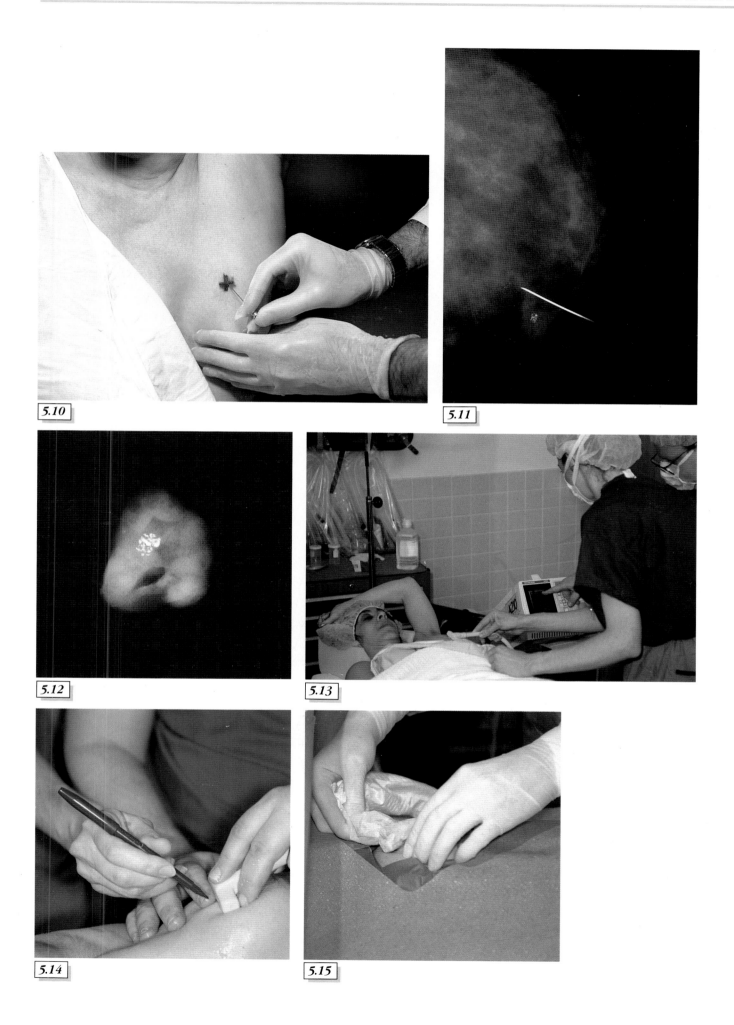

5.10

5.11

5.12

5.13

5.14

5.15

CENTRAL DUCT EXCISION

CENTRAL DUCT EXCISION

INDICATIONS • abnormal nipple discharge (bloody or spontaneous) with or without associated mass
• recurrent abscess or mastitis due to ductal ectasia

ANESTHESIA • local, with or without intravenous sedation (must be certain to anesthetize entire nipple–areola complex)

POSITIONING
PREP } same as for routine breast biopsy (see page 5.2)

PROCEDURE

The central duct area (retroareolar tissue) is approached through a circumareolar incision (Fig. 5.16). The areola is then undermined using hooks or a retracting suture at the skin edge (Fig. 5.17), and the lactiferous ducts (sinuses) are isolated (Fig. 5.18). The end of the major duct system is then transected at the base of the nipple (Fig. 5.19). The central ducts are excised together with a core of surrounding breast tissue (Fig. 5.20), and the entire specimen is submitted for histologic evaluation. The wound is inspected for hemostasis and then closed in a fashion similar to that for routine breast biopsy (see Fig. 5.8 and accompanying description). Fluff gauze dressings are placed over the incision and secured with two 6-inch Ace wraps around the chest wall (see Fig. 5.9).

MASTECTOMIES
STAGING OF BREAST CANCER

Staging of breast carcinoma refers to categorizing of patients by extent of disease. It is used to determine treatment options, estimate prognosis, and evaluate results of various treatment protocols. Patients are categorized according to clinical and pathologic staging. The Columbia Clinical Classification system (Table 5.1) is of historical importance. The most widely used system is currently based on the TNM (tumor, nodes, metastases) classification and is adopted by the Union Internationale Contre le Cancer (UICC) and the American Joint Committee on Cancer (AJCC) (Table 5.2). A schematic survey for treatment of breast cancer is given in Table 5.3. (Tables 5.2 and 5.3 appear on pages 5.8 and 5.9.)

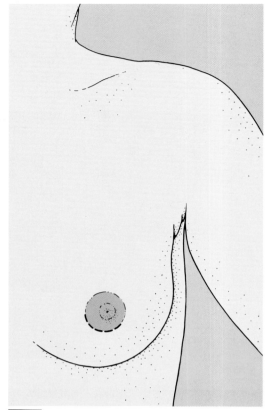

5.16

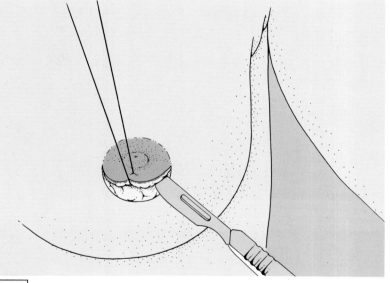

5.17

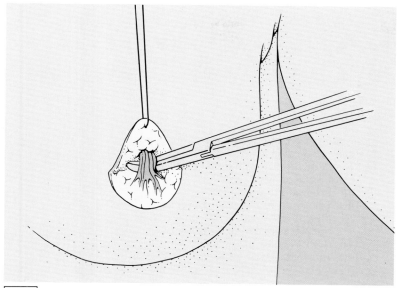

5.18

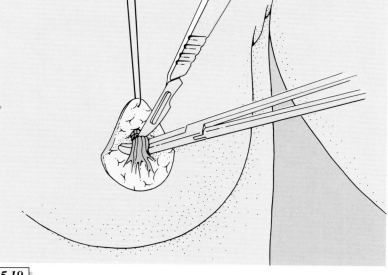

5.19

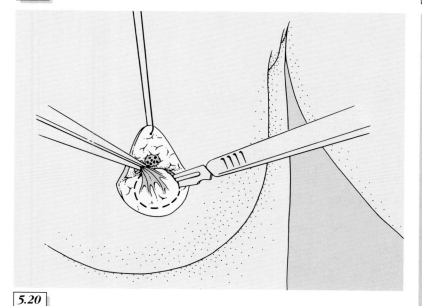

5.20

TABLE 5.1 COLUMBIA CLINICAL CLASSIFICATION OF BREAST CANCER*

STAGE A
No skin edema, ulceration, or solid fixation of the tumor to the chest wall. Axillary nodes are not clinically involved.

STAGE B
No skin edema, ulceration, or solid fixation of the tumor to the chest wall. Axillary nodes are clinically involved, but they are < 2.5 cm in transverse diameter and are not fixed to overlying skin or to deeper structures of the axilla.

STAGE C
Any one of the five grave signs of advanced breast carcinoma:
(1) edema of the skin of limited extent (involving less than one third of the skin over the breast)
(2) skin ulceration
(3) solid fixation of the tumor to the chest wall
(4) massive involvement of axillary lymph nodes (measuring 2.5 cm or more in transverse diameter)
(5) fixation of axillary nodes to overlying skin or deeper structures of axilla.

STAGE D
All other patients with more advanced breast carcinoma, including:
(1) a combination of any two or more of the five grave signs listed under Stage C
(2) extensive edema of the skin (involving more than one third of the skin over the breast)
(3) satellite skin nodules
(4) inflammatory type of carcinoma
(5) clinically involved supraclavicular lymph nodes
(6) internal mammary metastases as evidenced by a parasternal tumor
(7) edema of the arm
(8) distant metastases.

* From Haagensen, 1986.

TABLE 5.2 UICC–AJCC CLINICAL STAGING SYSTEM FOR BREAST CANCER*
REGIONAL LYMPH NODES (N)

PRIMARY TUMOR (T)

TX Primary tumor cannot be assessed
T0 No evidence of primary tumor
Tis Carcinoma in situ: intraductal carcinoma, lobular carcinoma in situ, or Paget's disease of the nipple with no tumor[a]
T1 Tumor ≤2 cm in greatest dimension
  T1a Tumor ≤0.5 cm in greatest dimension
  T1b Tumor >0.5 cm but ≤1 cm in greatest dimension
  T1c Tumor >1 cm but ≤2 cm in greatest dimension

T2 Tumor >2 cm but ≤5 cm in greatest dimension
T3 Tumor >5 cm in greatest dimension
T4 Tumor of any size with direct extension to chest wall[b] or skin
  T4a Extension to chest wall
  T4b Edema (including peau d'orange) or ulceration of skin of breast or satellite skin nodules confined to same breast
  T4c Both T4a and T4b
  T4d Inflammatory carcinoma

[a] Paget's disease associated with a tumor is classified according to size of the tumor.
[b] Chest wall includes ribs, intercostal muscles, and serratus anterior muscle but not pectoral muscle.

NX Regional lymph nodes cannot be assessed (eg, previously removed)
N0 No regional lymph node metastasis
N1 Metastasis to movable ipsilateral axillary lymph node(s)
N2 Metastasis to ipsilateral axillary lymph node(s) fixed to one another or to other structures
N3 Metastasis to ipsilateral internal mammary lymph node(s)

MX Presence of distant metastasis cannot be assessed
M0 No distant metastasis
M1 Distant metastasis present (including metastasis to ipsilateral supraclavicular lymph node[s])

DISTANT METASTASIS (M)

CLINICAL STAGE GROUPING

STAGE 0	Tis	N0	M0
STAGE I	T1	N0	M0
STAGE IIA	T0	N1	M0
	T1	N1	M0
	T2	N0	M0
STAGE IIB	T2	N1	M0
	T3	N0	M0
STAGE IIIA	T0, T1	N2	M0
	T2	N2	M0
	T3	N1, N2	M0
STAGE IIIB	T4	Any N	M0
	Any T	N3	M0
STAGE IV	Any T	Any N	M1

*From Beahrs OH, Henson DE, Hutter RVP, Myers MH (American Joint Committee on Cancer). *Manual for Staging of Cancer*, 3rd ed. Philadelphia, Pa: JB Lippincott Co; 1988.

TABLE 5.3 SCHEMATIC SURVEY FOR TREATMENT OF BREAST CANCER

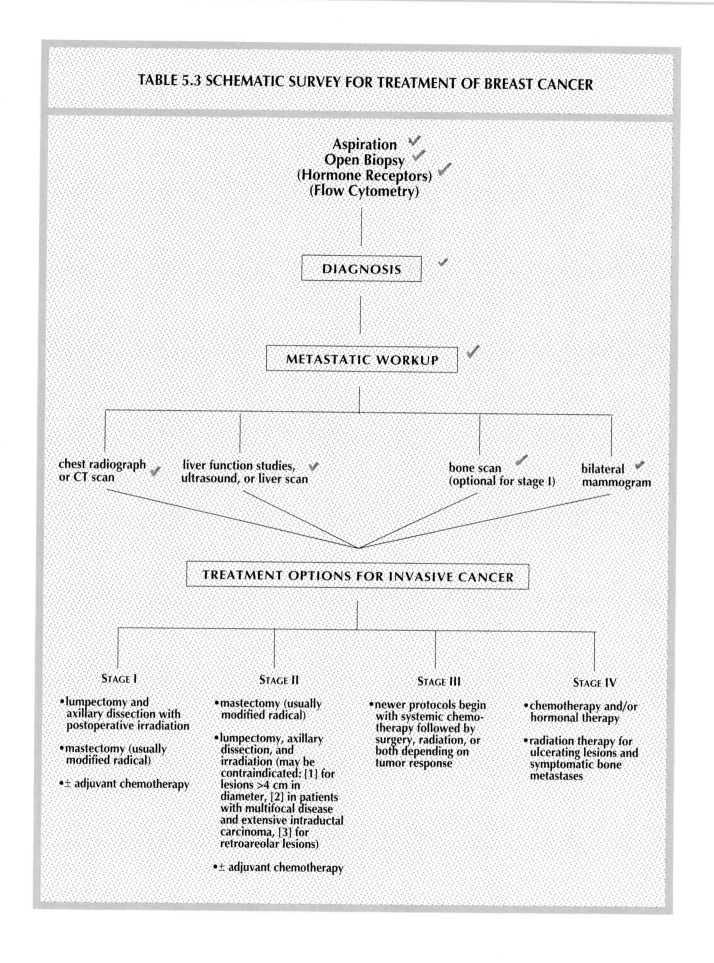

Aspiration
Open Biopsy
(Hormone Receptors)
(Flow Cytometry)

DIAGNOSIS

METASTATIC WORKUP

chest radiograph or CT scan

liver function studies, ultrasound, or liver scan

bone scan (optional for stage I)

bilateral mammogram

TREATMENT OPTIONS FOR INVASIVE CANCER

STAGE I
- lumpectomy and axillary dissection with postoperative irradiation
- mastectomy (usually modified radical)
- ± adjuvant chemotherapy

STAGE II
- mastectomy (usually modified radical)
- lumpectomy, axillary dissection, and irradiation (may be contraindicated: [1] for lesions >4 cm in diameter, [2] in patients with multifocal disease and extensive intraductal carcinoma, [3] for retroareolar lesions)
- ± adjuvant chemotherapy

STAGE III
- newer protocols begin with systemic chemo-therapy followed by surgery, radiation, or both depending on tumor response

STAGE IV
- chemotherapy and/or hormonal therapy
- radiation therapy for ulcerating lesions and symptomatic bone metastases

RADICAL MASTECTOMY

Removal of the Breast with Nipple–Areola Complex, Axillary Nodes (Levels I–III), and Pectoralis Major and Minor Muscles

RADICAL MASTECTOMY	
INDICATIONS	• breast carcinomas involving the pectoralis fascia and/or pectoralis muscle • stage III breast cancers following chemotherapy • chest wall sarcoma
ANESTHESIA	• general endotracheal
POSITIONING	• patient at edge of operating table on operative side, with arms abducted at 90° • electrocautery (if used) on the contralateral thigh • ipsilateral thigh kept available for harvesting a skin graft, if needed • hips and arms secured to avoid patient slipping • after induction of anesthesia, table is rotated away from surgeon approximately 30°, and head of table is raised to 45° to 60°
PREP	• usually Betadine solution is used unless there is an allergy to iodine • the field extends from the contralateral nipple or midclavicular line to the abdominal wall inferiorly, the neck superiorly, and posteriorly to the operative table, including the entire breast and axilla • the arm is prepped circumferentially down to the wrist and draped to allow movement in the operative field (Fig. 5.21)

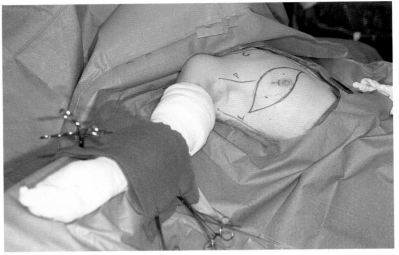

5.21

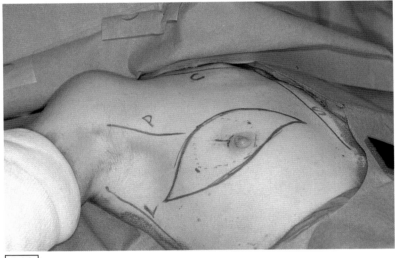

5.22

PROCEDURE

Once the patient is positioned and prepped, the incision is planned (Fig. 5.22). Either a transverse (Stewart) or vertical (Halsted–Haagensen) incision is chosen. The latter is often necessary with larger lesions. A 3- to 5-cm margin is allowed around the tumor or previous biopsy incision. The mastectomy incision is made with a #10 or #21 knife blade. Hemostasis is obtained at the level of the dermis. To facilitate retraction, a surgeon's cap is sewn to the edges of the specimen (Fig. 5.23).

Dissection is performed in the plane superficial to the superficial fascia of the breast (Fig. 5.24). Haagensen hooks are placed along the flaps for perpendicular traction, with the breast itself serving as countertraction (Fig. 5.25). The medial flap, the boundaries of which are the clavicle superiorly, the sternum medially, and the costal margin and rectus fascia inferiorly, is developed first. The platysma is included with the specimen, because it lies within the superficial fascia (Fig. 5.26).

The lateral flap is then developed after the Haagensen hooks are replaced along the inferior aspect of the flap. The boundaries of the lateral flap include the costal margin and rectus fascia inferiorly, the clavicle superiorly, and the latissimus dorsi muscle laterally (Fig. 5.27).

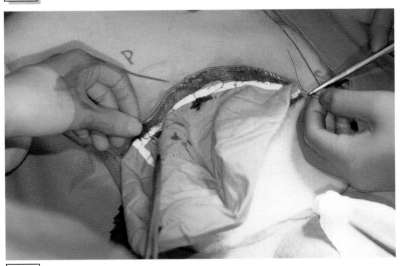

5.23

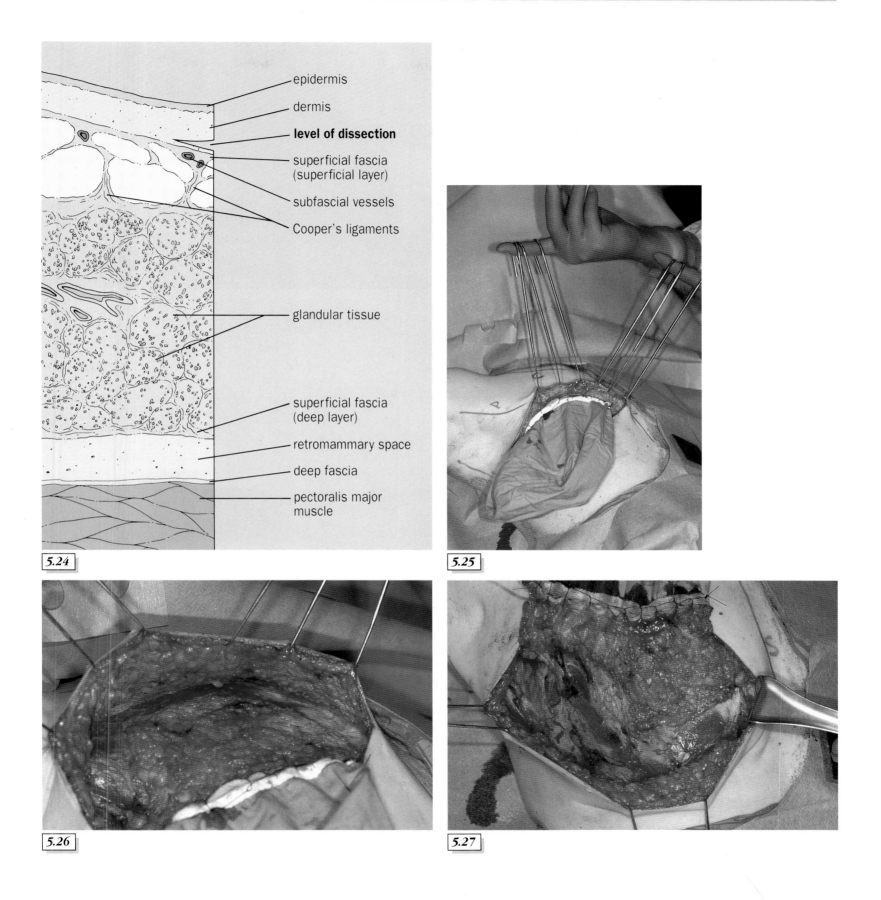

epidermis

dermis

level of dissection

superficial fascia
(superficial layer)

subfascial vessels

Cooper's ligaments

glandular tissue

superficial fascia
(deep layer)

retromammary space

deep fascia

pectoralis major
muscle

5.24

5.25

5.26

5.27

Attention is now directed to the bridge of tissue across the axilla. The axillary dissection is performed in its entirety using a #15 knife blade and fine DeBakey forceps. The latissimus should be followed until it becomes white tendon and one can identify the point at which the axillary vein crosses it; this marks the lateralmost margin of the dissection (Fig. 5.28). The intercostal nerves are identified along the inferior aspect of the axillary vein. It may be necessary to sacrifice these due to their course through the axillary nodes and lymphatic vessels.

The cephalic vein is identified in the deltopectoral groove, and care must be taken to avoid injury to this vessel. The inferior surface of the pectoralis major is dissected to allow division of the muscle approximately 2 cm from its insertion on the humerus (Fig. 5.29).

Vessels in the stump of the muscle are individually cauterized, or clipped and divided (Fig. 5.30). The thoracoacromial vessels and the inferior thoracic nerves supplying the pectoralis major are clipped and divided and then the muscle (with the breast) is dissected from the chest wall (Fig. 5.31). The clavicular head of the muscle is spared, leaving only enough muscle along the clavicle and sternum to allow hemostasis to be obtained. The muscle is allowed to fall laterally, and the dissection stops when the medial edge of the pectoralis minor is encountered.

Intercostal perforating vessels are individually clipped and divided. Inferiorly, the rectus fascia is included with the specimen. The intercostal spaces are cleared of all fat and areolar tissue. The pectoralis minor is now divided by first incising the costocoracoid fascia along the medial and lateral edges of the muscle. After circumferential control of the muscle is obtained, it is divided approximately 2 cm from its insertion on the coracoid process (Fig. 5.32).

The pectoralis minor is turned back over the axillary structures and divided from its attachments to the third, fourth, and fifth ribs, sacrificing the serratus fascia but sparing the muscle. The nerves and vessels to the pectoralis minor are ligated and divided, and the muscle is allowed to fall laterally (Fig. 5.33).

Using the fine forceps and a #15 knife blade, the axillary dissection is now continued by incision into the costocoracoid fascia parallel and cephalad to the brachial plexus. The fat and areolar tissue are dissected in a caudal direction, bringing the axillary vein into view. The inferior surface of the axillary vein is cleared from the lateralmost margin of the dissection (where the vein crosses the white tendon of the latissimus dorsi) to the apex of the axilla (where the vein passes beneath the subclavius muscle to enter the chest) (Fig. 5.34). Tributaries along the inferior aspect of the vein are individually ligated and divided. The axillary contents should be marked so that the pathologist can orient the specimen and separate the tissue into "apex of axilla," and levels I, II, and III nodes.

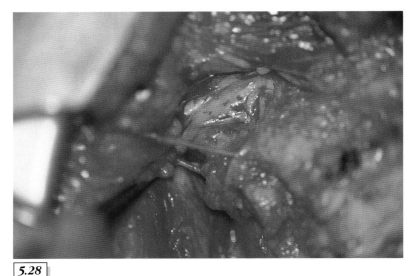

5.28

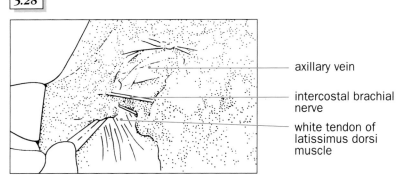

axillary vein

intercostal brachial nerve

white tendon of latissimus dorsi muscle

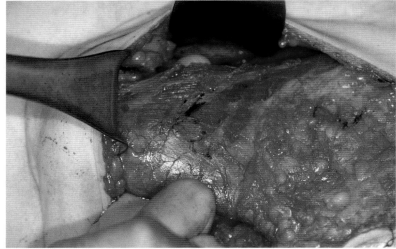

5.29

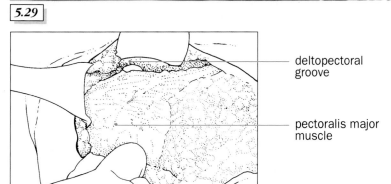

deltopectoral groove

pectoralis major muscle

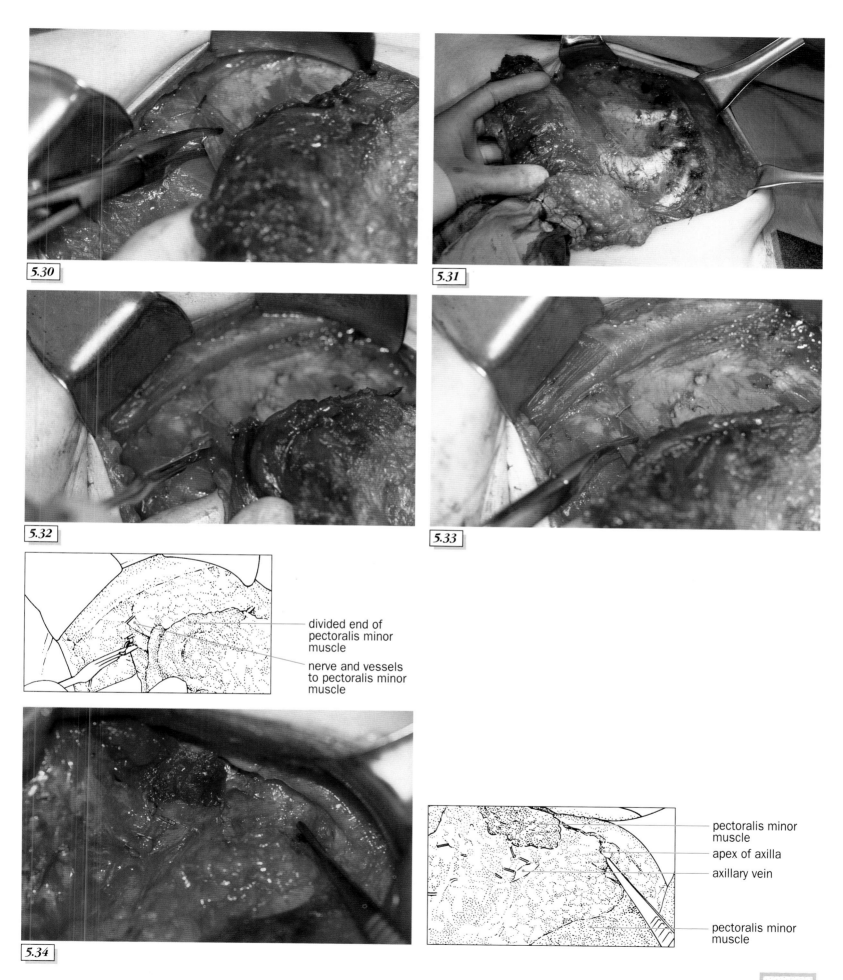

5.30

5.31

5.32

5.33

divided end of
pectoralis minor
muscle

nerve and vessels
to pectoralis minor
muscle

5.34

pectoralis minor
muscle

apex of axilla

axillary vein

pectoralis minor
muscle

Dissection is continued in the cleft along the chest wall, in the area bounded by the subscapularis muscle and teres major muscle. The long thoracic nerve is identified, skeletonized, and carefully preserved along its course (Fig. 5.35). The thoracodorsal nerve and vessels are identified where they emerge from beneath the axillary vein. It may be necessary to sacrifice the thoracodorsal nerve and vessels since they course through the axillary nodes and lymphatic vessels.

To excise the specimen, an incision is made in a longitudinal plane along the anterior surface of the latissimus dorsi muscle. The wound is inspected for hemostasis (Fig. 5.36), and is then irrigated with sterile water to kill any free-floating tumor cells. Two Jackson–Pratt drains are placed through stab wounds in the inferior flap. The medial one drains the flaps and the lateral one drains the axilla.

The flaps are revised to allow closure without tension and to avoid dog-ears. If a skin graft is to be used, the flaps are sewn to the chest wall and the recipient site prepared for the graft (Fig. 5.37). The dermis is closed with 5–0 Vicryl or Dexon, and skin staples are then placed.

A split-thickness skin graft can be harvested from the ipsilateral thigh using an entirely separate set of instruments and drapes. The surgeon should change gown and gloves to minimize tumor seeding. The donor site is then dressed, and the skin graft is secured in place over the chest-wall defect (Fig. 5.38).

A nonadherent dressing is placed over the incision, and fluff gauze dressings are then applied for gentle pressure. They are secured in place with three 6-inch Ace wraps around the chest wall. The hand and forearm are free to protrude from between the folds of the bandages (Fig. 5.39).

MODIFIED RADICAL MASTECTOMY

Auchincloss—Removal of the Breast, with Nipple–Areola Complex and Level I Axillary Lymph Nodes

Patey—Removal of the Breast, with Nipple–Areola Complex and Levels I, II, and III Axillary Lymph Nodes and Pectoralis Minor Muscle

MODIFIED RADICAL MASTECTOMY

INDICATIONS	• Stage I and II carcinomas of the breast based on the following conditions: 　• lesions over 4 cm in diameter 　• multicentric lesions 　• retroareolar lesions • suboptimal cosmetic result following biopsy (eg, deformity in breast due to size of lesion relative to size of breast) • inadequate radiation facility or noncompliant patient • patient preference
ANESTHESIA	• general endotracheal
POSITIONING PREP	same as for radical mastectomy (see page 5.10)

PROCEDURE

Once the patient has been prepped and positioned the incision is planned, with the surgeon choosing between a transverse (Stewart) or vertical (Halsted–Haagensen) approach. Using a #10 or #21 knife blade,

an incision is made down to the dermis (Fig. 5.40). Hemostasis is obtained along the edges of the incision, and a surgeon's cap is sewn to the edges of the specimen to facilitate retraction of the specimen during the procedure (see Fig. 5.23).

Using the Haagensen hooks for traction and the breast for counter-traction, the flaps are developed in the plane superficial to the superficial fascia of the breast in order that this fascia may be included with the specimen.

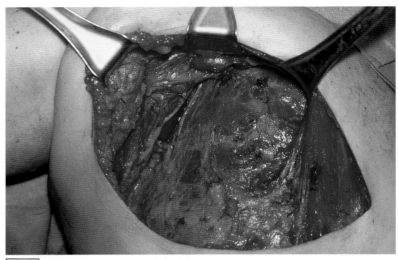

5.35

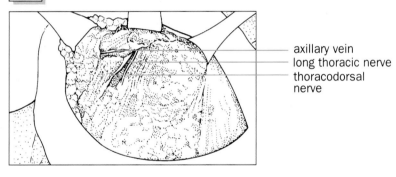

axillary vein
long thoracic nerve
thoracodorsal nerve

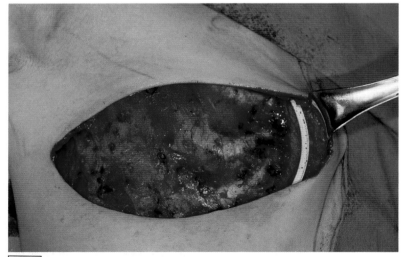

5.36

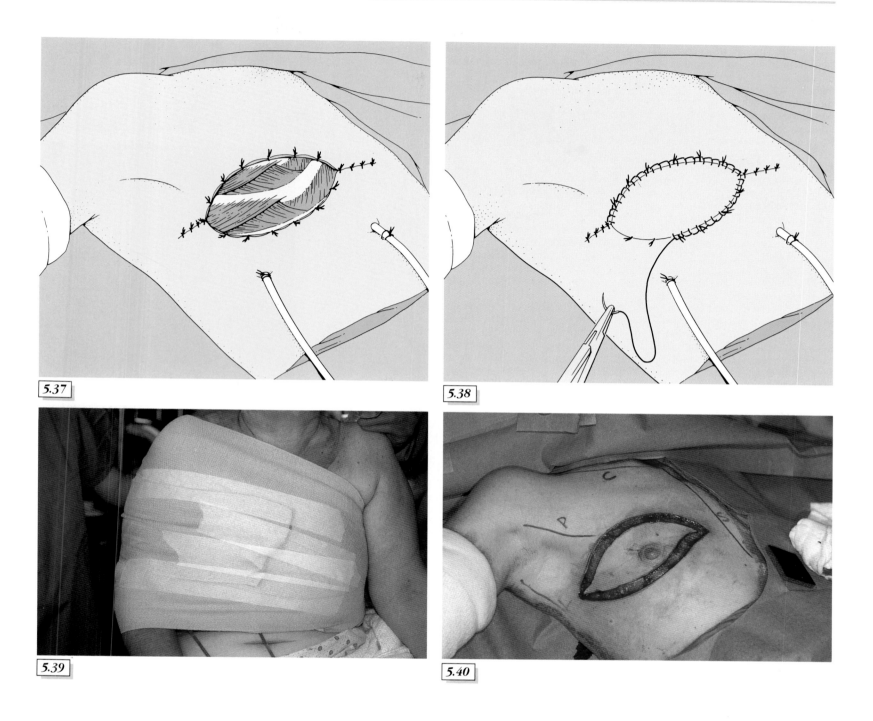

5.37

5.38

5.39

5.40

The boundaries of the superior flap extend to the clavicle superiorly, the sternum medially, and the edge of the pectoralis major and latissimus dorsi muscles laterally. The platysma, which lies within the superficial fascia, is included with the specimen (Fig. 5.41). The hooks are then placed along the inferior flap, which is developed in the same superficial plane, the boundaries being the sternum medially, the costal margin and rectus fascia inferiorly, and the serratus anterior and latissimus dorsi muscles laterally. The bridge of tissue across the axilla is left undisturbed at this time (Fig. 5.42).

The breast is now dissected away from the pectoralis major muscle; the fascia of the muscle is included with the specimen (Fig. 5.43).

The dissection is carried from the superomedial corner toward the inferolateral edge of the pectoralis major muscle. Perforating vessels are individually controlled.

With the breast reflected laterally, the axillary dissection is then performed in its entirety using a #15 knife blade and fine DeBakey forceps. The axillary vein is identified by incising the costocoracoid fascia parallel to and cephalad to it (Fig. 5.44). The fat and areolar tissue are dissected in a caudal direction, and the vein is brought into view. The point at which the axillary vein crosses the white tendon of the latissimus dorsi is the lateralmost margin of the dissection.

If only the level I nodes are to be dissected (Auchincloss), the pectoralis minor muscle is not released from its attachment to the coracoid process. The axillary dissection is carried medially only to the lateral edge of the pectoralis minor muscle (Fig. 5.45). If all three levels of axillary nodes are to be dissected (Patey), then the pectoralis muscle must be removed or at least taken down from its attachment to the coracoid.

First, Rotter's fascia (interpectoral) is excised by dissecting the tissue from between the posterior surface of the pectoralis major muscle and the anterior surface of the pectoralis minor muscle. The pectoralis major is retracted medially to facilitate the excision (Fig. 5.46). Rotter's fascia is submitted as a separate specimen.

To divide the pectoralis minor, the costocoracoid fascia is incised along its medial and lateral edges. After circumferential control of the pectoralis minor is obtained, the muscle is divided approximately 2 cm from its attachment to the coracoid (Fig. 5.47). The muscle is reflected laterally and divided from its attachments to the third, fourth, and fifth ribs. The muscle is allowed to fall laterally with the specimen. The lateral pectoral nerve will likely be sacrificed if the pectoralis minor muscle is detached from the coracoid.

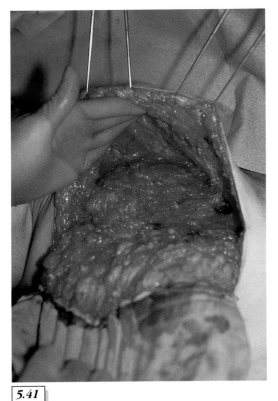

5.41

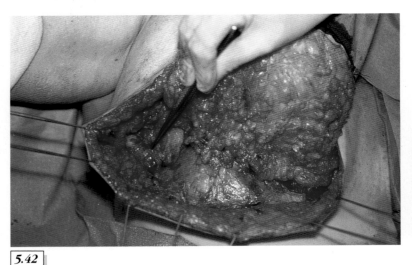

5.42

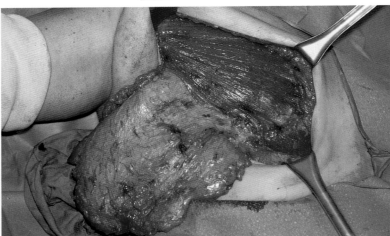

5.43

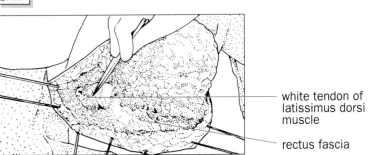

white tendon of latissimus dorsi muscle

rectus fascia

5.16

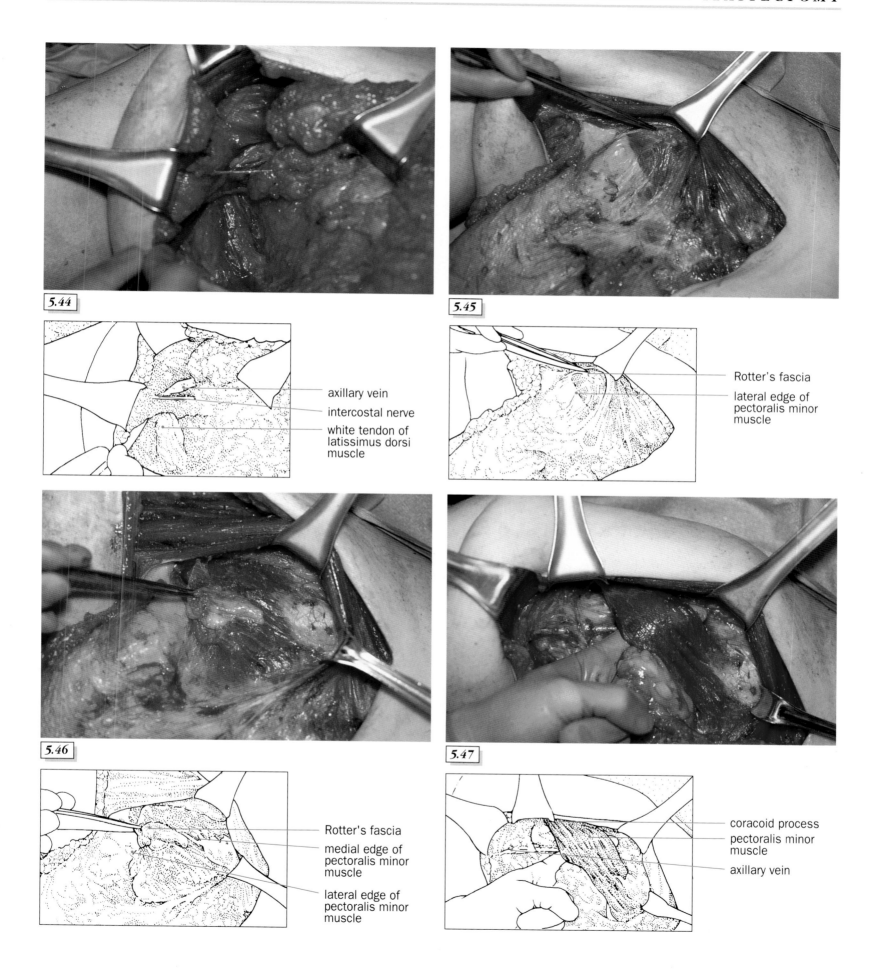

5.44

axillary vein
intercostal nerve
white tendon of
latissimus dorsi
muscle

5.45

Rotter's fascia
lateral edge of
pectoralis minor
muscle

5.46

Rotter's fascia
medial edge of
pectoralis minor
muscle
lateral edge of
pectoralis minor
muscle

5.47

coracoid process
pectoralis minor
muscle
axillary vein

The dissection along the axillary vein is now continued in a medial direction until the point at which the vein goes beneath the subclavius muscle to enter the chest (Fig. 5.48). Tributaries along the inferior aspect of the vein are individually clipped and divided. The intercostal nerves are encountered along the inferior surface of the axillary vein. It may be necessary to sacrifice these nerves since they run through the axillary nodes and lymphatic vessels (Fig. 5.49).

After dissection along the vein is completed, the dissection is continued in the cleft along the chest wall. The long thoracic nerve is identified as it runs along the chest wall; it is carefully skeletonized and preserved along its course (see Fig. 5.35). The thoracodorsal nerve and vessels are then identified where they emerge from behind the axillary vein. The thoracodorsal nerve may also need to be sacrificed if its course runs through the axillary nodes and lymphatic vessels.

The specimen should be tagged at its medial and lateral edges to allow the pathologist to orient it for evaluation. It is then removed by incision in a longitudinal plane along the latissimus dorsi muscle. The wound is irrigated with sterile water to kill any free-floating tumor cells. Two 3/16-inch Jackson–Pratt drains are placed through stab wounds in the inferior flap, the medial one to drain the flaps and the lateral one to drain the axilla (Fig. 5.50).

The flaps are replaced on the chest wall and fashioned to allow closure without tension and to avoid dog-ears. The incision is closed with interrupted 5–0 Vicryl or Dexon in the dermis and then skin staples are placed (Fig. 5.51). A nonadherent dressing is placed over the incision, and then fluff gauzes are applied for gentle pressure. These are secured in place with three 6-inch Ace wraps around the upper arm and chest wall. The hand and forearm are free to protrude between the folds of the bandages (see Fig. 5.39).

SIMPLE MASTECTOMY

Removal of the Breast, Nipple, and Areola

SIMPLE MASTECTOMY

INDICATIONS
- in-situ ductal carcinoma
- local recurrence following a lumpectomy, axillary dissection, and irradiation
- high-risk patients with lobular neoplasia (bilateral simple mastectomy)
- prophylaxis for high-risk patients (questionable)

ANESTHESIA
- general endotracheal
- local, with intravenous sedation, in patients at poor medical-surgical risk

POSITIONING
PREP
same as for radical mastectomy (see page 5.10)

PROCEDURE

Once the patient has been positioned and prepped, the incision is planned (Fig. 5.52). A transverse (Stewart) incision is usually used. A 3-cm margin is taken around the biopsy incision, including the nipple–areola complex. The incision is taken down to the dermis and hemostasis is effected. To facilitate retraction of the specimen during the procedure, a

surgeon's cap is sewn to the edges of the specimen. Skin hooks are used for perpendicular traction as the flaps are developed, with the breast serving as countertraction (Fig. 5.53).

The boundaries of the superior flap are the clavicle superiorly, the sternum medially, and the edges of the pectoralis major and latissimus dorsi muscles laterally. The flap is developed in the plane superficial to the superficial fascia of the breast so that the facia is included with the specimen.

The hooks are placed to allow development of the inferior flap in the same superficial plane. The boundaries of the flap are the sternum medially, the costal margin and rectus fascia inferiorly, and the serratus anterior and latissimus dorsi muscles laterally. Although no attempt is made to perform a formal axillary dissection, a few of the low-lying level I axillary nodes are included in the tail of Spence (Fig. 5.54).

The breast is now dissected free from the pectoralis major muscle, including the fascia of the muscle with the specimen (see Fig. 5.43). The wound is inspected for hemostasis and irrigated with sterile water to kill free-floating tumor cells.

The wound is drained with two Jackson–Pratt drains (closed suction), which are brought out through the inferior flap. The medial one drains the flap, and the lateral one drains the axilla (see Fig. 5.50). The flaps are fashioned to allow closure without tension and to avoid "dog-ears." The incision is closed with interrupted 5–0 Vicryl or Dexon in the dermis and skin staples (see Fig. 5.51).

A nonadherent dressing is placed and fluff gauze dressings are applied for gentle pressure. The upper arm is wrapped with the dressings by three 6-inch Ace wraps around the chest wall, leaving the hand and arm to protrude between the folds (see Fig. 5.39).

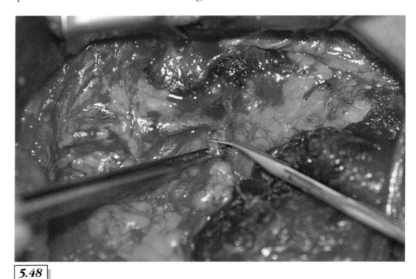

5.48

apex of axilla
axillary vein
cut end of pectoralis minor muscle

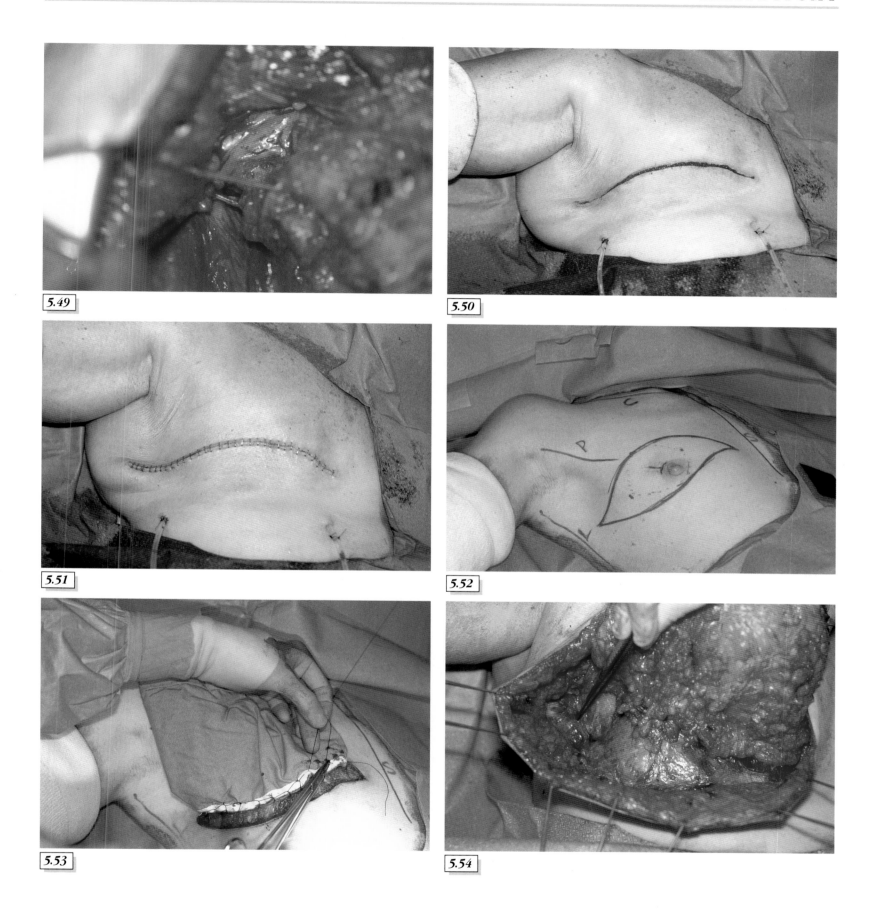

5.49

5.50

5.51

5.52

5.53

5.54

LUMPECTOMY WITH AXILLARY LYMPHADENECTOMY

Excision of a Primary Tumor with a Small Rim of "Normal" Tissue, Dissection of Level I and II Axillary Lymph Nodes

---

LUMPECTOMY WITH AXILLARY LYMPHADENECTOMY

INDICATIONS
- Stage I and II breast carcinomas based on the following conditions:
  - tumor size less than 4 cm (with some exceptions)
  - lack of multicentricity
  - patient preference
  - tumor location (contraindicated if retroareolar)
  - breast size and deformity following lumpectomy
  - patient compliance
  - adequate radiation facility

ANESTHESIA
- general endotracheal

POSITIONING
PREP
same as for radical mastectomy (see page 5.10)

If a level I axillary lymphadenectomy is performed and the nodes are negative, 10% of patients will have skip metastases to level II and III nodes. If a level I and II axillary lymphadenectomy is performed, the incidence of skip metastases to level III nodes is 1.5% (Fig. 5.55). When a lumpectomy is performed, all gross tumor must be excised to ensure the lowest rate of local recurrence.

PROCEDURE

AXILLARY LYMPHADENECTOMY

The incision is planned in a skin crease in the lower portion of the hair-bearing area of the axilla. It extends posteriorly from the lateral edge of the pectoralis major muscle to the edge of the latissimus dorsi muscle, measuring approximately 5 cm in length (Fig. 5.56).

Skin hooks and then retractors are used to develop the flaps. The caudal flap is developed first. The margins of dissection are the edge of the pectoralis major anteriorly, the fifth intercostal space inferiorly, and the latissimus dorsi posteriorly (Fig. 5.57). The cephalad flap is then developed, the margins being the pectoralis major muscle anteriorly, the latissimus posteriorly, and the axillary vein superiorly (Fig. 5.58).

The axillary dissection is performed using a #15 knife blade and fine DeBakey forceps in a manner similar to that used in a radical mastectomy. The axillary vein is cleared medially until the lateral edge of the pectoralis minor is encountered (Fig. 5.59). This constitutes a level I dissection.

With retraction of the pectoral muscles medially, dissection along the axillary vein can be continued until the medial edge of the pectoralis minor is encountered. A single large clip can be placed here to mark, for subsequent radiography, the most medial point of dissection (Fig. 5.60). The long thoracic and thoracodorsal nerves are identified and the former

is carefully preserved (Fig. 5.61). The thoracodorsal nerve may be sacrificed if it courses through the axillary lymphatics. The intercostal nerves, located along the inferior surface of the axillary vein, may also be sacrificed if necessary.

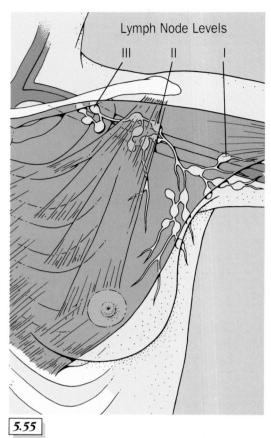

Lymph Node Levels

III   II   I

5.55

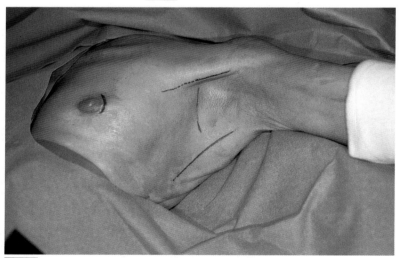

5.56

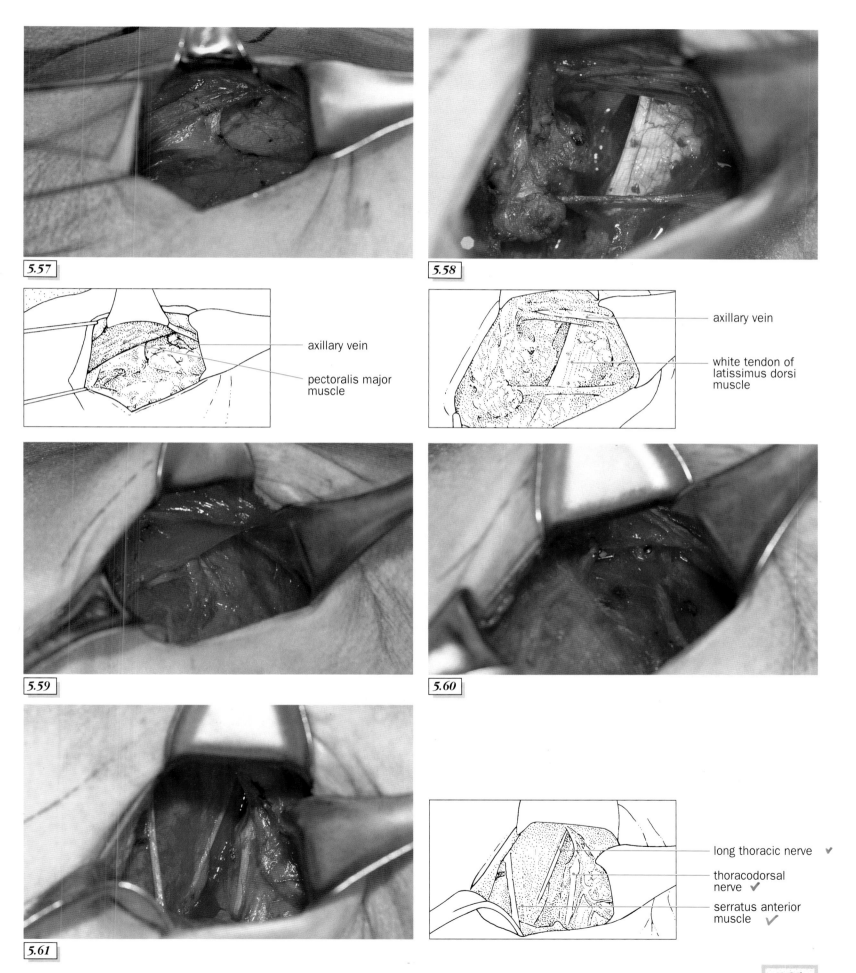

5.57

5.58

axillary vein

pectoralis major
muscle

axillary vein

white tendon of
latissimus dorsi
muscle

5.59

5.60

5.61

long thoracic nerve

thoracodorsal
nerve

serratus anterior
muscle

The wound is drained with a Jackson–Pratt drain brought out through a stab wound in the inferior flap. This stab wound or exit site is an area that will be covered by the patient's bra, and is included within the radiation field. (The specimen should be divided by the surgeon into its component parts and then submitted to the pathologist.) The wound is irrigated with sterile water to kill any free-floating tumor cells and then is closed with interrupted 5–0 Vicryl or Dexon in the fascia and a running intracuticular 5–0 Vicryl in the skin (Fig. 5.62).

LUMPECTOMY

After covering the axillary incision with a sterile nonadherent dressing and a sterile towel to exclude it from the field, the biopsy site in the breast is reopened (Fig. 5.63). The "lump" is reexcised with a small margin (1 cm) of grossly normal tissue. Hemostasis is effected. The inferior, medial, superior, and lateral margins of the wound, as well as its base, are marked with small metallic clips for subsequent radiographic localization. Biopsies from each of these locations may also be obtained to check the surgical margins (Fig. 5.64).

The wound is then closed in a similar fashion to that for routine breast biopsy and is dressed with fluff gauze over the breast and axilla. The dressing is secured in place with three 6-inch Ace wraps. The forearm and hand are free to protrude between the folds of the bandages.

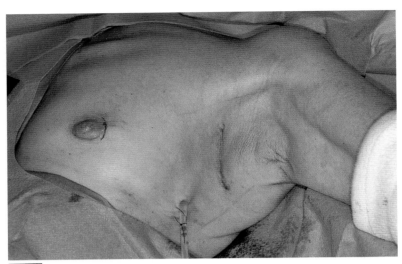

5.62

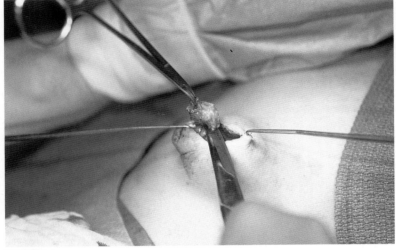

5.63

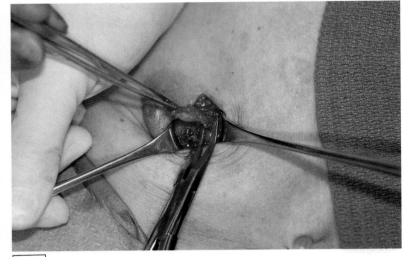

5.64

BIBLIOGRAPHY

Haagensen CD. *Diseases of the Breast*, 3rd ed. Philadelphia, Pa: WB Saunders Co; 1986.

Harris JR, Hellman S, Henderson C, Kinne D, eds. *Breast Diseases.* Philadelphia, Pa: JB Lippincott Co; 1987.

Strombeck JO, Rosato FE, eds. *Surgery of the Breast.* New York, Thieme; 1986.

6

Surgery of the Stomach, Duodenum, and Small Bowel

Jerome J. Vernick • Diane R. Gillum

SURGICAL ANATOMY

A precise knowledge of the arterial blood supply (Fig. 6.1) and the venous and lymphatic drainage (Fig. 6.2) to the upper abdominal viscera is essential for surgical treatment. Figure 6.3 shows the blood supply of the stomach, duodenum, spleen, and pancreas. Figure 6.4 shows the zonal lymphatic drainage of carcinoma of the stomach. The arterial supply to the small intestine is shown in Fig. 6.5.

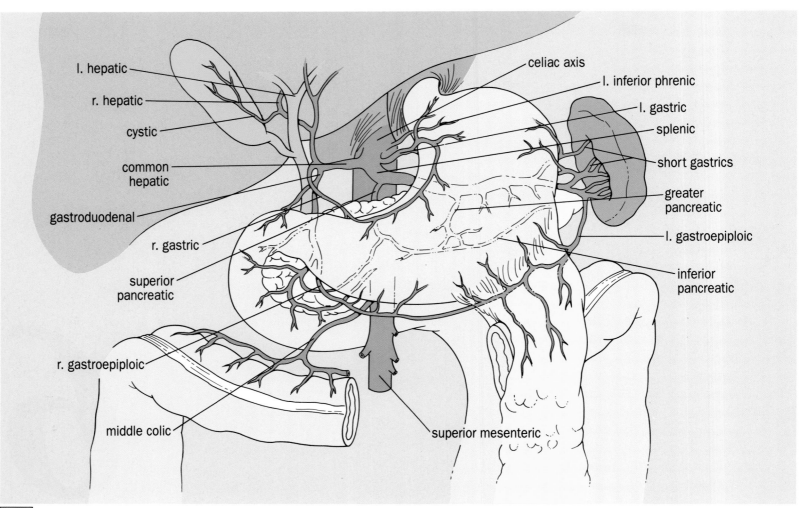

6.1

6.2

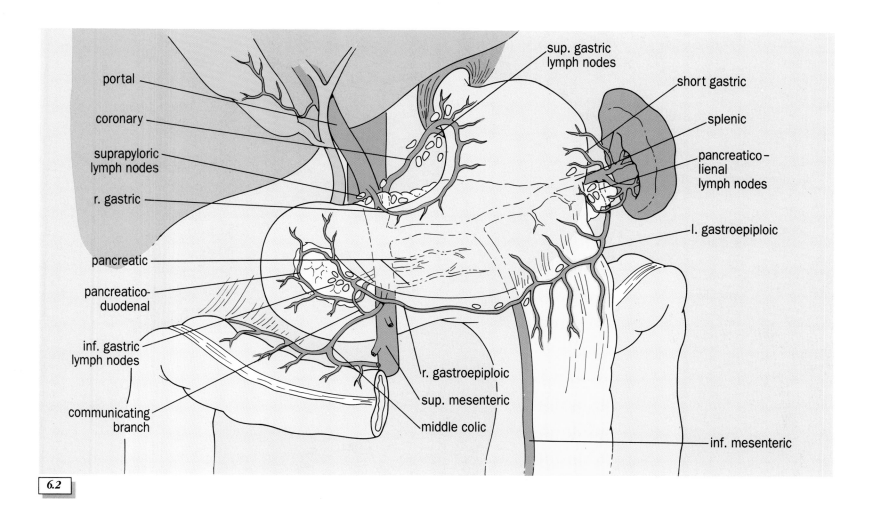

portal

coronary

suprapyloric
lymph nodes

r. gastric

sup. gastric
lymph nodes

short gastric

splenic

pancreatico-
lienal
lymph nodes

l. gastroepiploic

pancreatic

pancreatico-
duodenal

inf. gastric
lymph nodes

communicating
branch

r. gastroepiploic

sup. mesenteric

middle colic

inf. mesenteric

6.2

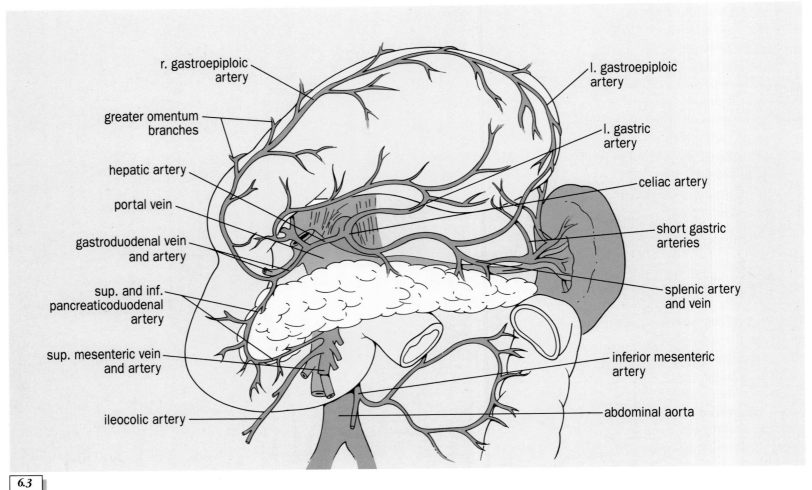

r. gastroepiploic
artery

l. gastroepiploic
artery

greater omentum
branches

l. gastric
artery

hepatic artery

celiac artery

portal vein

short gastric
arteries

gastroduodenal vein
and artery

sup. and inf.
pancreaticoduodenal
artery

splenic artery
and vein

sup. mesenteric vein
and artery

inferior mesenteric
artery

ileocolic artery

abdominal aorta

6.3

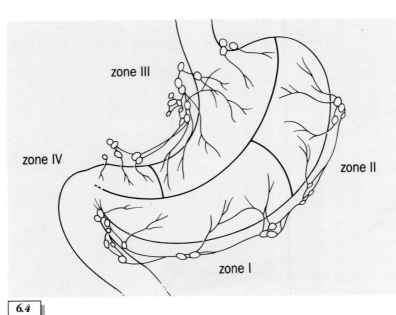

zone III

zone IV

zone II

zone I

6.4

6.4

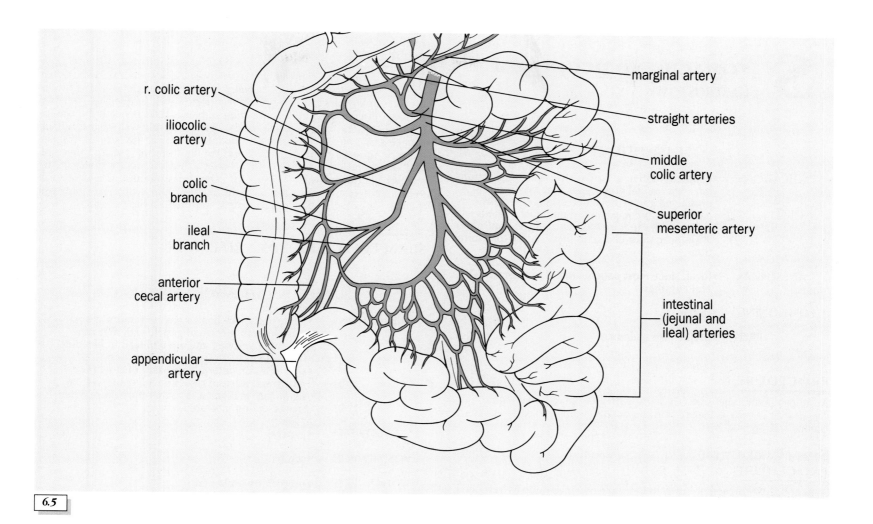

r. colic artery

iliocolic artery

colic branch

ileal branch

anterior cecal artery

appendicular artery

marginal artery

straight arteries

middle colic artery

superior mesenteric artery

intestinal (jejunal and ileal) arteries

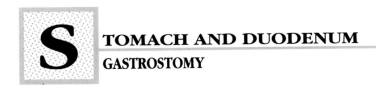

STOMACH AND DUODENUM

GASTROSTOMY

GASTROSTOMY

INDICATIONS	• good alternative to nasogastric tube after major intra-abdominal procedures that may require prolonged gastric decompression, especially for patients with compromised pulmonary status • patients who require long-term enteral nutritional support; poor choice in those at risk for aspiration
ANESTHESIA	• local, since most patients too ill to tolerate general anesthesia
POSITIONING	• supine
PREP	• prep entire abdomen

PROCEDURE

An upper midline incision (Fig. 6.6) is made from xyphoid to the umbilicus. The linea alba is incised and the peritoneum is grasped between two clamps and opened.

STAMM GASTROSTOMY
PROCEDURE

A temporary stoma that seals rather quickly once tube is removed, a Stamm gastrostomy requires placement of two concentric pursestring sutures of 2–0 silk or Vicryl (Fig. 6.7). A gastrotomy is then made using the cautery. A 24-French mushroom catheter is placed into the stomach and the pursestring sutures tied so that the gastric wall is inverted around the tube (Fig. 6.8). The tip of the mushroom catheter should be cut off to facilitate clearing blockages and changing the tube over a wire. Foley catheters should be avoided as gastrostomy tubes, since the inflated balloon tip may lodge in the pylorus creating a gastric outlet obstruction. The tube is then brought out through a stab wound in the anterior abdominal wall (Fig. 6.9). The gastric wall is then secured to the abdominal wall around the exit site with several sutures of 2–0 silk (Figs. 6.10, 6.11).

JANEWAY GASTROSTOMY
PROCEDURE

A more permanent form of gastrostomy since a mucosa-lined tract is formed from stomach to skin, a Janeway gastrostomy is facilitated by the use of stapling devices. The anterior stomach wall is grasped with two Babcock forceps and the linear cutting stapler is fired beneath the clamps (Fig. 6.12A). This creates a tube of the anterior gastric wall (Fig. 6.12B). It is necessary to leave an adequate amount of tissue at the base of this gastric tube to ensure an adequate blood supply from the greater curvature. The distal end of the tube is then brought out through a stoma in the anterior abdominal wall (Fig. 6.12C). The tip is amputated and the full thickness of gastric wall is sewn to the dermis of the skin. The stoma can then be intubated with an appropriately sized red rubber catheter.

SUBMUCOSAL LEIOMYOMA RESECTION

SUBMUCOSAL LEIOMYOMA RESECTION

INDICATIONS	• leiomyomas are benign gastric tumors arising from smooth muscle of gastric wall that can ulcerate overlying mucosa and lead to bleeding (Fig. 6.13) • size of lesion determines extent of resection: <4 cm submucosal resection adequate; >4 cm, significant malignant risk, therefore more extensive resection indicated
ANESTHESIA	• general
POSITIONING	• supine
PREP	• prep entire abdomen
INCISION	• upper midline incision

PROCEDURE

The stomach is palpated and the tumor located. The overlying serosa is incised and the tumor "shelled out," leaving the mucosa intact (Fig. 6.14). The serosal incision is then closed with multiple interrupted seromuscular sutures of 3–0 silk. The mucosa is often ulcerated over a portion of this mucosa and the serosa can be stapled (Fig 6.15).

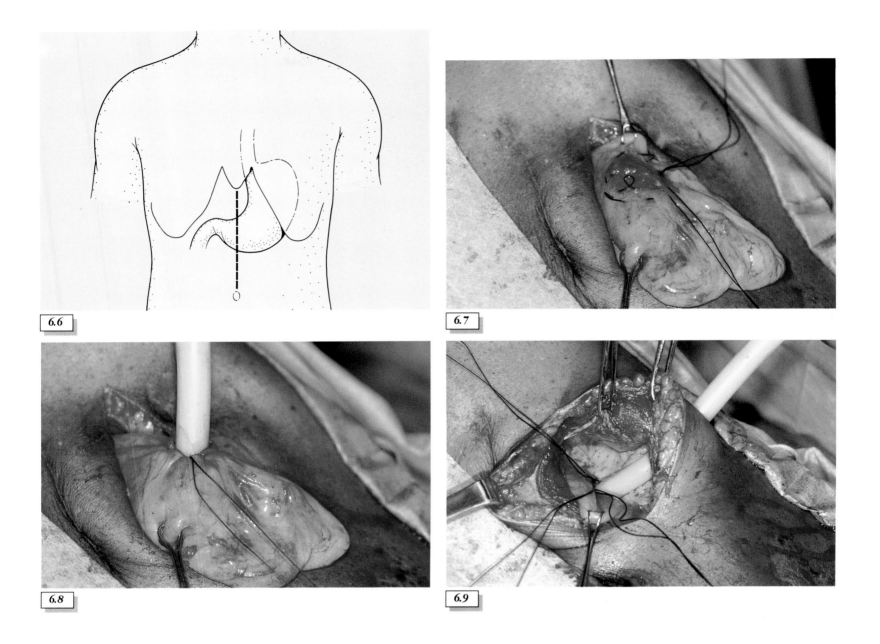

6.6

6.7

6.8

6.9

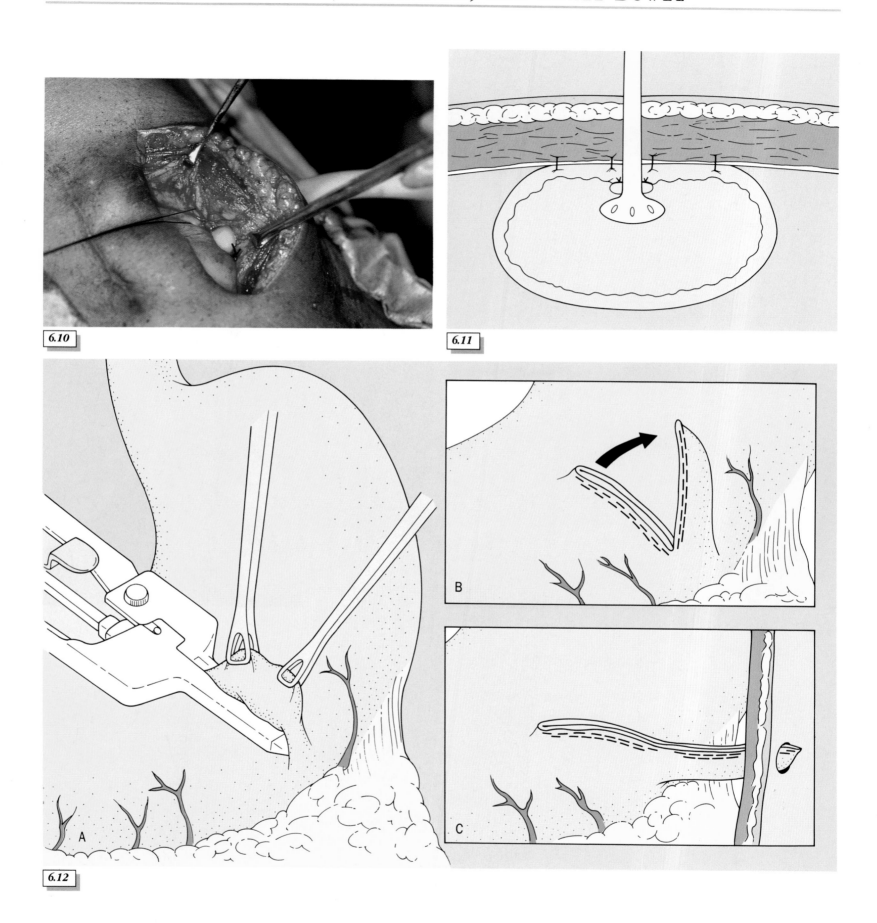

6.10

6.11

6.12

A

B

C

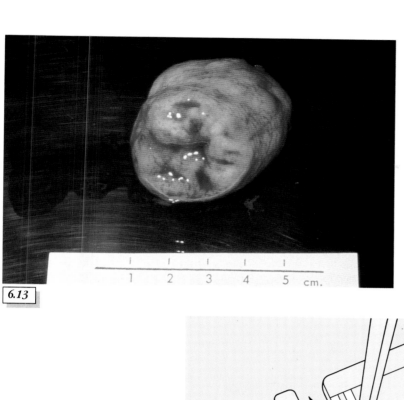

6.13

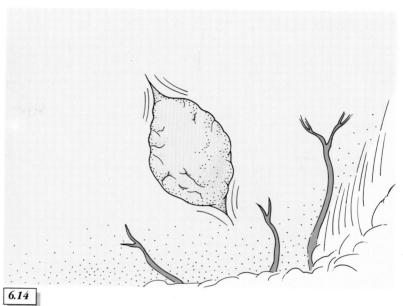

6.14

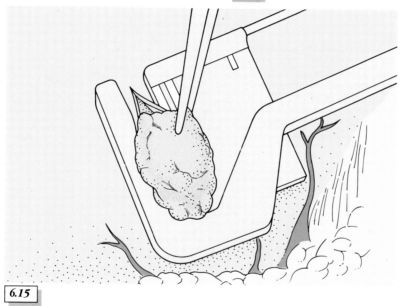

6.15

VAGOTOMY

Antrum of stomach secretes gastrin which stimulates HCl production from gastric fundus. Acetylcholine release from vagal stimulation causes gastrin secretion, depending on pH of antrum. Vagotomy interrupts this pathway of gastrin release. Extent of vagal denervation determines effectiveness and side effects.

VAGOTOMY

INDICATIONS	• treatment of peptic ulcer disease to lower acid output (Fig. 6.16)
	truncal vagotomy
	• lowest recurrence rates but also denervates entire abdominal viscera resulting gastric atony requires drainage procedure (pyloroplasty or gastro-jejunostomy)
	selective vagotomy
	• preserves celiac and hepatic branches of vagal trunks
	• entire stomach is denervated so gastric drainage procedure also required
	• not commonly used today because of more effective alternatives
	highly selective vagotomy
	• preserves vagal innervation to pylorus so gastric drainage procedure not necessary
	• higher ulcer recurrence rates (some estimate as high as 15%) but lowest morbidity and mortality may reduce acid output to degree where H2 blockers are effective, procedure of choice if intractable ulcer disease indication for surgery
ANESTHESIA	• general
POSITIONING	• supine
PREP	• prep entire abdomen
INCISION	• midline incision; use of self-retaining retraction may be helpful

TRUNCAL VAGOTOMY
PROCEDURE

The peritoneum overlying the esophagus is incised. With gentle traction on the esophagus to the patient's left, the posterior right trunk is identified. A segment of the nerve is excised after hemoclips are placed on the proximal and distal ends (Fig. 6.17). With gentle traction downward on the stomach, the anterior (left) trunk is tethered, which aids in identifying it. A segment of this trunk is then excised. Alternatively, the esophagus can be encircled with a Penrose drain. This is not as effective though, as pulling down on the stomach to put the right trunk on stretch and aid in identifying it.

HIGHLY SELECTIVE VAGOTOMY
PROCEDURE

For good results, attention to technical detail is mandatory. The "crow's foot" is identified and the dissection begun to the patient's left, approximately 6 cm from the pylorus (Fig. 6.18). The anterior leaf of the lesser omentum and the neurovascular bundles within it are carefully divided. This dissection is continued cephalad (Fig. 6.19). The posterior leaf of the gastrohepatic ligament is then similarly divided (Fig. 6.20). The esophagus must be denervated for approximately 6 cm, taking care not to divide the main trunks (Fig. 6.21). It may be helpful to isolate the main vagal trunks with tapes to aid in this dissection and avoid injury to them. It is also important to be sure to divide any transverse fibers from the posterior trunk (nerves of Grassi). The main nerves of Latarjet, the "crow's foot," and one or two additional terminal branches must be left intact with this procedure (Fig. 6.22).

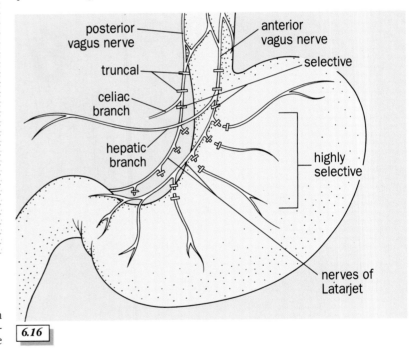

6.16

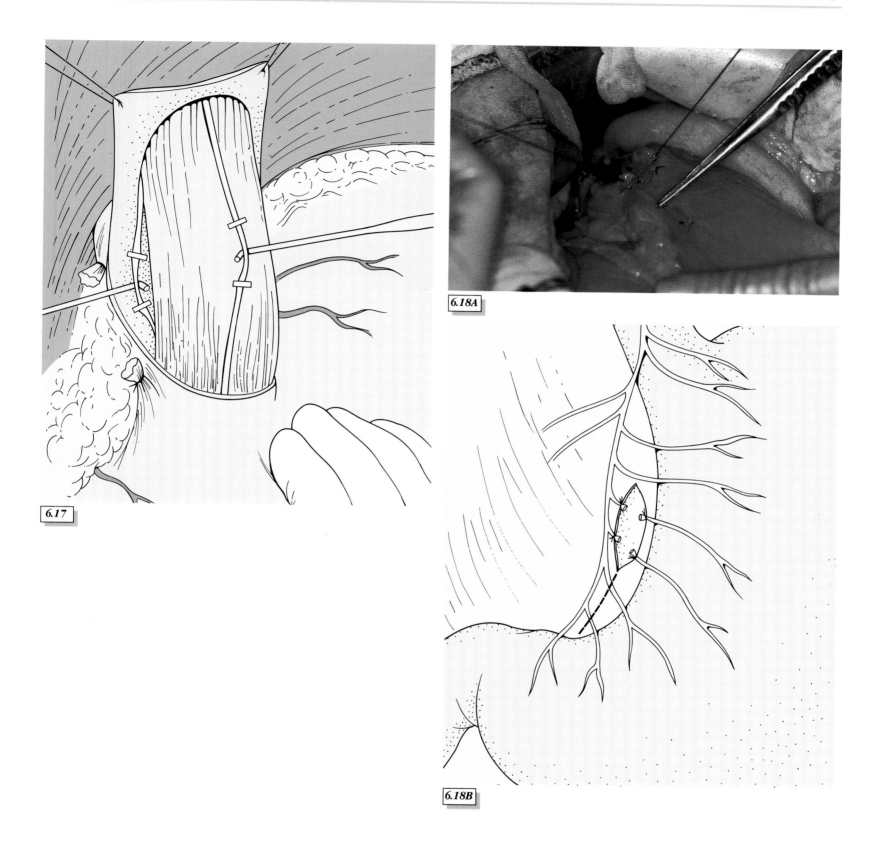

6.17

6.18A

6.18B

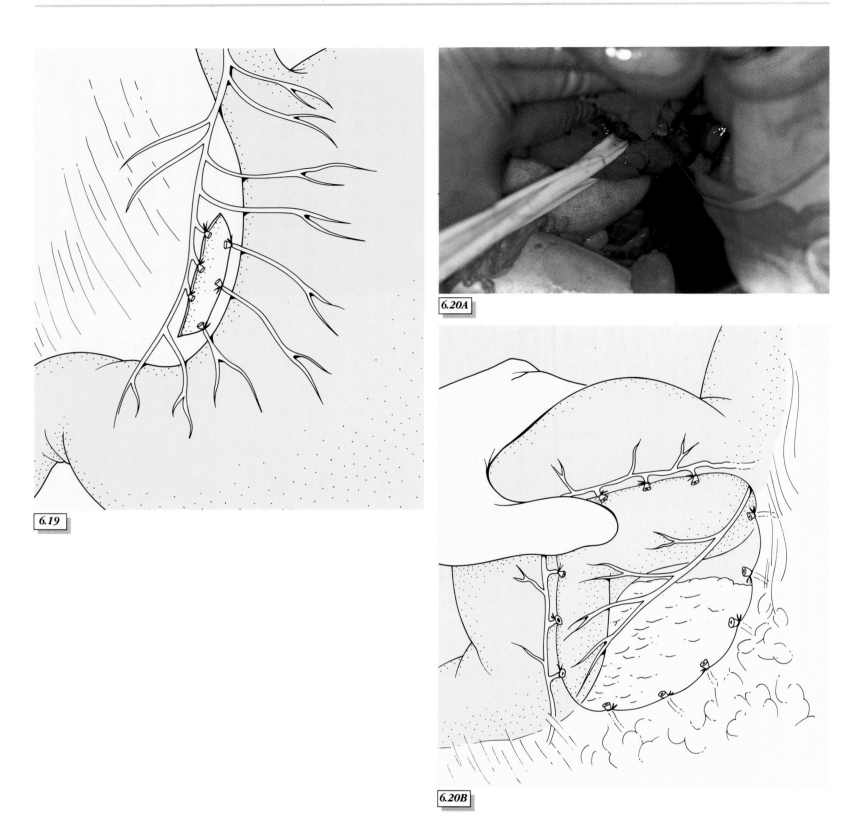

6.19

6.20A

6.20B

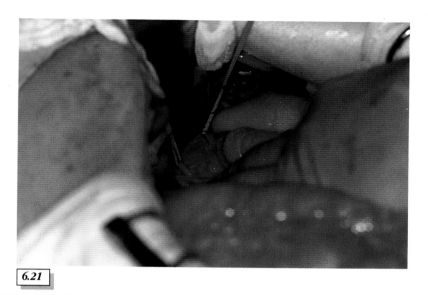

6.21

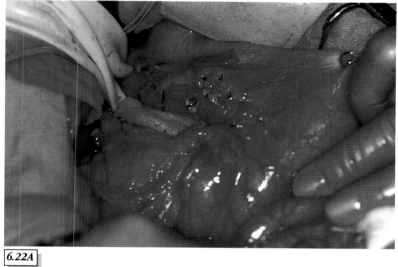

6.22A

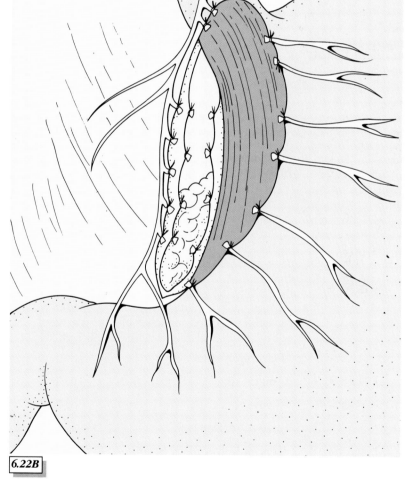

6.22B

PYLOROMYOTOMY

PYLOROMYOTOMY	
INDICATIONS	• infants with hypertrophic pyloric stenosis • ancillary procedure after esophagogastric mobilization and resection
ANESTHESIA	• general
POSITIONING	• supine
PREP	• prep entire abdomen
INCISION	• for infants, use a right upper quadrant transverse incision; the hypertrophied pyloric mass ("olive") is palpated through the abdominal wall in the infant and the incision is made overlying this • anterior rectus fascia is incised and the rectus muscle is divided using the cautery; posterior fascia and peritoneum are then opened (Fig. 6.23) • in adults, use a midline abdominal incision or other incision depending on the main procedure

PROCEDURE

In performing a pyloromyotomy, the pylorus is grasped between the thumb and index finger (Fig. 6.24). It is identified by the vein of Mayo crossing over it. A longitudinal incision approximately 2 cm long is then made over the hypertrophied pylorus (Fig. 6.24) through the serosa only. A curved hemostat is then used to spread the serosa and muscle apart, allowing the mucosa to bulge through (Fig. 6.25). Care must be taken at the duodenal end of the incision because it is easiest here to inadvertently enter the lumen. If this should happen, the safest reaction is to convert the pyloromyotomy into a pyloroplasty.

PYLOROPLASTY

PYLOROPLASTY	
INDICATIONS	• whenever normal mechanisms of gastric emptying are disturbed • usually related to vagotomy • extensive scarring and inflammation may preclude use of traditional Heineke-Mikulicz pyloroplasty, in which case a Jaboulay gastroduodenostomy is indicated
ANESTHESIA	• general
POSITIONING	• supine
PREP	• prep entire abdomen
INCISION	• same as for vagotomy (see page 6.15)

HEINEKE-MIKULICZ PROCEDURE

A Kocher maneuver is performed first by incising the peritoneum along the lateral aspect of the duodenum and then reflecting the duodenum medially (see Fig. 8.41). A 3-cm longitudinal incision is made through the anterior wall across the pylorus (Fig. 6.26). Stay sutures placed superiorly and inferiorly on the pylorus prior to making the incision facilitate closure. The incision is then closed in the opposite direction from which it was made (Fig. 6.27). Closure is in one layer using a modified Gambee stitch (Fig. 6.28).

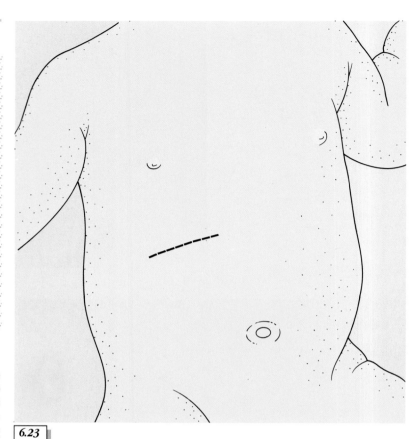

6.23

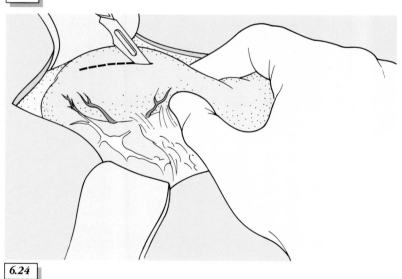

6.24

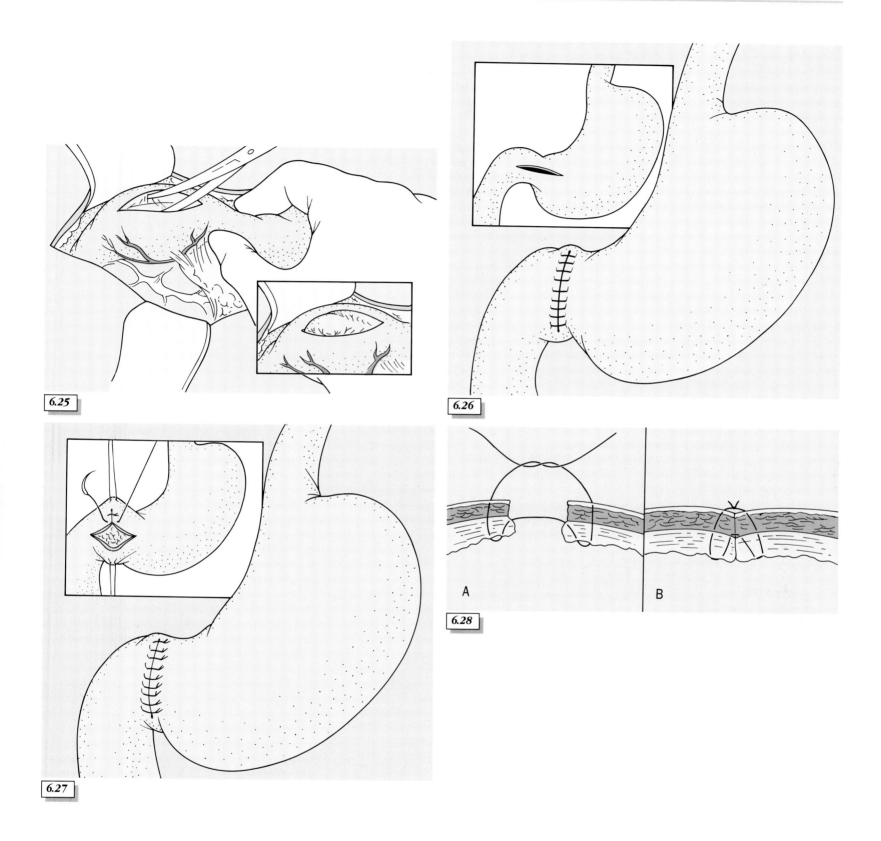

6.25

6.26

6.27

6.28

A   B

JABOULAY GASTRODUODENOSTOMY
PROCEDURE

The Jaboulay gastroduodenostomy (Fig. 6.29) is constructed by a two-layer anastomosis between the stomach and the second portion of the duodenum. The anastomosis, approximately 6 cm long, is made as close to the pylorus as possible. Incisions are then made in the stomach and duodenal wall. Posteriorly, the seromuscular layer is approximated with continuous suture of 3–0 silk (Fig. 6.30). The second layer posteriorly of full-thickness 3–0 Vicryl is then placed and continued on the anterior wall as a running Connell suture (Figs. 6.30, 6.31). The second layer anteriorly is completed with interrupted seromuscular Lembert sutures of 3–0 silk (Fig. 6.32). A closed suction drain may then be placed in the area of the pyloroplasty.

ANTRECTOMY

ANTRECTOMY	
INDICATIONS	• treatment of complicated peptic ulcer disease, particularly for bleeding secondary to duodenal ulcer or pyloric outlet obstruction from ulcer disease, combined with truncal vagotomy • lowest recurrence rates (approximately 1%) compared to vagotomy and pyloroplasty or highly selective vagotomy, but morbidity and mortality higher Reconstruction: Bilroth I (gastroduodenostomy) • preferable when technically possible (when duodenum can be mobilized enough to create a tension-free anastomosis) Bilroth II (gastrojejunostomy) • disadvantages include marginal ulceration, afferent loop syndromes, but usually technically easier to create anastomosis without tension antecolic • jejunal loop is anterior to transverse colon; preferably used in resections for carcinoma since recurrences at base of transverse mesocolon can lead to obstruction with retrocolic gastrojejunostomy retrocolic • jejunal loop through an avascular area in transverse mesocolon
ANESTHESIA	• general
POSITIONING	• supine
PREP	• prep entire abdomen
INCISION	• upper midline abdominal incision

PROCEDURE

The gastrocolic omentum is opened to enter the lesser sac (Fig. 6.33). Care is taken to identify and avoid injury to the middle colic artery (Fig. 6.33). Branches of the right gastroepiploic artery are divided and the dissection is carried cephalad along the greater curve. For an antrectomy, the greater curvature is divided at the point where the left and right gastroepiploic vessels meet. The dissection along the greater curve is then carried

distally toward the pylorus to 2 cm beyond it. Small branches from the gastroduodenal artery can be encountered in this area (Fig. 6.33). The posterior gastric wall is then freed in the avascular plane between it and the transverse mesocolon. Next the gastrohepatic omentum is opened to free the lesser curve. The right gastric vessels are dissected free and ligated (Fig. 6.34). The point of division of the lesser curve is at an avascular

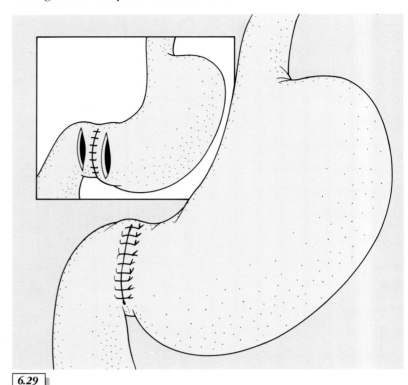

6.29

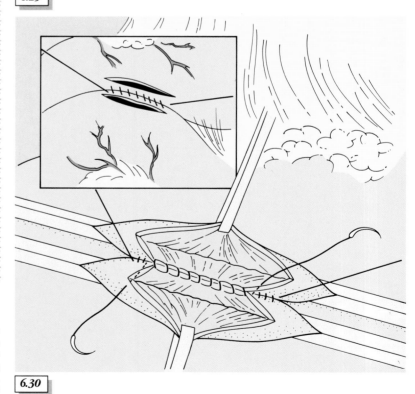

6.30

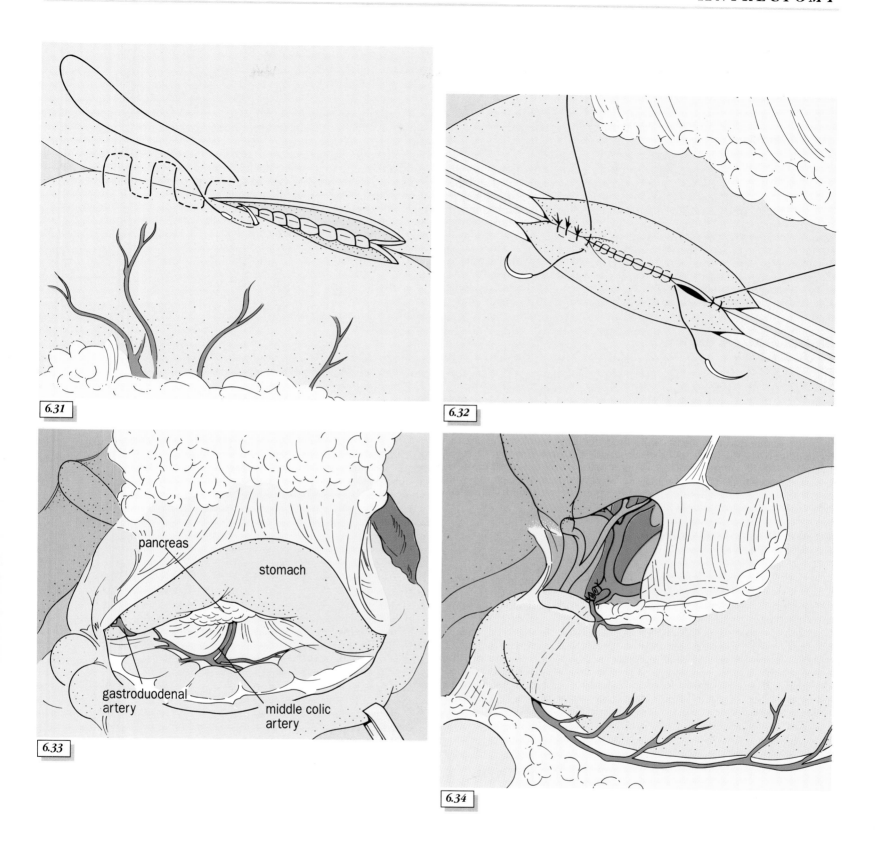

6.31

6.32

pancreas

stomach

gastroduodenal
artery

middle colic
artery

6.33

6.34

point approximately 2 cm from the gastroesophageal junction. The stomach is then transected using the linear gastric stapler with a Kocher clamp across the distal stomach (Fig. 6.35). Antrectomy removes approximately one-third or more of distal stomach and all gastrin-producing cells.

DUODENAL CLOSURE (BILROTH II RESECTION)
PROCEDURE

The duodenum must be dissected free 2 cm beyond the pylorus. The gastroduodenal artery is ligated and divided. Care must be taken around the duodenum to avoid injury to the structures of the portal triad and the pancreas (Fig. 6.36). Once the duodenum is sufficiently freed, closure is performed if a Bilroth I anastomosis is not planned. The duodenum is transected using a linear stapler (Fig. 6.37). This closure can also be accomplished with a two-layer suture technique (Fig. 6.38). Duodenal closure can be difficult if there is extensive scarring due to the ulcer. In these cases it may be necessary to suture the anterior duodenal wall to the ulcer bed, followed by another layer that sutures the duodenal wall to the pancreatic capsule, inverting the first suture line (Fig. 6.39). With any closure, the duodenal stump should be drained with a closed suction drain.

BILROTH I RECONSTRUCTION
PROCEDURE

The gastroduodenostomy can be performed using staplers or a hand-sewn technique. If the stapler is used, a triangulation technique is employed. On the greater curvature side, a portion of the staple line is excised. With the help of stay sutures the linear stapler is fired along the posterior row (Fig. 6.40). The anterior edge of the stomach and duodenum are bisected by a stay suture and the linear stapler fired twice to complete the anastomosis (Fig. 6.41). To hand sew the anastomosis, a posterior row of seromuscular 3–0 silk sutures is placed. This is followed by full-thickness continuous sutures of 3–0 Vicryl, which are continued onto the anterior wall as an inverting Connell suture. The anastomosis is completed with interrupted Lembert sutures of 3–0 silk.

BILROTH II RECONSTRUCTION
PROCEDURE

POLYA. Entire cut margin of stomach is anastomosed to jejunum.

HOFMEISTER. More commonly used; lesser curve side of gastric resection closed and anastomosis made along greater curve.

The gastrojejunostomy should be performed on the most dependent portion of the greater curve as possible. There is no proven advantage of a retrocolic versus an antecolic anastomosis, although for resections for carcinoma, an anterior anastomosis is preferred for the reasons mentioned previously. If a retrocolic configuration is chosen, care must be taken to suture the edges of the transverse mesocolon to the posterior wall of the stomach after the anastomosis is complete. This prevents the jejunal limb from obstructing by herniation through the defect in the mesocolon. The

limb between the duodenum and the gastrojejunostomy should be kept as short as possible while still allowing a tension-free anastomosis.

The gastrojejunostomy can also be performed using staplers or a hand-sewn technique. To staple the anastomosis, a corner of the gastric staple line on the greater curve is excised. The antemesenteric side of the jejunal limb is held in place with stay sutures and an enterostomy is made with the cautery. The linear cutting stapler is inserted and fired (Fig. 6.42). Care must be taken to visualize the entire staple line and ensure hemostasis. The remaining opening is closed with the linear stapler (Fig. 6.43). A 3–0 silk suture is used to reinforce the apex of the anastomosis. Using a similar technique, the anastomosis can be performed on the anterior or posterior gastric wall as long as the anastomosis is at least 2.5 cm from the gastric staple line. This prevents ischemia of the intervening gastric wall, which can occur if the staple lines are placed any closer together (Fig. 6.44). To hand sew the gastrojejunostomy, a similar two-layer technique is used, as previously described. The stoma should be at least 5 cm long. Seromuscular Lembert sutures of 3–0 silk are placed on the posterior wall first, approximating the gastric and jejunal walls. An incision is then made in the stomach and jejunum and a second layer posteriorly of full-thickness 3–0 Vicryl is placed. This is continued along the anterior wall as an inverting Connell suture. The anastomosis is completed with Lembert sutures on the anterior wall (Fig. 6.45).

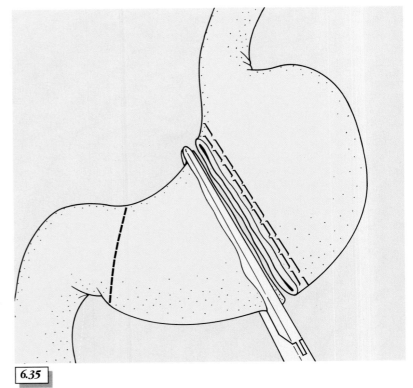

6.35

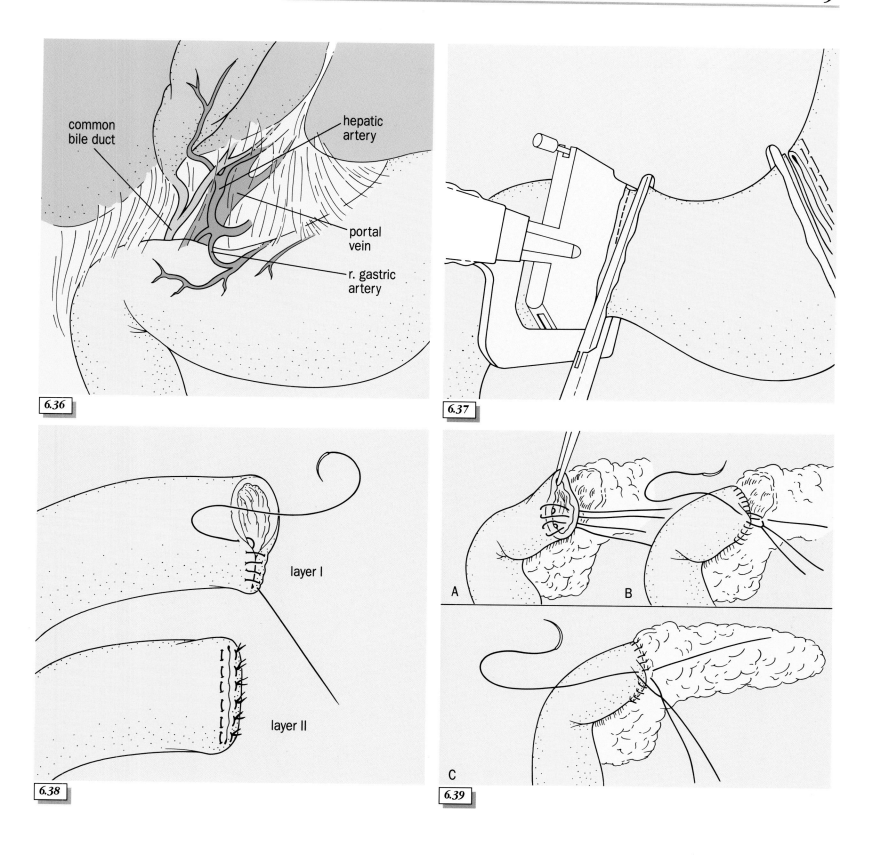

common bile duct

hepatic artery

portal vein

r. gastric artery

6.36

6.37

layer I

layer II

6.38

A

B

C

6.39

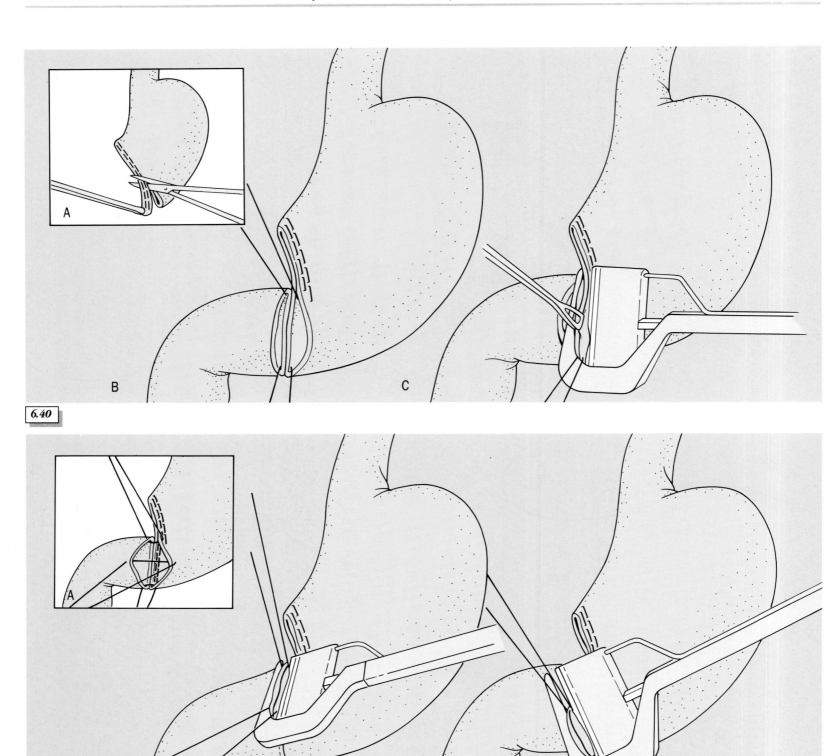

6.40

6.41

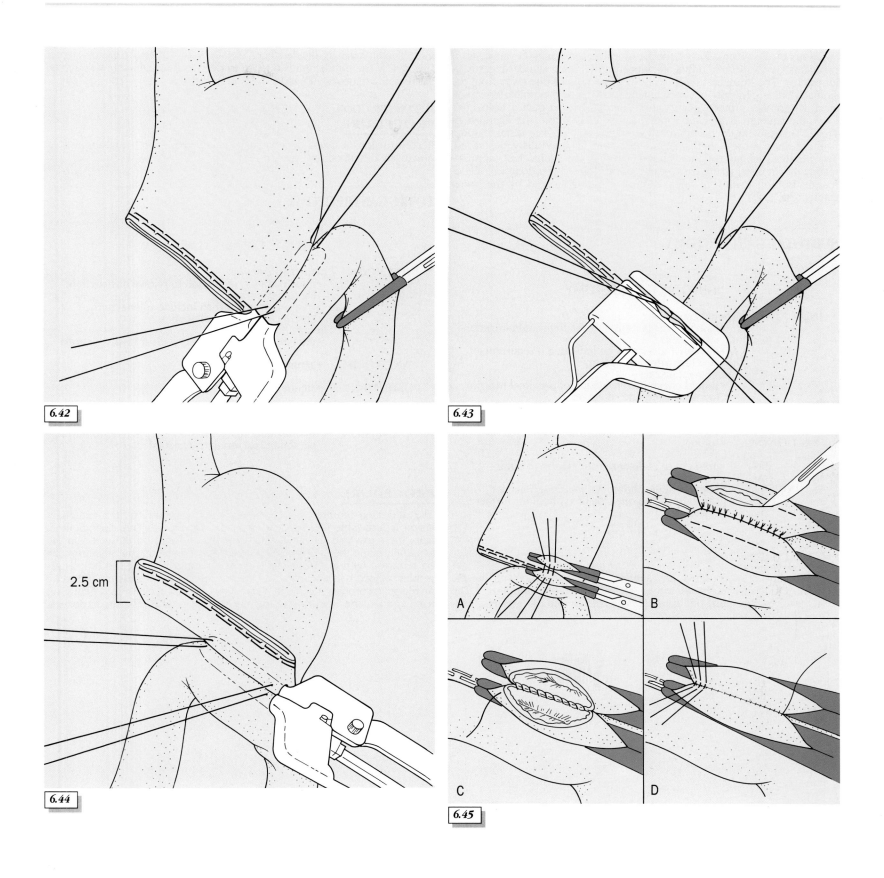

6.42

6.43

2.5 cm

6.44

A   B   C   D

6.45

A Roux-en-Y construction of the gastrojejunostomy may be indicated if problems develop with reflux alkaline gastritis after standard gastrojejunostomy. The Roux-en-Y loop will divert the flow of bile away from the stomach but is generally not recommended at the time of initial operation since it can also promote marginal ulceration. To construct a Roux-en-Y loop, the jejunum is divided approximately 10 cm from the ligament of Treitz. This can be done with a linear cutting stapler. The distal jejunum is then anastomosed to the gastric remnant as previously described. The proximal jejunum is then anastomosed to the jejunal limb approximately 40 cm distal to the gastrojejunostomy. This can be done in an end-to-side fashion using the linear cutting stapler followed by the linear stapler (Fig. 6.46).

ture. The stomach is divided here usually with the linear gastric stapler (Fig. 6.47). The duodenum is divided as described for antrectomy. Subtotal gastrectomy removes 70% to 80% of distal stomach.

RECONSTRUCTION
PROCEDURE

Reconstruction is usually accomplished with a Bilroth II anastomosis as previously described (see page 6.18).

TOTAL GASTRECTOMY

SUBTOTAL GASTRECTOMY

SUBTOTAL GASTRECTOMY

INDICATIONS	benign disease • gastric ulcer (extent of resection should include ulcer itself) • duodenal ulcer may be indicated if recurrence develops after antrectomy malignant disease • should check frozen section of proximal margin to insure adequate resection
ANESTHESIA	• general
POSITIONING	• supine
PREP	• prep entire abdomen from nipples to pubis
INCISION	• upper midline abdominal incision; if needed, can extend it to one side of xyphoid for further exposure

PROCEDURE

The technique of resection is very similar to antrectomy, except that the stomach, especially the greater curvature, must be further mobilized. The short gastric vessels must be ligated and divided to free the greater curva-

TOTAL GASTRECTOMY

INDICATIONS	malignant disease • most common indication to relieve obstruction, bleeding source • treatment should then include splenectomy, omenectomy, nodal dissection benign disease • uncommon indication; eg, if ulcer involves cardia
ANESTHESIA	• general
POSITIONING	• supine
PREP	• prep nipples to pubis and chest
INCISION	• midline abdominal incision; may extend to thoraco-abdominal incision if needed

PROCEDURE

The abdomen is entered and explored for resectability. If a malignant lesion is resectable for cure, the first step is to free the greater omentum from the transverse colon. This is done sharply right on the colon in the avascular plane there (Fig. 6.48). Once this is complete, the omentum can be removed with the stomach. The peritoneum overlying the esophagus is then opened using scissors and the left lobe of the liver is mobilized by dividing its coronary ligament. This allows the left lobe to fold gently on itself, and using a self-retaining retractor allows for better exposure.

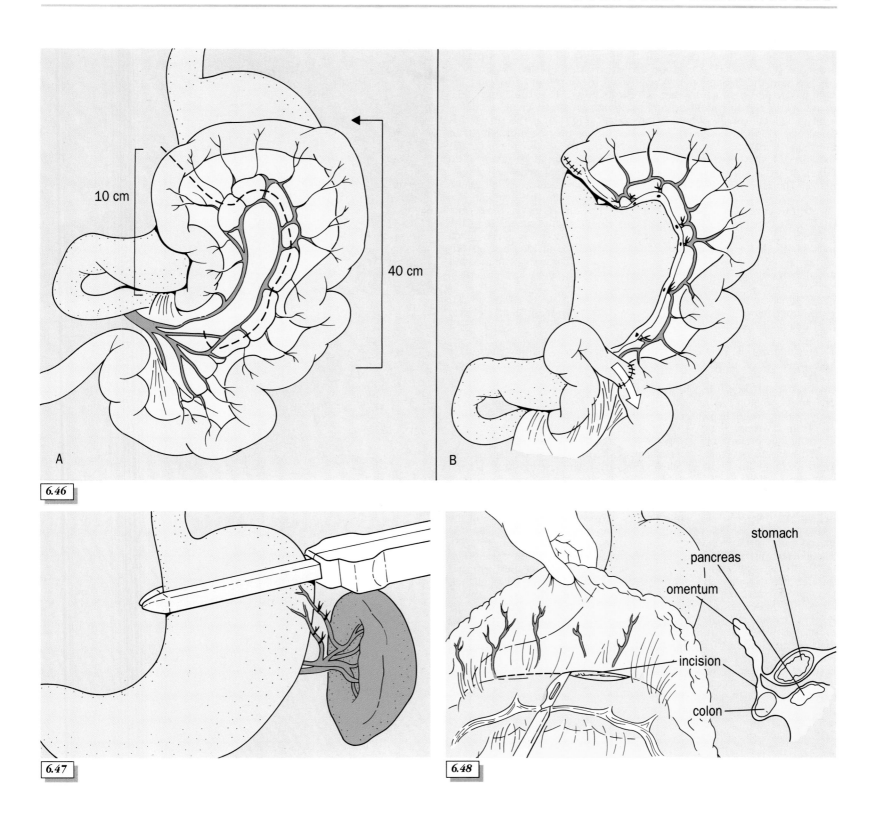

10 cm

40 cm

A

6.46

B

6.47

pancreas

stomach

omentum

incision

colon

6.48

The esophagus is freed circumferentially and a Penrose drain placed around it (Fig. 6.49). The vagi are divided. Next, the lesser omentum is opened and the dissection proceeds toward the pylorus, dividing the right gastric and right gastroepiploic near its origin (Fig. 6.50). Any nodal tissue in this region should be removed with the specimen. The duodenum is divided, usually with a linear stapler (Fig. 6.51). The stomach is freed posteriorly in the lesser sac, where tumor may be adherent to or invading the pancreas or transverse mesocolon. The greater curve is then mobilized. If the resection is for cure, the spleen should be removed en bloc (Fig. 6.52A). It is mobilized by dividing the lateral peritoneal attachments. The splenic artery and vein are then ligated and divided at the hilus just beyond the tail of the pancreas. If the spleen is left behind, the short gastric vessels must be divided to free the greater curve (Fig. 6.52B). At this point, the stomach can be lifted and retracted to the patient's left, exposing the left gastric artery and vein (Fig. 6.53). Each must be divided and the left gastric artery should be divided near its origin at the celiac axis. This leaves only the esophagus to be transected and the entire specimen removed (Fig. 6.54).

RESECTIONS

ESOPHAGODUODENOSTOMY. It is usually not technically feasible to mobilize duodenum adequately.

ESOPHAGOCOLOSTOMY. This is an extensive procedure with multiple suture lines, and is rarely used.

ESOPHAGOJEJUNOSTOMY

The most common reconstructions used are end-to-side esophagojejunostomy with or without jejunojejunostomy, Roux-en-Y esophagojejunostomy, Hunt-Lawrence pouch—which actually creates a gastric reservoir—is the technique preferred by these authors.

The jejunum is divided approximately 20 cm distal to the ligament of Treitz using the linear cutting stapler (Fig. 6.55). The distal jejunum is used to create a reservoir. Care must be taken to preserve the vascular arcade supplying blood to it. A 10-cm limb of the distal jejunum is folded onto itself and the walls between the two loops obliterated by firing linear cutting stapler (Fig. 6.56). The anastomosis between the esophagus and the jejunal reservoir is then performed. A "whip-stitch" pursestring suture is placed in the distal esophagus using an 0-Prolene suture (Figs. 6.56, 6.57). The pursestring device can make placement of this suture easier (Fig. 6.58). The end of an end-to-end anastomosis stapler is then inserted through the remaining opening in the jejunal reservoir and brought out through an enterostomy in the apex of the reservoir. This can be facilitated by first passing a red rubber catheter through the pouch to guide the stapler through (Figs. 6.59, 6.60). The anvil is opened and the distal esophagus is tied down over the center rod (see Fig. 6.59). The stapler is then closed and fired. The stapling device is removed and the remaining enterostomy closed with a linear stapler (Figs. 6.61, 6.62). The procedure is completed by anastomosing the proximal jejunum to the side of the distal jejunum well below the jejunal pouch. This can be done using the linear cutting stapler followed by the linear stapler as described elsewhere (Fig. 6.63). The completed procedure is seen in Fig. 6.64.

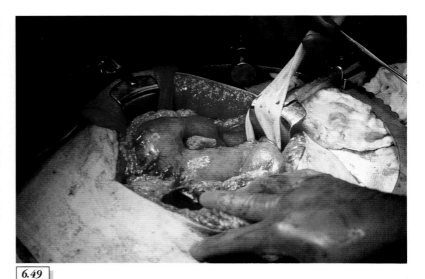

6.49

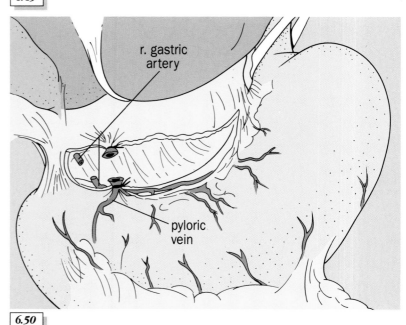

r. gastric artery

pyloric vein

6.50

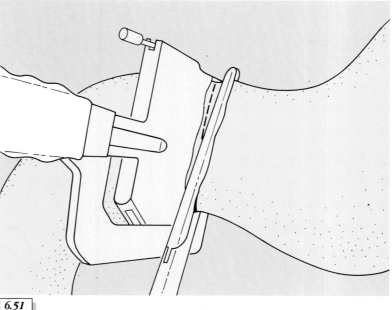

6.51

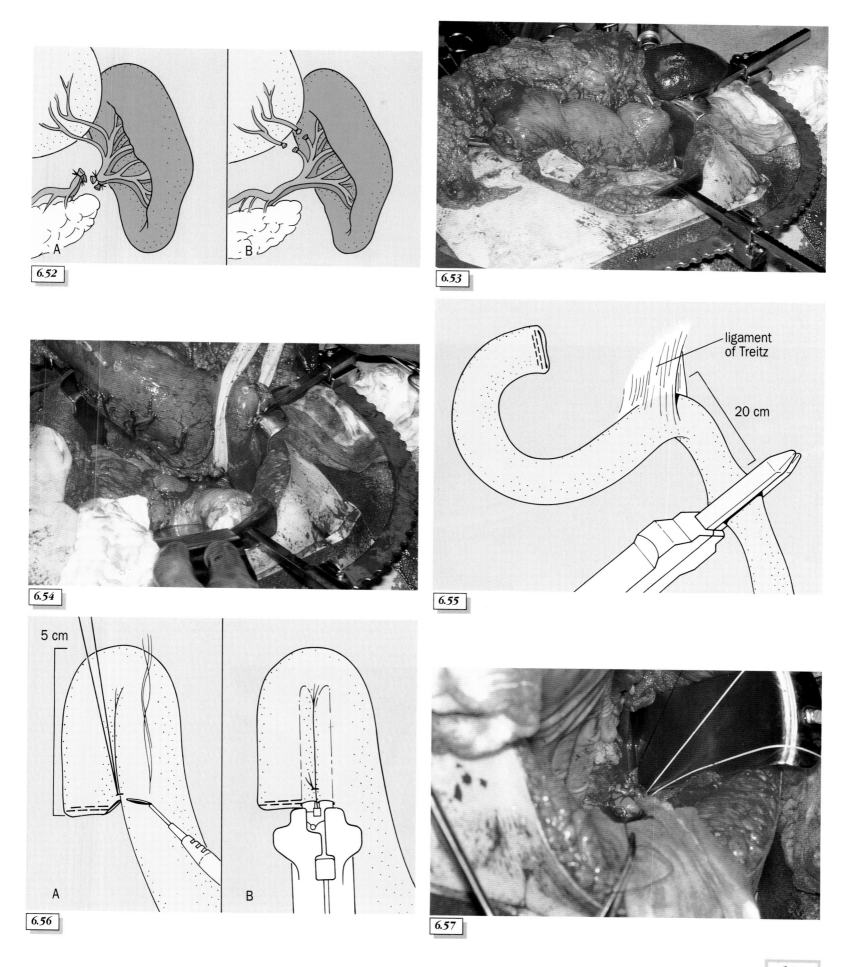

6.52

6.53

6.54

6.55

ligament of Treitz

20 cm

5 cm

A

B

6.56

6.57

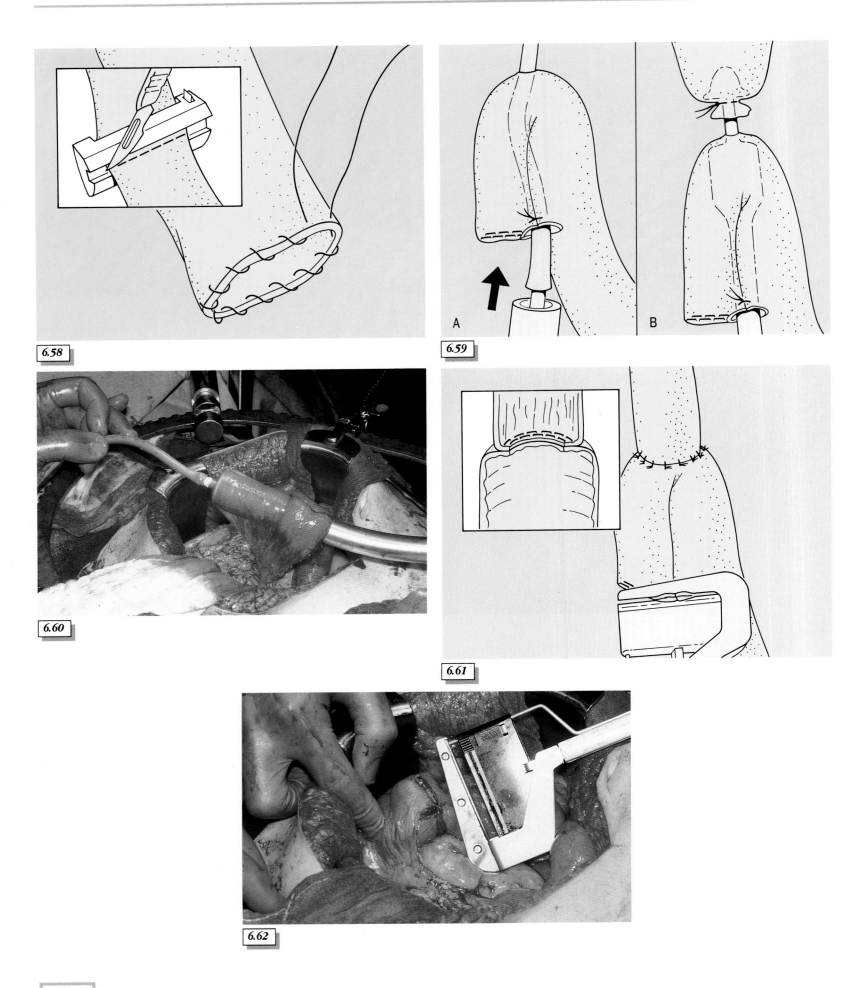

6.58

6.59

6.60

6.61

6.62

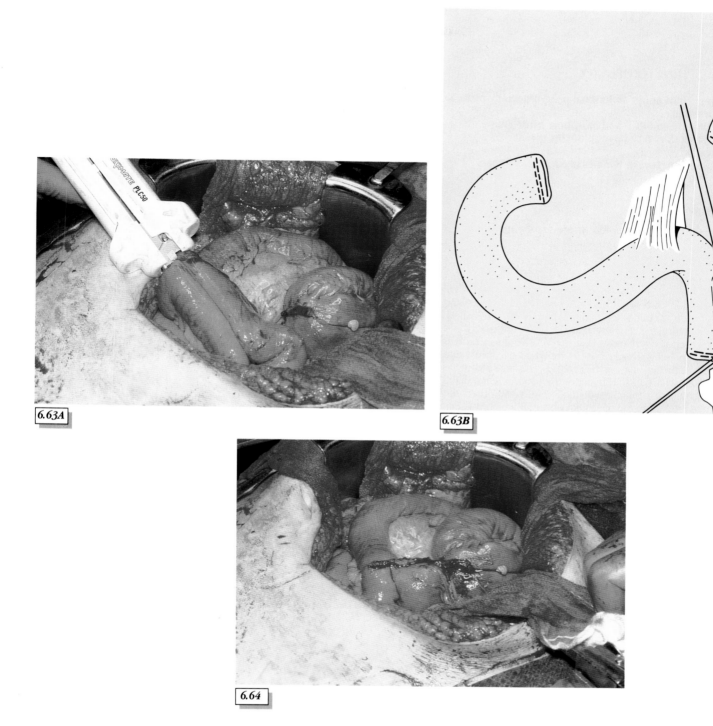

6.63A

6.63B

6.64

SPHINCTEROPLASTY

SPHINCTEROPLASTY	
INDICATIONS	•recurrent upper abdominal pain, especially post-prandial •patients on ERCP and morphine-prostigmine testing shown to have sphincter spasm (odditis) •usually occurs in females aged 20 to 50 years
ANESTHESIA	•general
POSITIONING	•supine
PREP	•right subcostal incision (if previously operated upon, old incision reopened)

PROCEDURE

Right upper quadrant adhesions are lysed and the common bile duct and duodenum are dissected free. A full Kocher maneuver is accomplished. Common duct exploration is done. A Fogarty balloon probe is passed into the duodenum through the choledochotomy (Fig. 6.65). The duodenum is opened over the papilla (Fig. 6.66). The Fogarty is modified as shown and used to elevate the papilla into the incision (Fig. 6.67). The papillotomy is performed over the catheter (Fig. 6.67). The pancreatic duct is cannulated (Fig. 6.68). The pancreaticobiliary septum is divided (Fig. 6.69). Then the ductal and duodenal mucosa are approximated with absorbable sutures (Fig. 6.70). The duodenum is closed with a linear stapler (Fig. 6.71). The choledochotomy is closed over a T-tube with interrupted absorbable sutures. An operative cholangiogram is obtained, primarily to rule out retroduodenal leak. Patients must be carefully chosen to obtain satisfactory results.

NISSEN FUNDOPLICATION

NISSEN FUNDOPLICATION	
INDICATIONS	•only indicated when intensive medical therapy has failed to control symptomatic hiatal hernial disease; preoperative esophagogastroscopy should be done to confirm reflux esophagitis and its degree, rule out any other pathology •esophageal manometry with pH monitoring to establish degree of reflux •Nissen fundoplication advocated most often (360° wrap of gastric fundus around esophagus) •usually abdominal approach
ANESTHESIA	•general
POSITIONING	•supine
PREP	•prep entire abdomen
INCISION	•midline abdominal incision

PROCEDURE

The triangular ligament of the liver is divided so that the left lobe can be folded under and gently retracted to allow good exposure of the hiatus. The peritoneum overlying the esophagus is divided and using blunt dissection the esophagus is surrounded by a Penrose drain. Gentle traction on this reduces the stomach into the abdominal cavity. Next the fundus must be adequately mobilized to allow a tension-free wrap. Once mobilization is complete, the diaphragmatic hiatus is reapproximated with several simple sutures of 0–Prolene (Fig. 6.72). Mobilization of the fundus is accomplished by dividing the gastrohepatic ligament. Care must be taken not to divide the vagus nerves. The greater curvature is then freed by carefully dividing the short gastric vessels. A 40-French nasogastric tube or Maloney dilator is then placed through the mouth into the stomach. This prevents a gastric wrap which is too tight. The gastric fundus is then

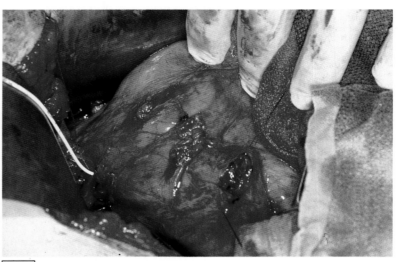

6.65

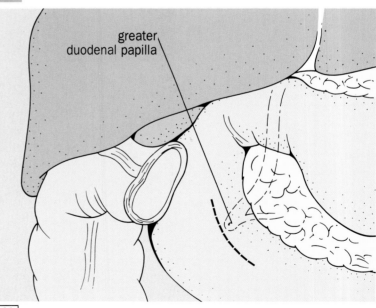

greater duodenal papilla

6.66

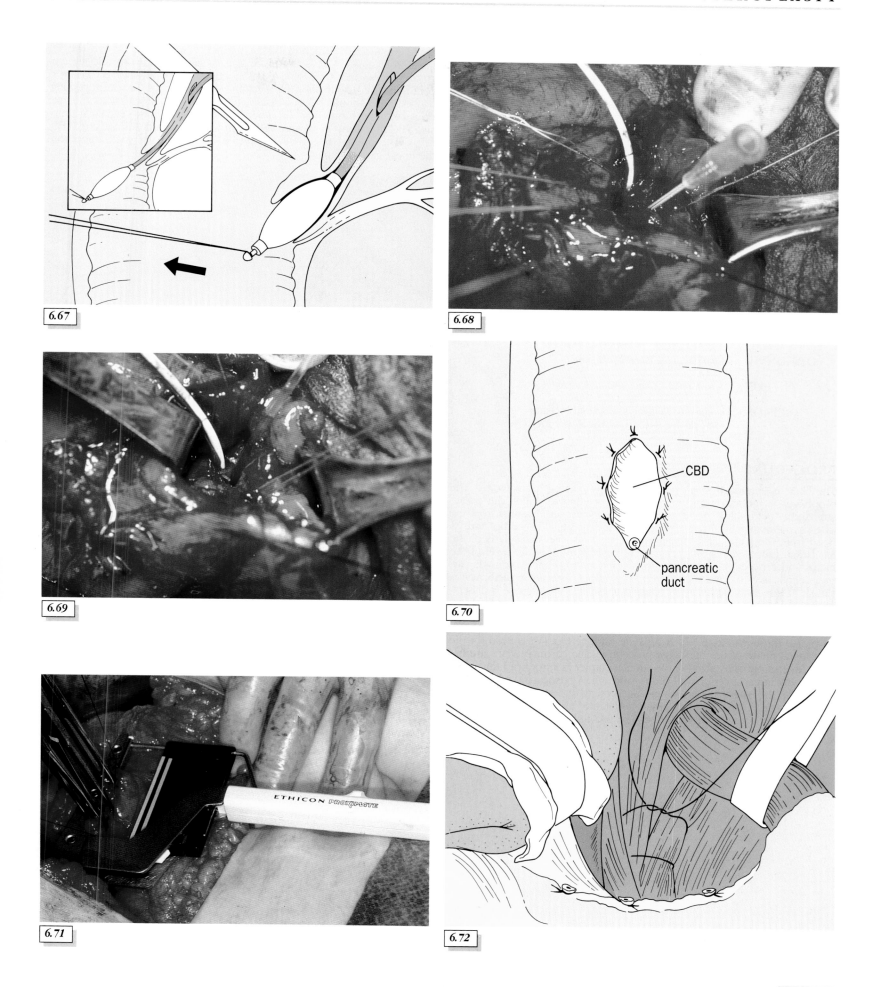

6.67

6.68

6.69

6.70

CBD

pancreatic
duct

6.71

ETHICON PROXIMATE

6.72

brought posteriorly around the distal esophagus using the right hand (Fig. 6.73). The gastric walls are then approximated anteriorly for 5–6 cm using multiple sutures of 2–0 silk. These sutures should also include a serosal bite of the esophagus so the wrap does not slip (Fig. 6.74). Additional assurance that the wrap will not slip can be obtained by securing the lower 2 or 3 sutures of the wrap to the median arcuate ligament.

ESOPHAGOGASTRIC DEVASCULARIZATION

ESOPHAGOGASTRIC DEVASCULARIZATION

INDICATIONS	• management of variceal bleeding (this procedure may be indicated over standard shunting procedures to avoid risks of encephalopathy) • may be indicated when shunting procedures (selective or nonselective) have failed
ANESTHESIA	• general
POSITIONING	• partial right lateral position
PREP	• prep entire chest and abdomen
INCISION	• separate midline abdominal incision • left posterolateral thoracotomy incision

PROCEDURE

The chest is entered through a standard posterolateral thoracotomy. The esophagus is mobilized and encircled with a Penrose drain. The paraesophageal "perforating" veins are divided between silk ligatures from the inferior pulmonary ligament to the esophageal hiatus. The esophagus is freed from the hiatus and brought into the chest. The muscularis of the left lateral esophagus is divided longitudinally starting at the level of the hiatus and proceeding cephalad 5–6 cm (Fig. 6.75). The myotomy is carried deeper until the mucosa is seen bulging out. The initial dissection is similar to that for a Heller esophagomyotomy. Next the mucosa is dissected free from the muscularis circumferentially for 2 cm using a right-angle clamp. Care is taken not to injure any of the submucosal varices. The right-angle clamp is then passed around the mucosa tube and a #1 silk tie pulled through (Fig. 6.76). A separate midline incision is used for the abdominal phase of the one-stage procedure. The coronary veins are ligated. An appropriately sized curve circular stapler is introduced through a gastrotomy in the anterior wall of the stomach. A nasogastric tube is then passed by the anesthesiologist and secured to the anvil of the stapler with a silk tie. This is used to guide the stapler as it is pulled cephalad into the newly created mucosal tube. The previously placed silk tie is fas-

tened around the armature of the opened stapler 2 cm above the EG junction (Fig. 6.77). It is fired, dividing esophageal mucosa and submucosal varices, and then removed. The completeness of the staple line is confirmed by examination of the transected tissue in the cartridge (Fig. 6.78). There should be one complete doughnut in contrast to the two rings of tissue formed by the device for the usual end-to-end anastomosis. The myotomy is closed with simple interrupted silk sutures (Fig. 6.79). The operation is then completed by closing the gastrotomy with the linear gastric stapler.

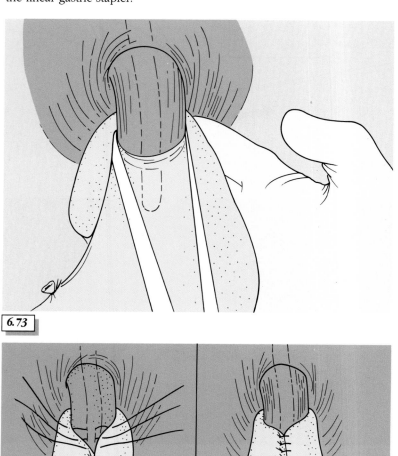

6.73

6.74

A   B

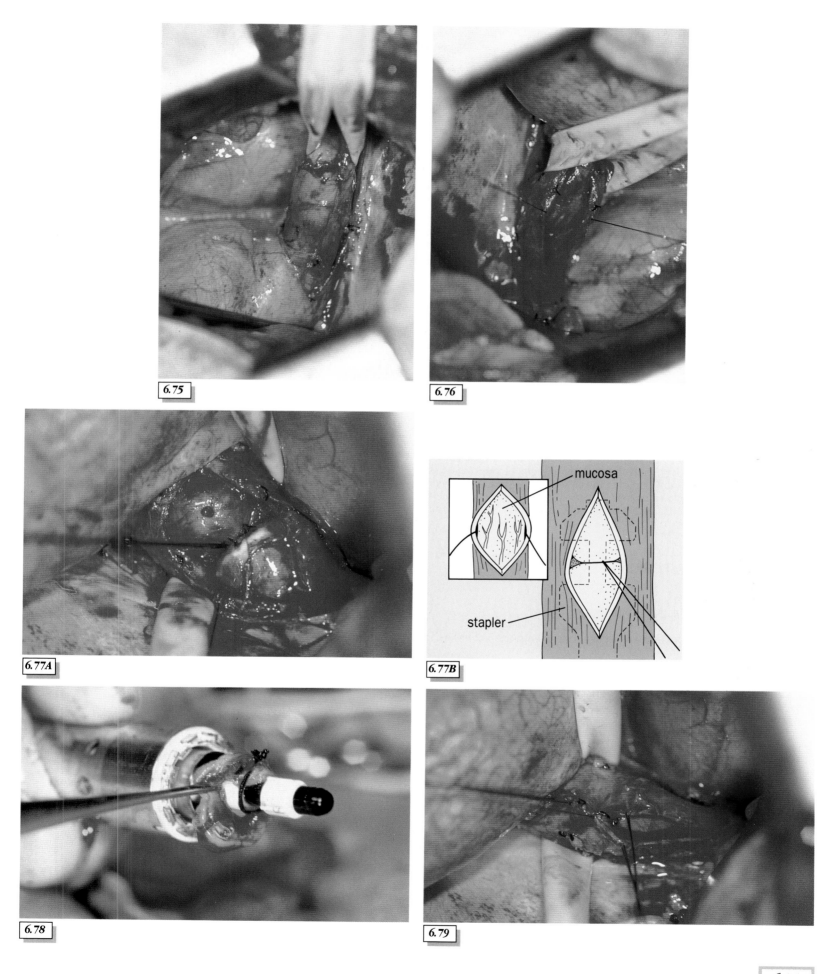

6.75

6.76

6.77A

mucosa

stapler

6.77B

6.78

6.79

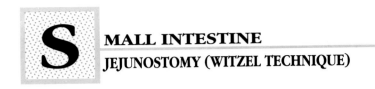

SMALL INTESTINE
JEJUNOSTOMY (WITZEL TECHNIQUE)

JEJUNOSTOMY (WITZEL TECHNIQUE)

INDICATIONS	• means to provide enteral nutritional support, usually on a long-term basis
	• preferable over gastrostomy only if history of aspiration and its complications precludes use of gastrostomy
ANESTHESIA	• local
POSITIONING	• supine
PREP	• prep entire abdomen
INCISION	• paramedian incision

PROCEDURE

The abdominal cavity is entered. A suitable loop of jejunum is identified to place the jejunostomy. A pursestring suture of 3–0 silk is placed on the antimesenteric side of the jejunum (Fig. 6.80). An enterotomy is made with the cautery. An 18-French red rubber catheter is inserted in the lumen and the pursestring suture tied. A "tunnel" for the tube is then formed with multiple seromuscular sutures of 3–0 silk for an approximately 6 cm distance (Fig. 6.81). The tube is then brought out through the anterior abdominal wall and secured to the inside of the abdominal wall at the exit site with multiple sutures of 3–0 silk (Fig. 6.82). The abdomen is then closed in standard fashion and the tube carefully secured to the skin with a suture.

SMALL INTESTINE RESECTION

SMALL INTESTINE RESECTION

INDICATIONS	• neoplasms and ischemic segments of small bowel
ANESTHESIA	• general
POSITIONING	• supine
PREP	• prep entire abdomen
INCISION	• midline abdominal incision

END-TO-END ANASTOMOSIS
ONE LAYER SUTURE TECHNIQUE
PROCEDURE

The bowel is transected proximally and distally. The ends of the resected bowel are approximated with two stay sutures superiorly and inferiorly. Simple sutures of 3–0 Vicryl are placed posteriorly through the entire thickness of the bowel wall, with larger bites through serosa and smaller bites through the mucosa. This helps to invert the suture line (Fig. 6.83). This same suture is used on the anterior layer with the assistant helping to invert the bowel wall (Fig. 6.84).

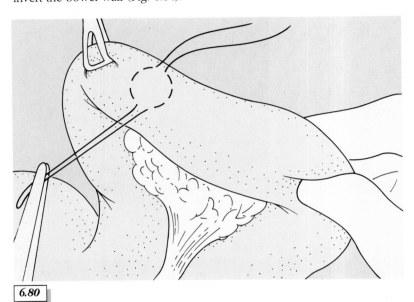

6.80

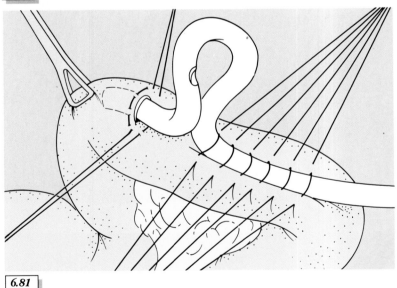

6.81

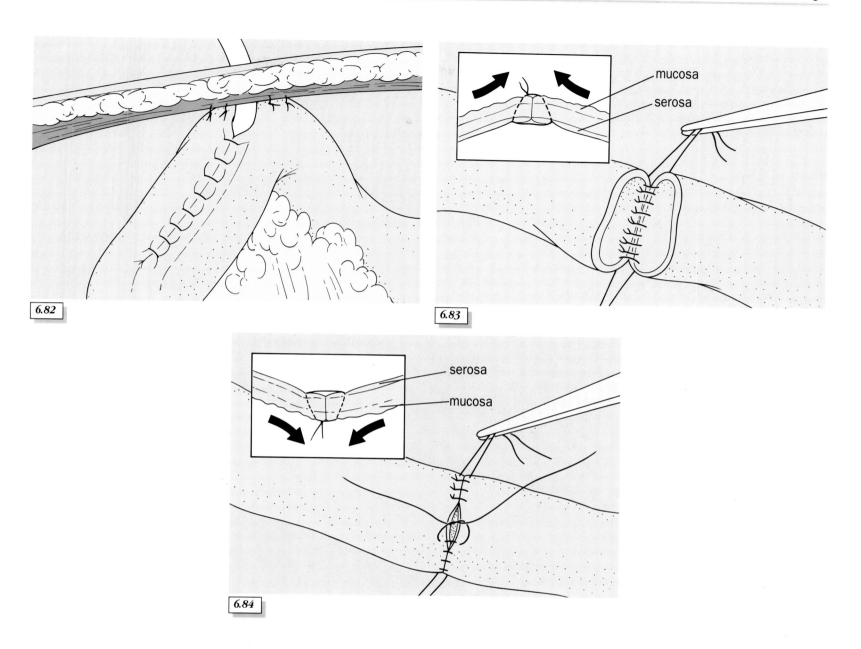

6.82

6.83

mucosa
serosa

serosa
mucosa

6.84

TWO LAYER. With the ends of the resected bowel approximated, the posterior row is completed with simple interrupted sutures of 3–0 silk on the seromuscular layer (Fig. 6.85). The second row posteriorly is then placed with 3–0 Vicryl and full-thickness bites through the bowel wall. This is then carried onto the anterior wall as a continuous inverting Connell suture (Fig. 6.86). The second row anteriorly is completed with seromuscular sutures of 3–0 silk (Fig. 6.87).

STAPLED TECHNIQUE (FUNCTIONAL END-TO-END)
PROCEDURE

The linear cutter stapler is used to transect the bowel proximally and distally (Fig. 6.88). This should be done at an oblique angle so the mesenteric side is longer than the antimesenteric side (Fig. 6.88). To create the anastomosis, the antimesenteric sides of the bowel are approximated and the linear cutting stapler fired (Fig. 6.89). The remaining opening in the bowel is closed with the linear staple (Fig. 6.89). The previous staple lines should be staggered when firing the linear stapler. A 3–0 silk Lembert suture should be placed to take tension off the "crotch" of the stapled anastomosis. Alternatively, without first dividing the bowel, the anastomosis can be done by approximating the antimesenteric borders of the two loops of small bowel to be resected (Fig. 6.90). Using the cautery, enterostomies are made on the antimesenteric side of each bowel segment and the linear cutting stapler is inserted and fired (Fig. 6.91). The common opening is then closed with the Linear cutter (Fig. 6.92). Again the "crotch" of the stapled anastomosis should be reinforced with a 3–0 silk suture. Regardless of the technique used to create the anastomosis, care must be taken to close the mesenteric defect created with the resection. This should be done with a 3–0 Vicryl suture. This prevents problems with internal herniation through the mesenteric defect.

SIDE-TO-SIDE ANASTOMOSIS
PROCEDURE

This creates an enterenterostomy without resecting any bowel. The two loops of bowel are approximated and enterotomies are made in each on the antimesenteric side using the cautery (Fig. 6.93). The linear cutting stapler is inserted and fired. The remaining opening is closed with the linear stapler (Fig. 6.94).

MECKEL'S DIVERTICULECTOMY

MECKEL'S DIVERTICULECTOMY	
INDICATIONS	•development of acute abdomen (perforation or obstruction) or bleeding •incidental finding at laparotomy
ANESTHESIA	•general
POSITIONING	•supine
PREP	•prep entire abdomen
INCISION	•usually midline abdominal incision

PROCEDURE

The most expeditious way to resect the diverticulum is with the use of the stapler. The diverticulum is grasped with Babcock forceps and amputated at the base after the linear stapler is fired (Fig. 6.95). Alternatively this can

be hand-sewn using a one- or two-layer closure technique as described elsewhere to close the defect in the intestinal wall. Occasionally resection of a small segment of ileum containing the diverticulum is more prudent and anastomosis then done as previously described.

ILEOSTOMY

ILEOSTOMY	
INDICATIONS	permanent •most often after total colectomy for ulcerative •colitis temporary •end-ileostomy—after resection for perforated cecum (unusual indication) •loop ileostomy—protect ileoanal anastomoses; provide viable stoma in obese patients
ANESTHESIA	•general
POSITIONING	•supine
PREP	•prep entire abdomen •preoperatively, the site for stoma in right lower quadrant should be marked by stomal therapist
INCISION	•midline abdominal incision

PERMANENT STOMA
PROCEDURE

A circular incision is made in the skin at the site of the stoma in the right lower quadrant (Fig. 6.96). The fascia over the rectus is divided, the muscle is split and the peritoneum entered. The stoma should admit two fingers easily to be of adequate size. The ileum should be well mobilized enough to allow 5–6 cm of ileum above the skin level. The ileum is brought through the stoma and nipple created. This is done by folding the ileum back on itself. Multiple sutures of absorbable suture are used to create the nipple by taking a bite through full thickness of cut edge of ileum wall, then a sero-muscular bite of ileum and then through skin dermis (Fig. 6.97). The mesentery of the ileum should then be tacked to the lateral peritoneal gutter to prevent internal herniation. A proper appliance is then fitted over the stoma.

LOOP ILEOSTOMY
PROCEDURE

A suitable loop of distal ileum for the stoma is identified. This loop needs to reach the skin without tension. An incision is made in the right lower quadrant for the stoma as just described. The loop of ileum is brought through the stoma and a straight connector brought through the mesentery under the loop (Fig. 6.98). A large Prolene suture is brought through the connector and tied to keep the connector in place (Fig. 6.99). An incision on the efferent side of the loop in the ileum is made (Fig. 6.99). This keeps the effluent draining inferiorly. Absorbable sutures are used to secure the full thickness of ileum wall to the dermis of the skin. Around the bar it may be necessary to take full-thickness bites of the skin (Fig. 6.100). An appropriate appliance is then applied. The bar can be removed approximately one week postoperatively.

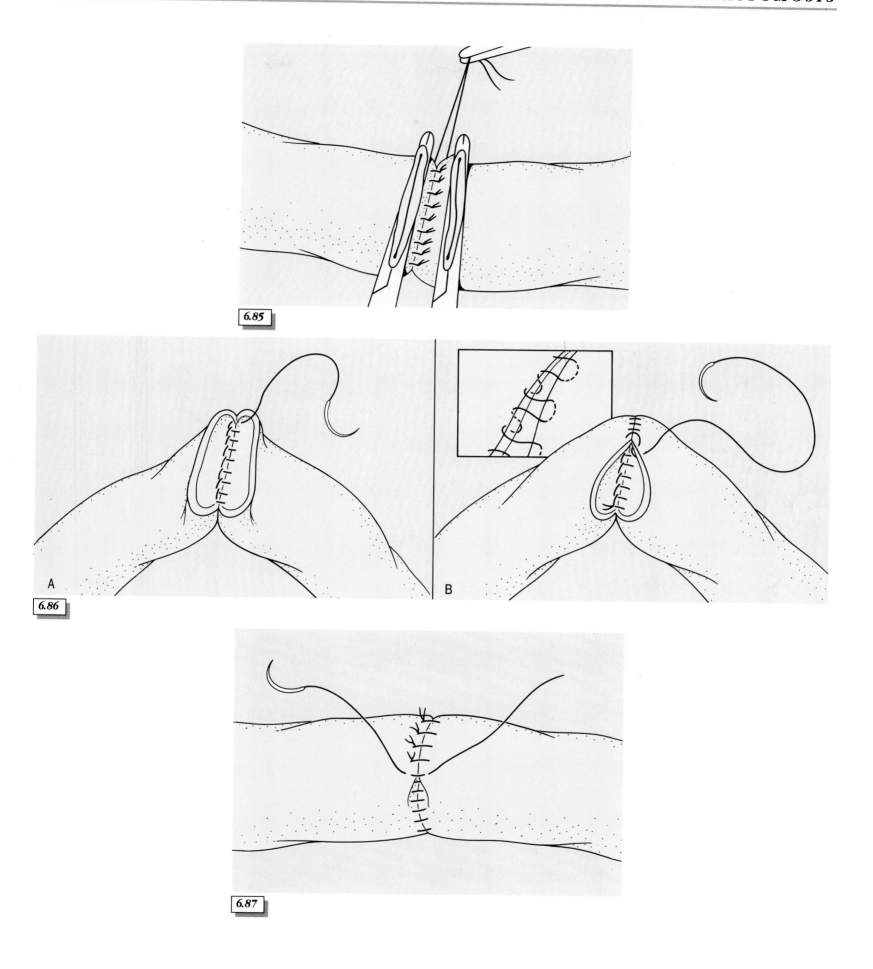

6.85

6.86

A

B

6.87

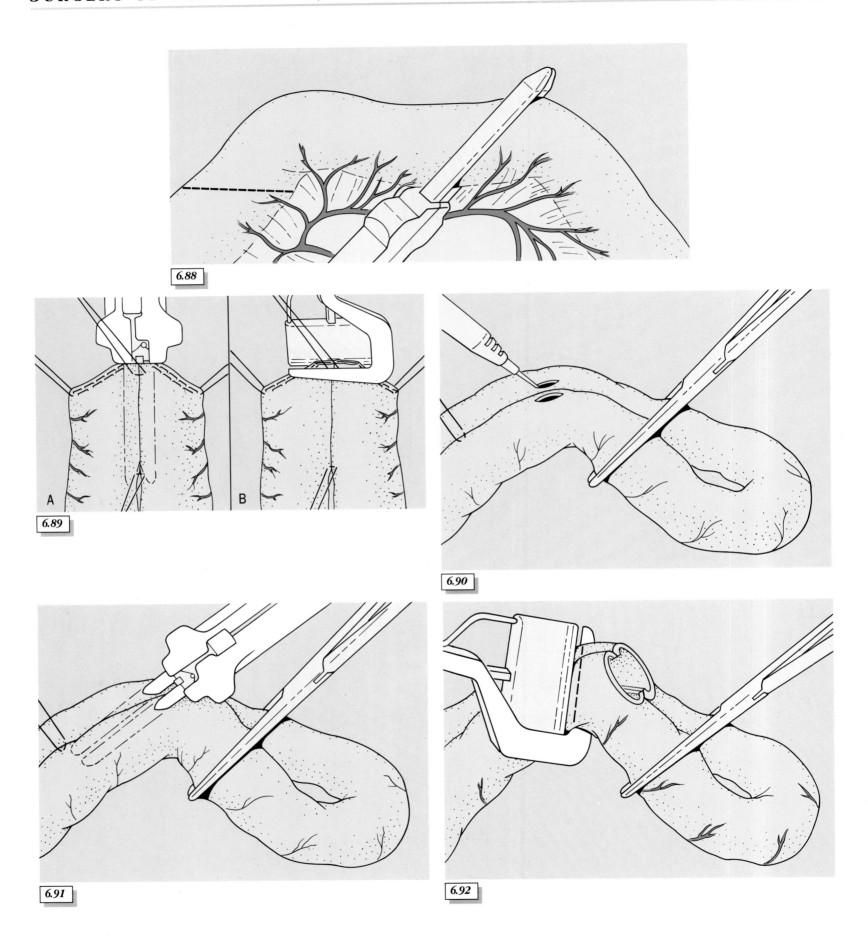

6.88

6.89

6.90

6.91

6.92

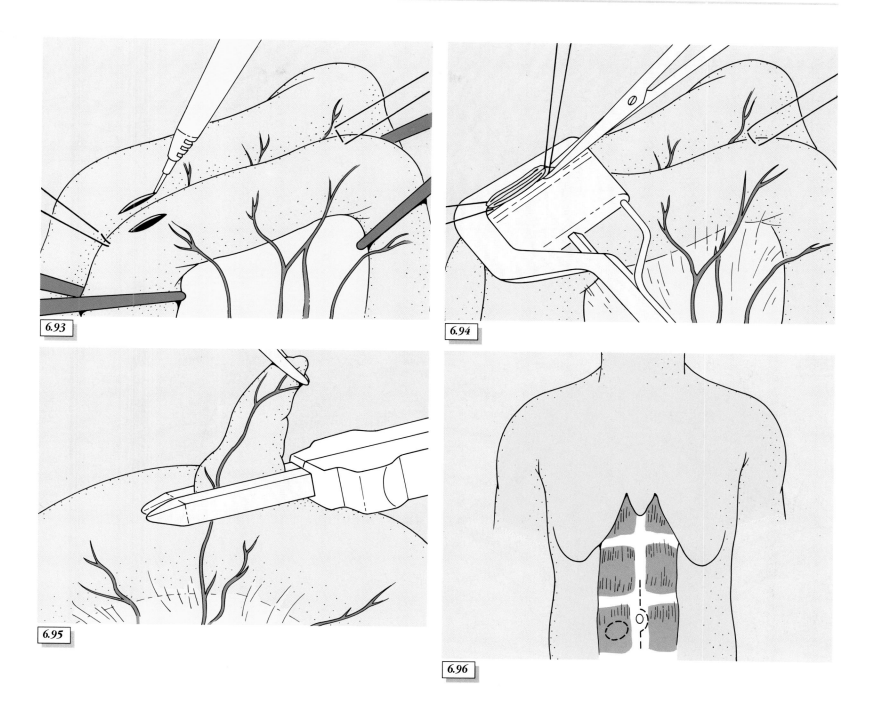

6.93

6.94

6.95

6.96

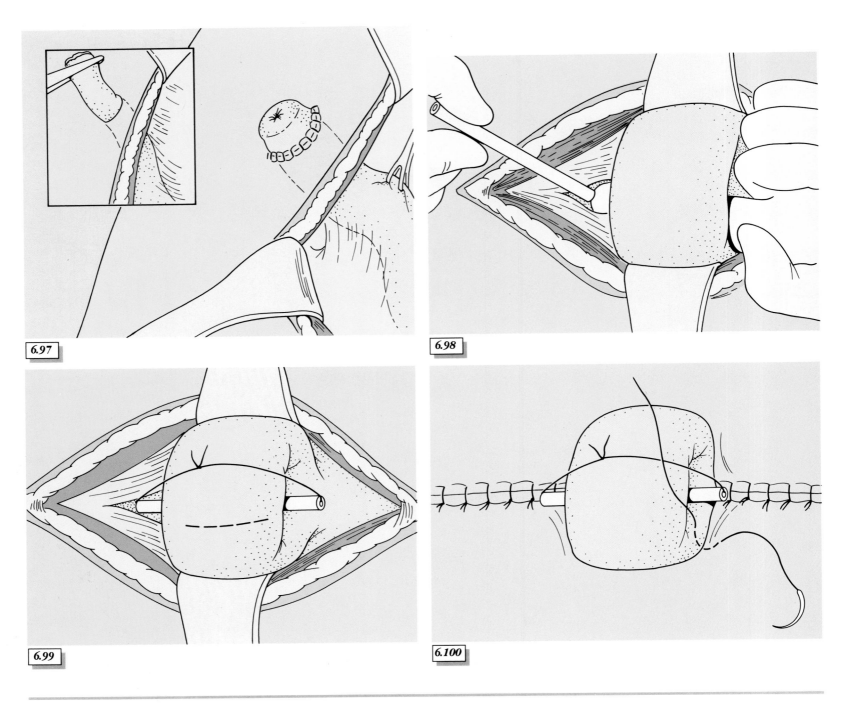

6.97

6.98

6.99

6.100

BIBLIOGRAPHY

Nora PF, ed. Operative Surgery: *Principles and Techniques*. Philadelphia, Pa: Lea and Febiger; 1980.

Shackelford RT, Zuidema GD. *Surgery of the Alimentary Tract*. Philadelphia, Pa: WB Saunders Co; 1978.

Zollinger RM, Zollinger RM, *Atlas of Surgical Operations*. New York: Macmillan; 1988.

7

Surgery of the Pancreas and Spleen

Francis E. Rosato • Donna J. Barbot • Jerome J. Vernick

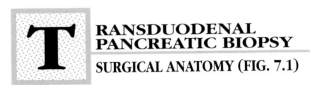

TRANSDUODENAL PANCREATIC BIOPSY

SURGICAL ANATOMY (FIG. 7.1)

TRANSDUODENAL PANCREATIC BIOPSY

INDICATIONS	• evaluation of pancreatic masses
ANESTHESIA	• general endotracheal
POSITIONING	• supine
PREP	• preoperative prep: broad-spectrum antibiotics, usually cephalosporin the day before, day of, and day after biopsy • Betadine (organic iodine solution) from nipple line to pubis and from table side to table side

PROCEDURE

Usually a subcostal incision is made extending from the anterior axillary line on the right, across the midline following the curve of the costal margin, onto the left side to the nipple line. The incision should be 2.5 to 3.0 cm below the costal margina (Fig. 7.2). Subcutaneous tissue is divided with electrocautery, the rectus muscle completely divided on the right and left sides. It is a simple matter to move the skin and subcutaneous tissue laterally on the left side to accomplish complete division of the left rectus muscle. The peritoneal cavity is entered after the posterior sheath and peritoneum are grasped with Kelly hemostats, raised ("tented") and incised. The round ligament is divided between Kelly hemostats to afford complete entry to the peritoneal cavity.

Next, the Kocher maneuver is performed to mobilize the duodenum completely (see Fig. 8.41). The peritoneal investing fibers at the juncture of the lateral margin of the duodenum and the posterior peritoneum are sharply incised with scissors, affording mobilization of the duodenum and the head of the pancreas. As the mobilization is continued, the vena cava can be seen posteriorly. With this maneuver, it is possible to palpate the entire thickness of the head of the pancreas anteriorly and posteriorly.

Traction sutures of 3–0 Vicryl are then placed on the anterior surface of the descending duodenum, which is opened by the middle portion of the electrocautery. With one hand grasping the duodenal tumor, a "Tru-Cut" biopsy needle can then be introduced through the duodenal mucosa directly into the pancreatic mass, taking care to avoid the ampulla, which is visible. At least two and sometimes three samples are taken, depending on the operating surgeon's evaluation of their quality. These are then submitted for frozen section analysis. Bleeding at the needle entrance site can be corrected by 3–0 silk "figure of 8" sutures placed over the needle entry site and/or the application of electrocautery current to the site.

It should be emphasized that when this technique fails to provide a definitive diagnosis, a direct-wedge biopsy of the pancreatic mass can be taken using the scalpel, with electrocautery for hemostasis. A generous wedge can be taken, the biopsy facilitated by the mobilization of the pancreatic head as previously described. No attempt is made to close the wedge defect in the pancreas but simply to assure its hemostasis. We have found that there are few, if any, complications pursuant to pancreatic biopsies, whether transduodenal needle biopsies or wedge biopsies, when the underlying condition is a tumor. There is an approximately 15% incidence of pancreatic complications, including fistula, pseudocysts, abscess or severe pancreatitis, when inflammatory underlying conditions are eventually identified. The duodenum is closed in two layers. If the procedure is to be terminated at this point, two Jackson–Pratt drains are placed. One of the drains is placed in the lesser peritoneal sac

and the other directly over the head of the pancreas in the region of the suprarenal pouch. These are left in place until oral alimentation has been resumed and the drainage is less than 10 cc in 24 hours.

PANCREATICO-DUODENECTOMY

THE WHIPPLE RESECTION

INDICATIONS	• removal of malignant and/or premalignant tumor of the head of the pancreas, duodenum, bile duct, or ampulla
ANESTHESIA	• general endotracheal
POSITIONING	• supine

PREP	• preoperative prep
	  • arteriogram required for basic anatomy reference and to rule out inoperability
	  • antibiotic coverage using broad-spectrum cephalosporin day before, day of and postoperatively for at least 5 days, or longer if patient has elevated white count, fever, or any systemic sign of infection
	  • Betadine—exactly as with transduodenal pancreatic biopsy

PROCEDURE

The incision is again an extended bilateral subcostal incision (see above) and the peritoneal cavity is entered in the same fashion. Standard maneuvers are performed to determine the operability of the patient. One of these maneuvers is the Kocher maneuver (see Fig. 8.41), mobilizing the head of the pancreas off the vena cava and underlying aorta.

Once it has been determined that the tumor is removable by the pancreatico-duodenal (Whipple) approach, the pancreas is exposed throughout its entire length by opening the gastrocolic omentum. This is best accomplished by maintaining a plane of dissection immediately adjacent to the colon since the vascular supply is minimal at that point. In separating the greater omentum from the superior–anterior surface of the transverse colon, care should be taken to avoid damage to the transverse mesocolon. The hepatic flexure of the right colon is mobilized by incising its lateral peritoneal attachments, allowing downward and medial reflection of that structure. The transverse colon is retracted downward and the stomach cephalad, allowing wide exposure of the pancreas. A cholecystectomy is next performed in a routine fashion (see page 8.2). At this point, we prefer to begin the operation by dividing the distal stomach in such a way as to encompass the distal 50% of the lesser curvature and 25% of the greater curvature; this minimizes problems with hyperacidity and postpancreatectomy ulcer (Fig. 7.3).

When the points on the greater and lesser curvature have been identified, serial application of small hemostats is used to free the distal greater and lesser curvature from the gastroepiploic and right gastric branches respectively. A TA-90 gastric stapler (staple height: 4.8 mm) is then introduced to divide the stomach. The dissection continues along the superior surface of the duodenum where the common bile duct is now identified as it passes beneath the pyloroduodenal area. We divide the common bile duct just above its juncture with the cystic duct. The position of the common bile duct in the portal triad facilitates division because it is most anterior. The duct is divided between Crile hemostats and the distal portion then tied with a heavy suture of 0–silk and the proximal clamped portion allowed to remain in place awaiting later anastomosis.

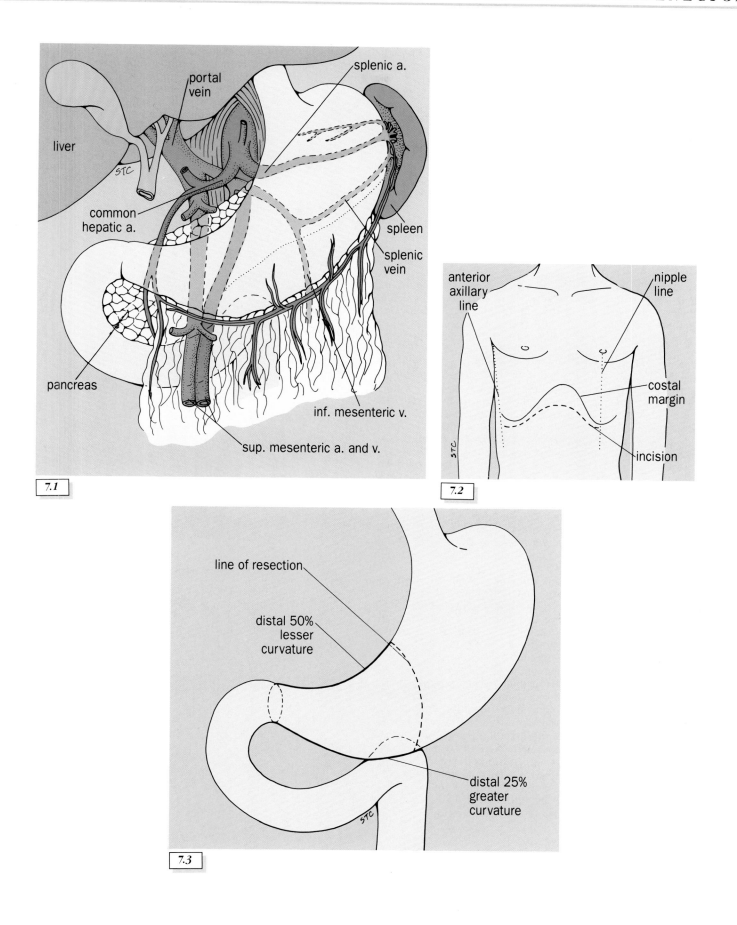

liver

portal vein

splenic a.

common hepatic a.

spleen

splenic vein

pancreas

inf. mesenteric v.

sup. mesenteric a. and v.

7.1

anterior axillary line

nipple line

costal margin

incision

7.2

line of resection

distal 50% lesser curvature

distal 25% greater curvature

7.3

We next divide the body of the pancreas just to the left of the mesenteric vessels. To accomplish this, we start with blunt dissection using a "pusher" (a small gauze pledgette in a Kelly hemostat) to identify and slightly elevate the inferior margin of the pancreas. The splenic vein is usually encountered along this inferior surface. If possible, the pancreas is dissected in the plane anterior to the splenic vein, leaving it intact to drain the spleen and residual distal pancreas. On the cephalad side of the pancreas attempts are made to conserve the splenic artery, and again the pancreas is dissected off the vessel by sharp dissection (Fig. 7.4).

Having gained this advantage, and with continued upward traction on the superior and inferior edges, the entire posterior portion of the gland can be exposed to allow the passage of a large Penrose drain. With upper traction on the Penrose drain, the gland is then divided by sharp knife dissection. Bleeding at this point is often vigorous, requiring manual compression of the splenic (distal) pancreas to allow suture ligature of major bleeding points. Usually at this juncture the duct can be easily visualized in the posterior portion of the body of the pancreas (Fig. 7.5).

Now the head of the pancreas can be elevated off the splenic and mesenteric veins. This is best accomplished by continued upward traction on the divided duodenal edge of the gland, allowing identification of the small anterior branches entering the posterior surface of the gland and then their division between 3–0 silk sutures, using a fine right-angle clamp (Fig. 7.6). In this fashion the entire head is elevated off the splenic–mesenteric confluence.

At this point the duodenojejunal juncture at the ligament of Treitz is divided with the use of the gastrointestinal anastomosis (GIA) stapler. The proximal retroperitoneal portion of the jejunum is delivered from beneath the transverse mesocolon after ligation of its mesentery. This is a difficult step not generally addressed in most texts, but we have found it of help to do a good deal of the mesenteric division from the caudad side of the transverse colon freeing up as much of the most distal duodenum from that approach before retracting it into the right retroperitoneal space above the transverse mesocolon. Having thus mobilized the distal duodenum and having elevated the pancreatic head off the mesenteric-splenic–portal confluence, we continue to follow the contour of the pancreas as it passes medial to the vena cava and then posterior into the retroperitoneal space as the uncinate process (Fig. 7.7). As this is followed, the glandular structure gradually is replaced by a tough fibrous band, which is divided by sharp dissection. When the sharp dissection is completed the entire specimen can be lifted.

Reconstitution of the GI biliary tract is now required. We prefer to do the pancreatico-intestinal anastomosis first. The jejunum is brought through the Treitz opening. If there has been a tough pancreatic capsule, then a first layer approximating the pancreatic capsule to the serosa of the most proximal portion of the antimesenteric jejunum is begun using 3–0 silk (Fig. 7.8). Following incision into the attached bowel wall, an incision matching in size the pancreatic duct, an interrupted 4–0 PDS anastomosis approximating the full thickness of the pancreatic duct to the small opening in the jejunum is then performed (Fig. 7.9). A fine red rubber tube 8- to 10-French in diameter is introduced through a separate, more distal, enterotomy and passed through the ductal intestinal anastomosis prior to completion of the ductal anastomosis. Again, if there is a firm capsule, a second inverting layer along the facing edge of the pancreas to the antimesenteric serosa is performed (Fig. 7.10). Where the pancreas is soft and the capsule nonexistent, the pancreatic ductal–jejunal mucosal anastomosis is done and tension taken off this suture line by approximating the serosa of the intestine to any portions of the peripancreatic tissue that are fibrous and dense enough to hold the sutures. Occasionally, no other tissue is available and the anas-

tomosis is dependent on the ductal–mucosal sutures alone for maintenance. The 10- to 12-French red rubber tube that is "stenting" the anastomosis is tunnelled using a Wetzel approach. Our preference is always for a direct ductal intestinal anastomosis and, where possible, a second protecting serosa to pancreatic capsule layer. Most importantly, we always protect the anastomosis with the stent tube.

Attention is generally given next to the choledocho-jejunal anastomosis. This is performed at any convenient distance along the course of the proximal jejunum, usually within 15 to 25 cm of the pancreatic anastomosis. It is done exactly as described in bile duct reconstruction (choledocho-jejunostomy; see page 8.18) and again with stenting.

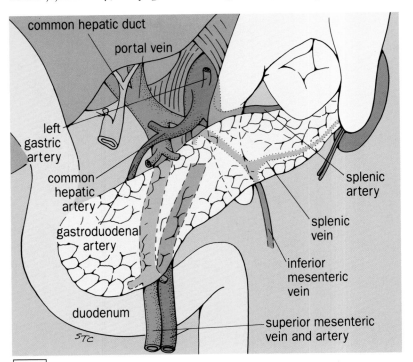

common hepatic duct
portal vein
left gastric artery
common hepatic artery
gastroduodenal artery
duodenum
splenic artery
splenic vein
inferior mesenteric vein
superior mesenteric vein and artery

7.4

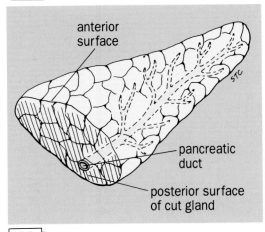

anterior surface
pancreatic duct
posterior surface of cut gland

7.5

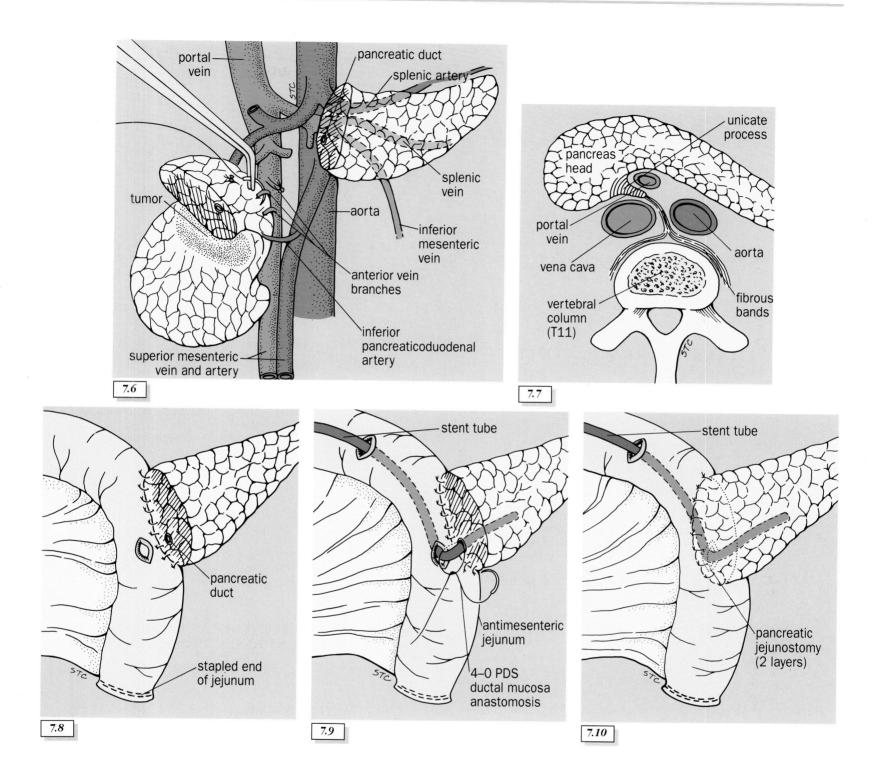

7.6

portal vein

pancreatic duct

splenic artery

tumor

splenic vein

aorta

inferior mesenteric vein

anterior vein branches

inferior pancreaticoduodenal artery

superior mesenteric vein and artery

7.7

unicate process

pancreas head

portal vein

aorta

vena cava

vertebral column (T11)

fibrous bands

7.8

pancreatic duct

stapled end of jejunum

7.9

stent tube

antimesenteric jejunum

4–0 PDS ductal mucosa anastomosis

7.10

stent tube

pancreatic jejunostomy (2 layers)

The final anastomosis performed is a gastro-jejunostomy again as close "downstream" as convenient and usually within 15 to 25 cm of the choledochojejunal anastomosis. The technique of gastrojejunostomy is described on page 6.18.

In final configuration the anastomoses are made in the following sequence, at the closest anatomically convenient interval:

1. Pancreatico-jejunostomy; retrocolic, through area of ligament of Treitz
2. Choledocho-jejunostomy; antecolic, with stent through anastomosis
3. Gastrojejunostomy; antecolic.

After thorough irrigation of the abdominal cavity, a Jackson–Pratt drain is exited from the area of the pancreatico-jejunostomy through a stab wound in the anterior abdominal wall. A second Jackson–Pratt, also from the retroperitoneal area, drains the suprarenal pouch, exiting through a right-side abdominal stab wound. The abdomen is closed in layers, the peritoneum with continuous 0–Vicryl, the fascial layer with continuous #1 PDS and the skin with staples.

TOTAL PANCREATECTOMY

TOTAL PANCREATECTOMY

INDICATIONS • malignant tumors of the pancreas
• nonlocalizable islet cell tumors, eg gastrinomas, insulinomas

ANESTHESIA • general endotracheal

POSITIONING • supine

PREP • preoperative prep: same as for Whipple (see page 7.2) except with addition of preoperative administration of pneumovax (in anticipation of splenectomy)
• Betadine—exactly as with transduodenal pancreatic biopsy

PROCEDURE

A total pancreatectomy represents only a relatively minor modification of the Whipple operation. All the steps are identical to those presented for the Whipple procedure up to the point where in the Whipple procedure the gland would be divided somewhat to the anatomical left of the mesenteric vessels. Such a division is not carried out in a total pancreatectomy. Instead, at that point the entire gland is mobilized from the splenic end toward the duodenal end.

Beginning with the point in the Whipple operation described in Fig. 7.3, the operator moves instead to the left upper quadrant where the ligaments retaining the spleen in place are fully mobilized (see page 7.16). In general, since this operation is done almost always for malignant tumors, we prefer to remove the spleen en bloc because of the concentration of nodes in the splenic hilum. However, for technical reasons, it is almost impossible to remove the entire distal pancreas and spare the spleen since the splenic artery and vein are usually in such close proximity to the pancreas that attempting to skeletonize them and leave them behind would be a serious breach in the tumor principles of wide en bloc dissection.

With the spleen mobilized, the pancreas is then lifted gently from its retroperitoneal attachments. This is usually a very easy step and can be managed by blunt dissection. Figure 7.11 shows elevation of the distal pancreas from its retroperitoneal setting.

As one approaches the celiac axis superiorly, the splenic artery is divided, the proximal end is tied with 3–0 silk suture and a suture ligature of 3–0 silk is placed distal to the free tie.

Inferiorly, as one approaches the mesenteric vessels, the splenic vein—usually along the inferior margin of the pancreas—is also ligated in a fashion similar to that of the artery. From this point the operation proceeds as has been described for the remainder of the Whipple operation, with the obvious exception of a pancreatico-jejunal anastomosis.

DISTAL PANCREATECTOMY WITHOUT SPLEEN PRESERVATION

DISTAL PANCREATECTOMY WITHOUT SPLEEN PRESERVATION

INDICATIONS • benign or malignant tumors
• distal pancreas
• isolated pseudocyst, distal pancreas
• post-traumatic pancreatitis confined to distal pancreas

ANESTHESIA • general endotracheal

POSITIONING • supine

PREP • preoperative prep: same as for Whipple (see page 7.2) except with addition of preoperative administration of pneumovax (in anticipation of splenectomy)
• Betadine—exactly as with transduodenal pancreatic biopsy

PROCEDURE

This operation commences with the step shown in Fig. 7.4. The point at which the pancreas is to be divided is chosen, and at that point the artery and vein are secured and the pancreas divided (Fig. 7.12). In dividing the pancreas, a stapler can be employed as long as there is no obstruction to the duodenal flow of pancreatic juice.

DISTAL PANCREATECTOMY WITH SPLEEN PRESERVATION

DISTAL PANCREATECTOMY WITH SPLEEN PRESERVATION

INDICATIONS • usually benign tumors of pancreas and/or chronic pancreatitis confined to distal pancreas, or isolated pseudocyst

ANESTHESIA • general endotracheal

POSITIONING • supine

PREP • same as for Whipple (see page 7.2)

PROCEDURE

This operation proceeds by identifying the most distal portion of the pancreas and proceeding gently by blunt and sharp dissection to raise it from a retroperitoneal position. Along the superior surface of the gland, all small branches from the splenic artery to the pancreas are individually ligated with 3–0 silk (Fig. 7.13). Inferiorly, the same is done for the vein. At the point of transsection, a stapler is applied as previously described.

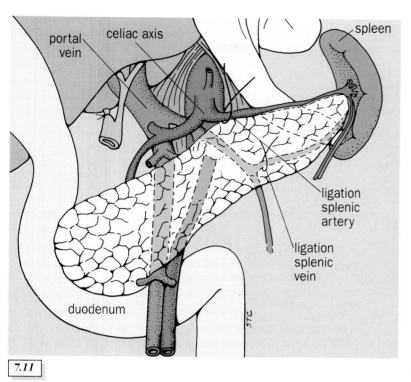

portal vein

celiac axis

spleen

ligation splenic artery

ligation splenic vein

duodenum

7.11

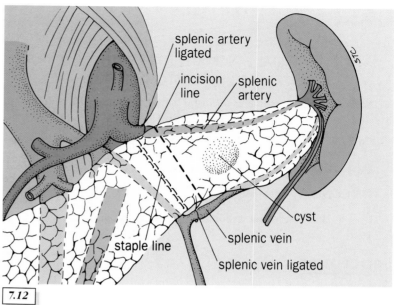

splenic artery ligated

incision line

splenic artery

cyst

staple line

splenic vein

splenic vein ligated

7.12

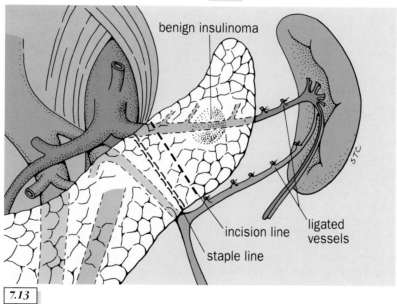

benign insulinoma

incision line

ligated vessels

staple line

7.13

DISTAL PANCREATECTOMY WITH PANCREATICO-JEJUNOSTOMY (DUVAL)

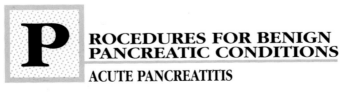

DISTAL PANCREATECTOMY WITH PANCREATICO-JEJUNOSTOMY (DUVAL)

INDICATIONS	•same as for distal pancreatectomy with or without spleen preservation (see page 7.6) but with suspected obstruction of remaining pancreatic duct
ANESTHESIA	•general endotracheal
POSITIONING	•supine
PREP	•same as for Whipple (see page 7.2)

PROCEDURE

This operation may be used for distal pancreatectomy with or without spleen preservation. The transsection of the pancreas is performed without the aid of a stapler. The distal duct can be identified, and then a Roux-en-Y loop of jejunum is brought to the pancreatic tail for anastomosis.

We prefer to divide the intestine about 45 cm from the ligament of Treitz and bring up the distal limb, providing a 60-cm length of defunctionalized bowel between the pancreatico-jejunostomy and the entero-enterostomy which reconstitutes gastrointestinal continuity (Fig. 7.14).

The stapler is used to divide the intestine at the point chosen approximately 45 cm from the ligament of Treitz. The GIA stapler with 3.5-mm staples is utilized. The distal limb is then brought to the posterior edge of the transsected pancreas whose duct has been identified and cannulated. The staples are excised, opening the bowel lumen. The objective is to invaginate the cut edge of the distal pancreas into the lumen of the distal limb of intestine. A posterior row of sutures joining the serosa of the intestine about 5 mm from its edge to the capsule of the pancreas are then placed (Fig. 7.15). An anterior layer of 3–0 silk sutures affixing the serosa 5 mm back from its edge to the pancreatic capsule is also placed. We prefer to have an 8- or 10-French red rubber tube as a stent into the duct. This is placed prior to the tying of the anterior row of sutures and its position fixed by suture fixation to the enterotomy site with a 3–0 Vicryl suture. This tube is exited through a separate stab wound in the abdomen and firmly fixed at the abdominal skin level as well. It affords the opportunity to obtain postoperative pancreatograms if required, and we believe it helps guarantee a patent pancreatico-jejunostomy. The tube is placed to straight drainage in a closed system. On the first or second office visit, 6 to 8 weeks after surgery, it can be removed.

PROCEDURES FOR BENIGN PANCREATIC CONDITIONS

ACUTE PANCREATITIS

Most episodes of acute pancreatitis resolve without sequelae. Exploration is occasionally undertaken in the patient with acute pancreatitis when the diagnosis is in doubt in a deteriorating patient. When acute hemorrhagic

pancreatitis is confirmed, sump drainage and postoperative irrigation may be helpful in patient stabilization. In acute necrotizing pancreatitis, pancreatic debridement and drainage are often necessary. The patient often requires multiple operative explorations in this circumstance. Peripancreatic debris is removed and sump drainage catheters are placed to drain the lesser sac. The cavity size can be followed to resolution by CT scan and contrast injection through the drainage catheters. Some infected lesser sac collections may be treatable by percutaneous drainage catheter placement. Figure 7.16 is a CT image of a patient with pancreatic phlegmon. This patient subsequently developed a pancreatic abscess (Fig. 7.17). This abscess was treated successfully by percutaneous drainage and catheter placement (Fig. 7.18), and no surgical intervention was required. The patient's overall condition will dictate the choice of operative versus nonoperative management.

The more severe the pancreatitis, the more likely it is that a complication will develop over the subsequent several weeks of recovery. Acute pancreatitis may resolve, progress to chronicity, or develop into lesser sac collections. Lesser sac processes often evolve into entities requiring surgical intervention. Lesser sac collections may become abscesses and require drainage and debridement of infected material.

Pancreatic pseudocysts can develop after an episode of acute pancreatitis or in chronic pancreatitis. Pseudocysts can also develop after traumatic disruption or tumor obstruction of the pancreatic duct. Many pancreatic pseudocysts will resolve spontaneously and should be observed for at least 6 weeks after the diagnosis is made. If no resolution is noted and the cyst remains 5 cm or larger, or is symptomatic, operative intervention is usually required. Persistent pseudocysts can cause pain, leukocytosis, occult blood loss, hyperamylasemia, biliary or duodenal obstruction, erosion into adjacent organs, infection, or hemorrhage.

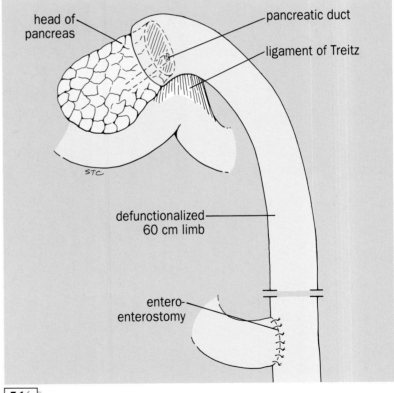

7.14

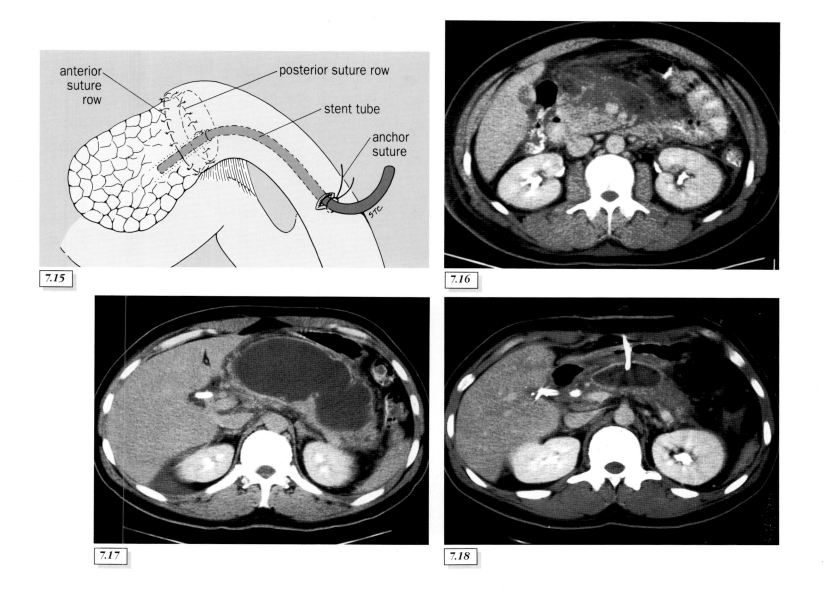

ACUTE PANCREATITIS

INDICATIONS	• hemorrhagic pancreatitis • necrotizing pancreatitis • pancreatic abscess • pancreatic pseudocyst
POSITIONING	• supine on an x-ray table
ANESTHESIA	• general with endotracheal intubation
PREP	• hemodynamic stabilization of the patient • may require invasive hemodynamic monitoring before, during, and after surgery • systemic antibiotics in most circumstances
INCISION	• midline or bilateral subcostal

PROCEDURES

EXTERNAL DRAINAGE

External drainage is always chosen for abscesses. Pancreatic pseudocysts which are infected or which do not have well-developed walls are also externally drained. These tend to be relatively acute. External drainage is performed with closed system drains or sump drains. The inevitable result is a controlled pancreatic fistula that can generally be expected to close. Closure often takes weeks and can be facilitated by the use of parenteral nutrition and somatostatin. Attempted internal drainage of immature pseudocysts results in leaks and major complications. All doubtful cases should be drained externally.

The collection may be entered through the gastrocolic (greater) omentum (Fig. 7.19) or via an infracolic approach through the transverse mesocolon. The infracolic approach avoids dense upper abdominal adhesions. We prefer to aspirate the collection with a large-gauge needle for Gram stain and culture (Fig. 7.20). A contrast film, cystogram, may also be obtained through a catheter passed through this needle if needed for delineation of extent of the collection and connections to the pancreatic duct.

If the collection is infected, the abscess is opened widely (Fig. 7.21) and drainage catheters are placed (Figs. 7.22, 7.23). An open packing technique can be used as well to treat pancreatic abscesses (Fig. 7.24). This technique requires frequent operative packing changes, and is reserved for the most severe cases of abscess and necrotizing pancreatitis.

INTERNAL DRAINAGE

Collections which remain free of infection and mature for 3 to 5 weeks are ultimately surrounded by organized reactive tissue arising from the surfaces of adjacent organs. The walls produced by this reactive tissue and the contained fluid constitute a pancreatic pseudocyst. If the pseudocyst has not spontaneously resolved in 6 weeks from its diagnosis, operative intervention is advisable. The choice of operation depends on the location and character of the pseudocyst. A few pseudocysts of modest diameter may be suitable for resection by distal pancreatectomy. The majority of mature pseudocysts are large and associated with surrounding inflammation and are best treated by internal drainage procedures. Infected pseudocysts are treated by external drainage.

Preoperative assessment includes upper GI (Fig. 7.25), CT scan (Fig. 7.26), and ERCP where appropriate to plan the surgical approach.

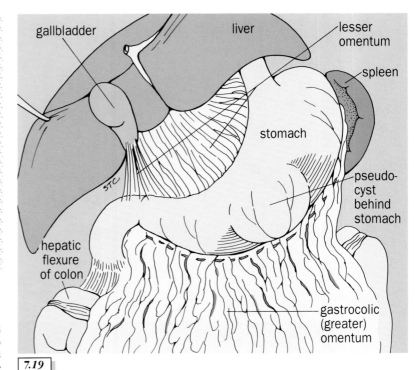

7.19

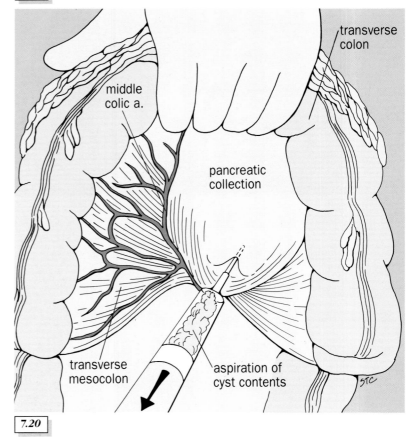

7.20

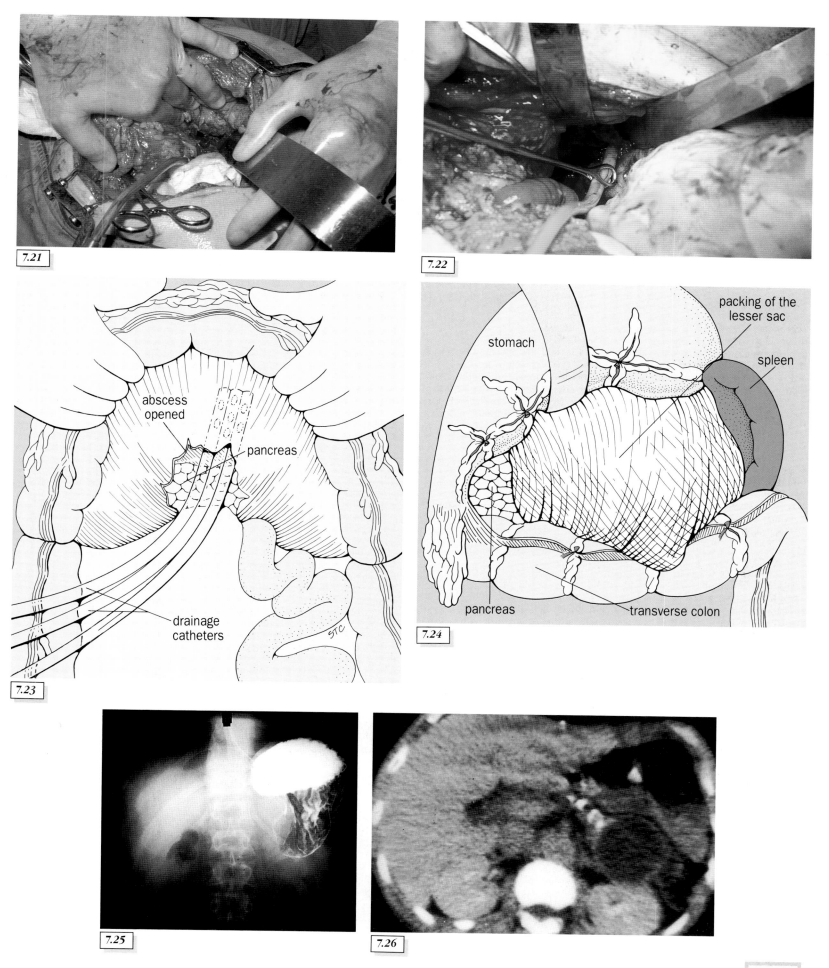

7.21

7.22

abscess
opened

pancreas

drainage
catheters

STC

7.23

stomach

packing of the
lesser sac

spleen

pancreas

transverse colon

7.24

7.25

7.26

The usual situation is for the posterior wall of the stomach to form the anterior wall of the pseudocyst (Fig. 7.27). Careful examination should assure that the attachment is a broad solid one. Naturally, internal drainage is best done by capitalizing on formed attachments. Figure 7.28 shows the stomach bulging anteriorly because of the large pseudocyst behind it.

The anterior wall of the stomach is entered in the mid-body by making an opening with cautery and inserting the forks of a linear cutting stapler. This produces a 50-cm opening with good hemostasis (Fig. 7.29).

The posterior wall of the stomach is inspected for the center of the pseudocyst. This is often manifested by a smooth, featureless area of mucosa which contrasts with the normal rugae of the rest of the stomach (Fig. 7.30).

The combination of the gastric wall and the process forming the wall of the pseudocyst may reach 2 cm in thickness. It is possible to stab directly into the cyst with a scalpel, but the thickness and vascularity of the wall and the uncertainty of cutting in the right place suggest an alternate method. A 16-gauge needle cannula may be used to localize the cyst (Fig. 7.31). Cautery may be used to cut down on the pseudocyst wall to enlarge the opening to accept a Kelly clamp. The extent of the cavity can be explored and the wall opened appropriately (Fig. 7.32). A wire can be inserted through the cannula to guide the clamp placement. A pacemaker insertion cannula can also help to dilate an extremely thick or edematous wall to gain entry into the cyst cavity. A generous core of the pseudocyst wall should be excised using electrocautery for frozen section pathological evaluation, to rule out malignancy before the internal drainage procedure is done (Fig. 7.33). Heavy silk or PDS suture is used to whipstitch the opening for hemostasis. The anterior stomach wall is closed using a 90-mm stapler (Fig. 7.34).

When the pseudocyst forms inferiorly and the mesocolon is the major contributor to the anterior cyst wall, a Roux-en-Y jejunal loop is the safest method of internal drainage. This is best done by using a continuous nonabsorbable suture to anastomose the side of the jejunum to the opening created in the inferior portion of the cyst (Figs. 7.35–7.37).

CHRONIC PANCREATITIS

Pancreatitis which progresses to chronicity may require surgical treatment for relief of pain. Alcoholic patients who continue to drink do not obtain good results from any of the procedures described below. The choice of operation depends primarily on the condition of the duct. This determination is best made by ERCP.

Unrelenting pain in chronic pancreatitis with a small strictured duct has no appealing therapeutic options. The alternatives include subtotal resection of up to 90% of the pancreas. This operation was described by Child. It is usually necessary to mobilize and include the spleen with the pancreatic resection. The chronically inflamed pancreas will probably be sufficiently adherent to the splenic vessels to preclude splenic preservation. (The technique of distal pancreatectomy is discussed on page 7.8.)

	CHRONIC PANCREATITIS
INDICATIONS	•unrelenting pain
ANESTHESIA	•general
POSITIONING	•supine
PREP	•preoperative ERCP •perioperative antibiotics •postoperative psychiatric assistance in the drug or alcohol-dependent patient

PROCEDURE

Although the operation is called a 95% resection, in most hands it is not more than a 65% resection. Care must be taken to avoid bile duct injury and interruption of the duodenal blood supply. When the resection is carried out to the superior mesenteric vein it is considered an 85% pancreatec-tomy (Fig. 7.38). To complete a 95% pancreatectomy the resection leaves only the small portion of tissue abutting the duodenal C-loop. This is accomplished with an extensive Kocher maneuver and mobilization of the uncinate process (Fig. 7.39). A biliary Fogarty should be placed through the common bile duct to prevent duct injury (Fig. 7.40). Extensive resections often result in brittle diabetes, which often causes death by ketoacidosis in alcoholic patients. These procedures are rarely performed and are mentioned for completeness.

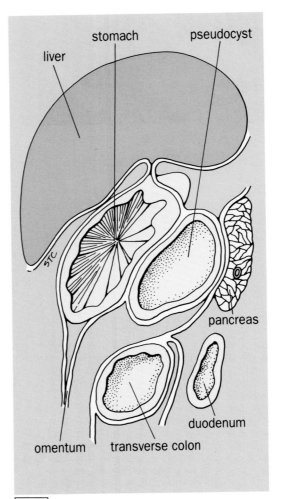

7.27

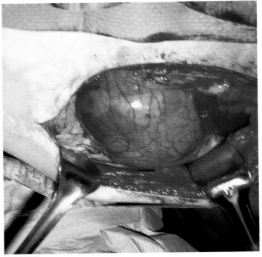

7.28

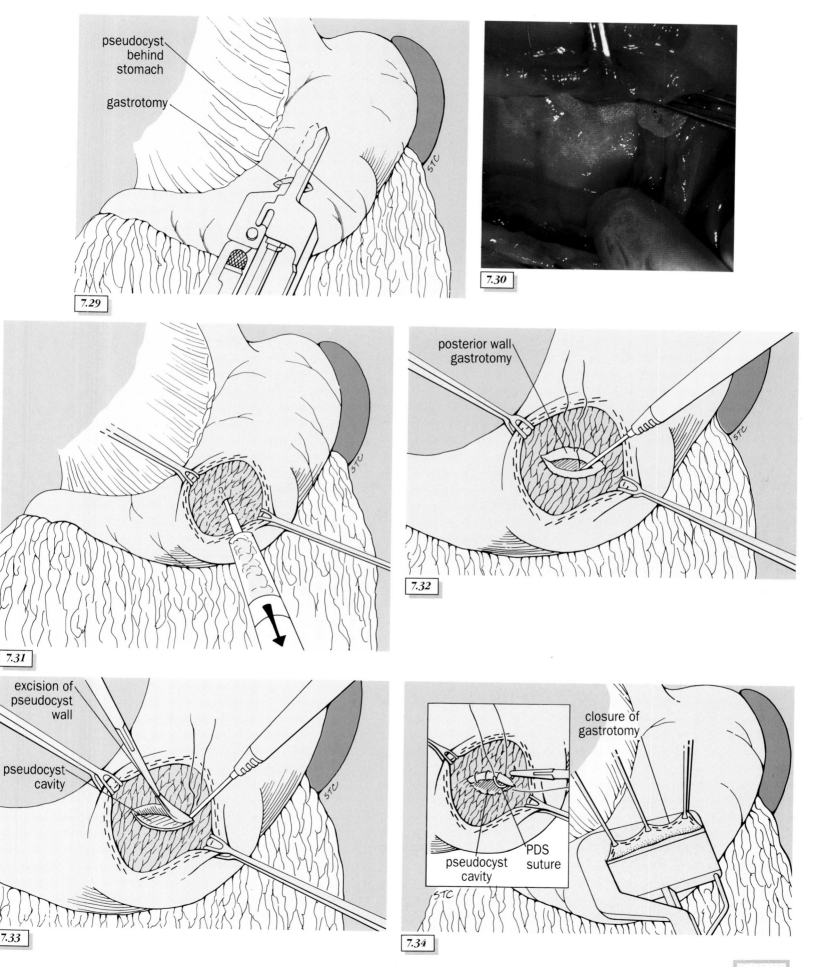

pseudocyst
behind
stomach

gastrotomy

7.29

7.30

posterior wall
gastrotomy

7.31

7.32

excision of
pseudocyst
wall

pseudocyst
cavity

7.33

closure of
gastrotomy

pseudocyst
cavity

PDS
suture

7.34

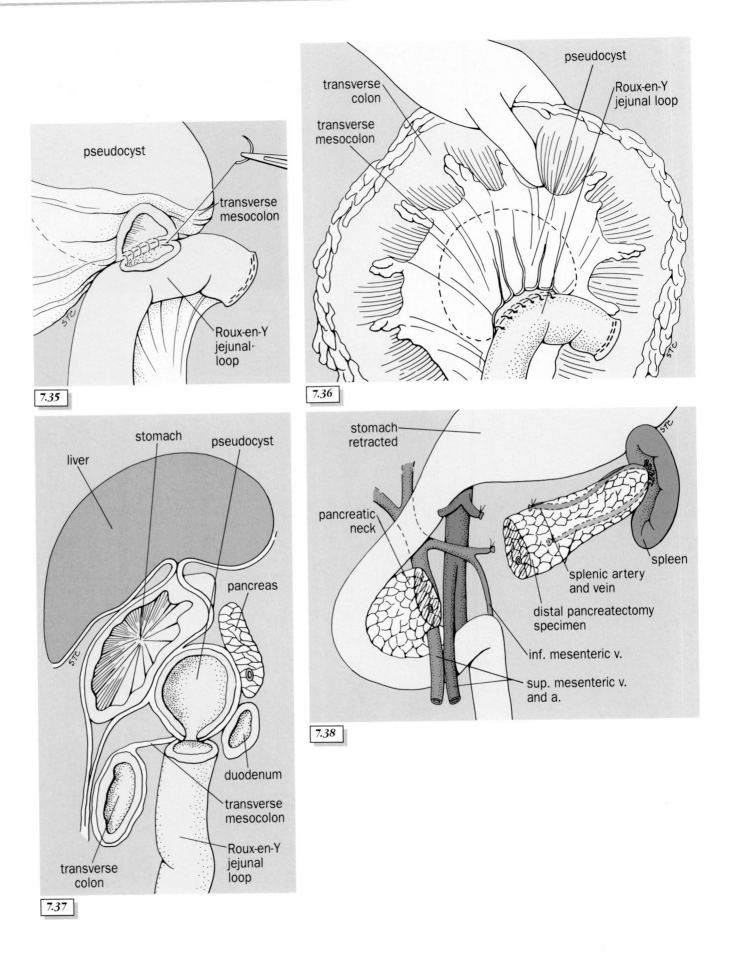

7.35

pseudocyst

transverse
mesocolon

Roux-en-Y
jejunal
loop

7.36

transverse
colon

transverse
mesocolon

pseudocyst

Roux-en-Y
jejunal loop

7.37

liver

stomach

pseudocyst

pancreas

duodenum

transverse
mesocolon

Roux-en-Y
jejunal
loop

transverse
colon

7.38

stomach
retracted

pancreatic
neck

spleen

splenic artery
and vein

distal pancreatectomy
specimen

inf. mesenteric v.

sup. mesenteric v.
and a.

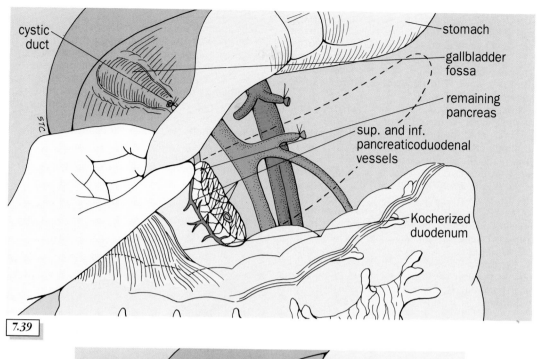

7.39

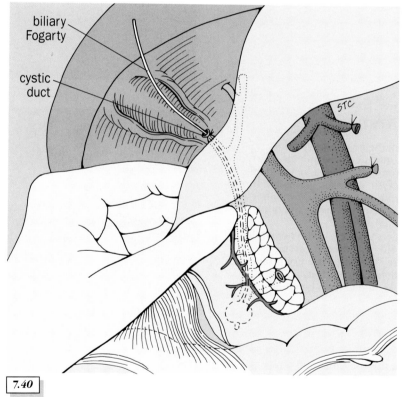

7.40

Patients with unrelenting pain from large duct chronic pancreatitis have a better outlook. Ducts shown by ERCP to be dilated with multiple strictures of the classical "chain of lakes" appearance may be internally drained with good results (Fig. 7.41).

Lateral side-to-side pancreatico-jejunostomy as described by Puestow and Gillespie is the procedure of choice. The pancreas is widely exposed by dividing the gastrocolic omentum (Fig. 7.42).

The duct can usually be palpated as a sulcus when the examining finger is passed over the body of the pancreas. Insertion of a 20-gauge needle will allow aspiration of the duct to confirm location and guide the opening of the duct in a longitudinal manner. Intraoperative ultrasound may also be helpful in delineating the pancreatic ductal anatomy. When the opening is adequate a right-angle clamp is inserted and the duct is opened with electrocautery to within 2 cm of the duodenum (Figs. 7.43, 7.44).

It is worthwhile to curette the thick mucoid material and calcium from the dilated side ducts. A Roux-en-Y loop is then created and anastomosed side to side to the pancreas using a single layer with full thickness bites of 3–0 nonabsorbable suture or two layers with an inner layer of running absorbable suture (Figs. 7.45, 7.46). Figures 7.47 and 7.48 show the completed pancreatico-jejunostomy. Retrograde drainage (Fig. 7.49), described by Duval, and sphincteroplasty have been described as alternatives to the Puestow operation in chronic pancreatitis. These procedures do not provide sufficiently extensive drainage, and thus, are not recommended in this condition.

SPLENECTOMY

SPLENECTOMY	
INDICATIONS	• irreparable traumatic or operative injury ✓ • hematologic disorders causing splenic enlargement, and or thrombocytopenia, neutropenia or anemia (hemolytic anemias, idiopathic thrombocytopenic purpura, thrombotic thrombocytopenic purpura, secondary hypersplenism, myeloid metaplasia) ✓ • metabolic disorders which result in hematologic abnormalities (Felty's syndrome, sarcoidosis, Gaucher's disease, and porphyria erythropoietica) • malignant disorders such as Hodgkin's disease, pancreatic tumors, and certain lymphomas and leukemias • splenic abscess
ANESTHESIA	• general ✓
POSITIONING	• supine; the table may be tilted into a reverse Trendelenberg to gain exposure ✓
INCISION	• midline or left subcostal (Fig. 7.50) (we generally use a midline incision, which gives optimum exposure, and should always be used in the trauma setting or staging laparotomy for Hodgkin's disease; a left subcostal incision is usually reserved for removal of a small spleen where no additional procedures are warranted at that time)

PROCEDURE

The patient is entered in the usual manner and the abdominal exploration is carried out. A self-retaining retractor such as the Buckwalter is very helpful for exposure of the left upper quadrant. It is advantageous to ligate the splenic artery first in most processes requiring splenectomy. The lesser sac is entered through the gastrocolic ligament and the artery found and ligated along the superior border of the pancreas. At this stage of the procedure this is not always possible and should not be forced until better exposure is obtained usually through ligation and division of the short gastric vessels. The lateral attachments of the stomach are then serially clamped, ligated and divided along its entire border, carefully preserving the right gastroepiploic vessels. Figure 7.51 shows the Buckwalter in place with the gastrocolic omentum being divided.

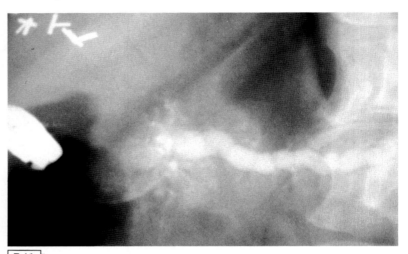

7.41

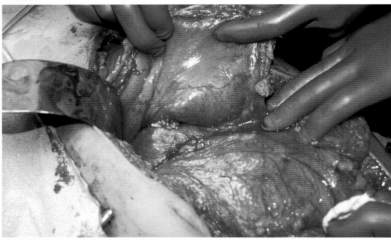

7.42

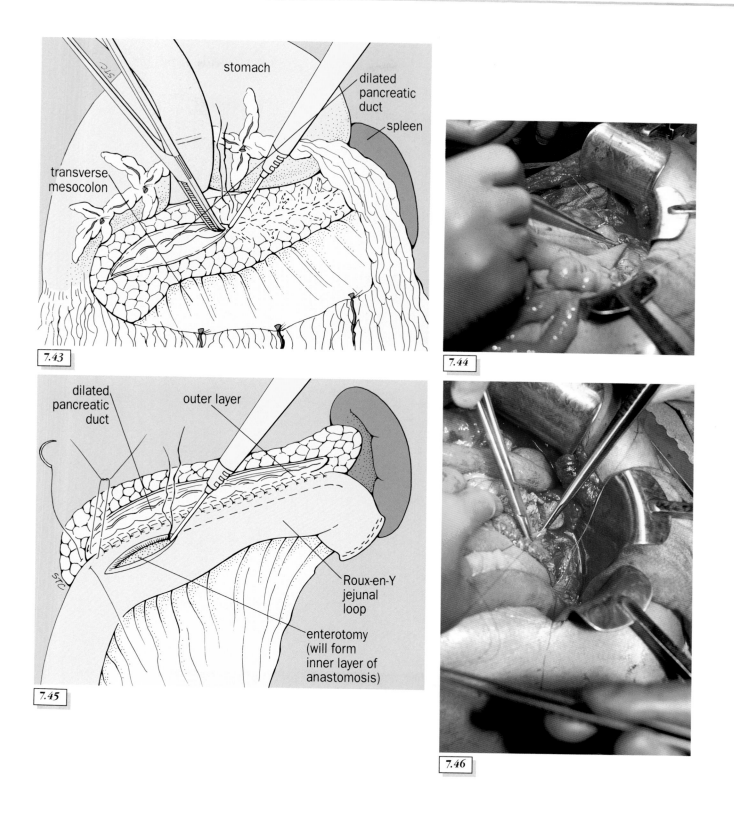

7.43

stomach

dilated pancreatic duct

spleen

transverse mesocolon

7.44

dilated pancreatic duct

outer layer

Roux-en-Y jejunal loop

enterotomy (will form inner layer of anastomosis)

7.45

7.46

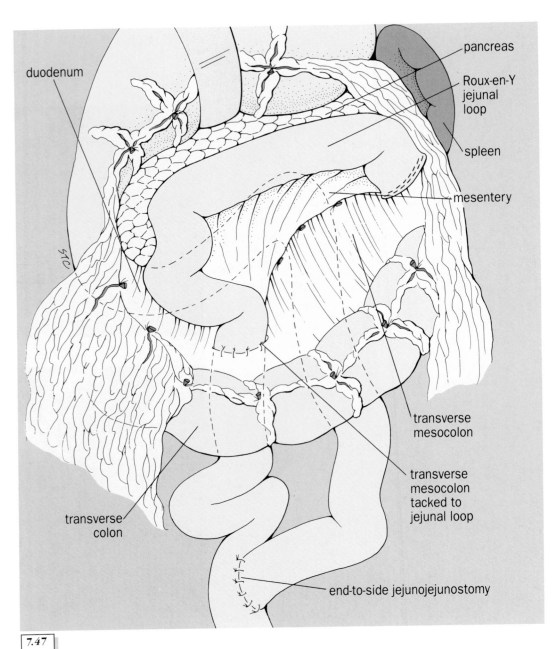

duodenum

pancreas

Roux-en-Y
jejunal
loop

spleen

mesentery

transverse
mesocolon

transverse
mesocolon
tacked to
jejunal loop

transverse
colon

end-to-side jejunojejunostomy

7.47

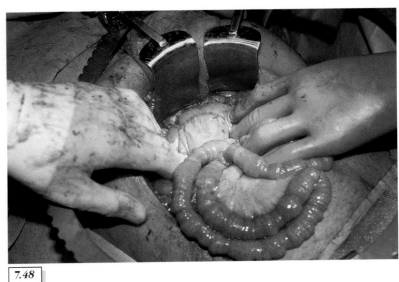

7.48

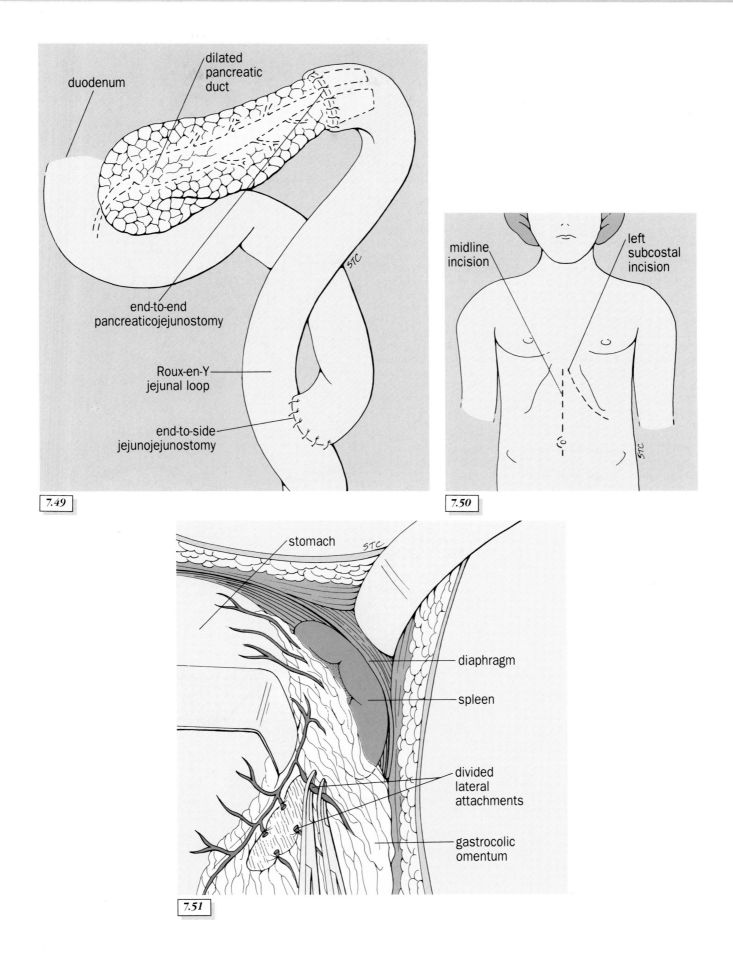

duodenum

dilated
pancreatic
duct

end-to-end
pancreaticojejunostomy

Roux-en-Y
jejunal loop

end-to-side
jejunojejunostomy

7.49

midline
incision

left
subcostal
incision

7.50

stomach

diaphragm

spleen

divided
lateral
attachments

gastrocolic
omentum

7.51

In the cephalad aspect of this dissection the short gastric vessels are encountered. It is helpful to place one to two wet packs (or a spleen roll) cephalad and posterior to the spleen to gain better exposure of these upper vessels (Figs. 7.52, 7.53).

There is occasionally a small vein in the peritoneal attachments connecting the upper medial spleen, stomach, and diaphragm (the splenophrenic ligament). This area should be ligated prior to division. In the patient with massive splenomegaly there may be large and tortuous vessels in this area. These should be carefully ligated or significant blood loss may be encountered (Fig. 7.54). If the splenic artery can be safely approached at this point a ligature should be placed and tied, if it has not already been ligated (Fig. 7.55).

It may be preferable to divide the vessel later when more length on the ends can be obtained. This maneuver allows an autotransfusion of splenic blood back to the patient. This can be a significant quantity in the patient with splenomegaly. The inferior peritoneal attachments to the spleen, the splenocolic ligament, are carefully divided. Additional exposure of the splenic hilar structures can be obtained by separating the posterolateral aspect of the spleen from its peritoneal attachments by sharp or electrocautery dissection. The surgeon rotates the spleen medially, and using a right angle to go under the peritoneal attachments, the assistant uses the Bovie electrocautery with long tip to divide the peritoneum (Fig. 7.56). This allows the spleen to be elevated and rotated medially, giving excellent exposure of the splenic hilar vessels (which are then actually visible in both their posterior and anterior aspects). It is easier, as well, to delineate the tail of the pancreas from the surrounding retroperitoneal and splenic hilar fatty tissues, avoiding inadvertent pancreatic tail injury (Fig. 7.57). This maneuver is helpful in the trauma setting to gain vascular control by manual compression until the injury can be inspected and splenic salvage attempted (Fig. 7.58).

The artery is ligated and divided first, then the veins (Fig. 7.59). Suture ligatures should be used on the major vessels that are ligated in this area.

The splenic bed is inspected for bleeding. The pancreatic tail is inspected for injury. In certain hematologic disorders a careful inspection for accessory spleen should be made and these small spleens removed. Accessory spleens have been reported in 14% to 30% of patients. The higher incidence is found in patients with hematologic disorders. The usual location for accessory spleens is quite close to the spleen itself, most commonly in the splenic hilus, the gastrosplenic, gastocolic and splenorenal ligaments, and the greater omentum. Other less common sites include the small bowel mesentery, pelvis, ovary, and testicle.

If warranted, a closed system drain is used and brought out of the abdomen through a separate stab wound. We would certainly use a drain in the following situations:

1. Difficult splenic hilar dissection
2. If abscess was the surgical indication
3. Potentially continuing coagulation defect
4. Inadvertent pancreatic injury.

The abdomen is closed in a standard fashion.

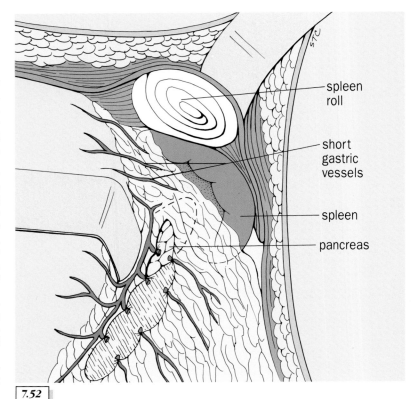

spleen roll

short gastric vessels

spleen

pancreas

7.52

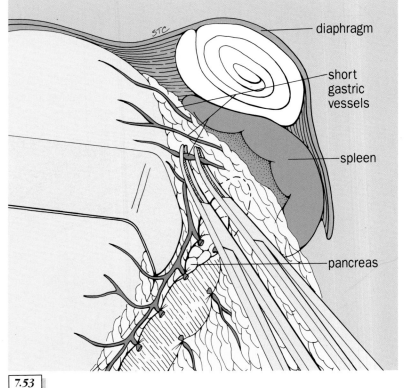

diaphragm

short gastric vessels

spleen

pancreas

7.53

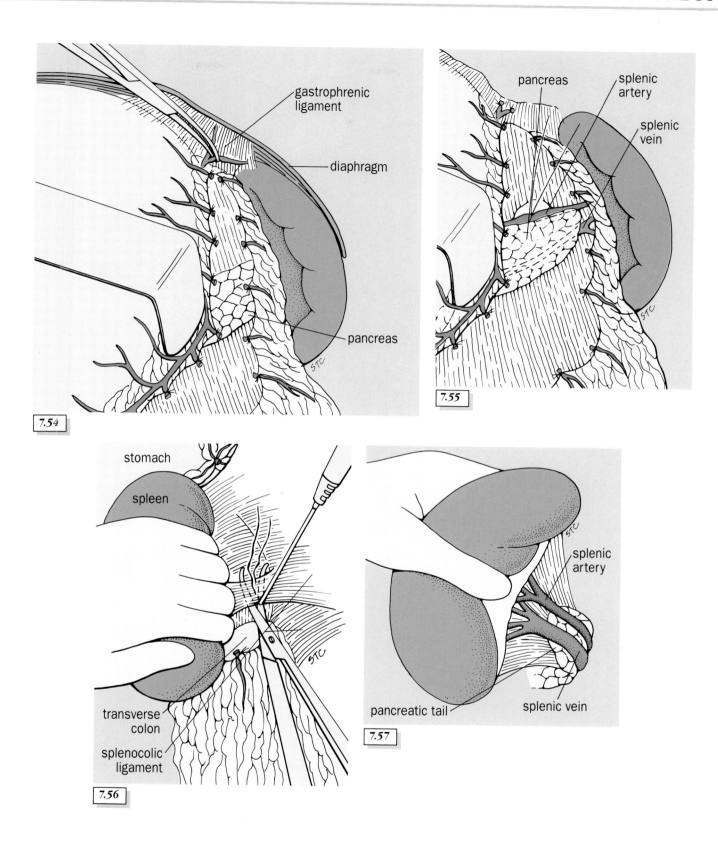

gastrophrenic ligament

diaphragm

pancreas

7.54

pancreas

splenic artery

splenic vein

7.55

stomach

spleen

transverse colon

splenocolic ligament

7.56

splenic artery

pancreatic tail

splenic vein

7.57

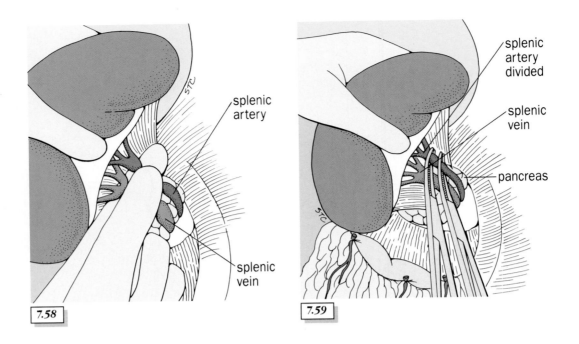

splenic
artery

splenic
vein

7.58

splenic
artery
divided

splenic
vein

pancreas

7.59

BIBLIOGRAPHY

Cameron J, et al. *Atlas of Surgery*, Vol. I. Philadelphia, Pa: Decker; 1990.

Nyhus L, et al. *Mastery of Surgery*. Boston, Ma: Little, Brown, & Co.; 1984.

Rosato FE, Mackie JA. Pancreatic cysts and pseudocysts. *Arch Surg* 1963; 86:551–556.

Weiss SM, Skibber J, Dobelbower R, Whittington M, Rosato FE. Operative pancreatic biopsy: ten year review of accuracy and complications. *Am Surgeon* 1982; 48(5):214–216.

8

Surgery of the Liver and Biliary Tree

Francis E. Rosato • Donna J. Barbot

CHOLECYSTECTOMY

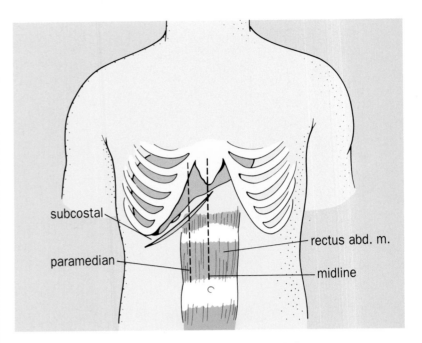

CHOLECYSTECTOMY ✓

INDICATIONS	•symptomatic calculous cholecystitis documented by ultrasonogram or oral cholecystogram •acute cholecystitis documented by hepatobiliary scan •acalculous cholecystitis •incidental with hepatic resections, at time of hepatic artery catheterization for chemotherapy, or at time of morbid obesity surgery with asymptomatic gallstones
ANESTHESIA	•usually general endotracheal, very rarely spinal or local
POSITIONING	•supine on an x-ray table; preoperative scout film may prevent later delays intraoperatively
PREP	•prep entire abdomen

PROCEDURE

A right subcostal incision is made (Fig. 8.1), following which the skin and subcutaneous tissues are incised sharply down to and through the external oblique fascia (Fig. 8.2). A long Kelly clamp is placed under the entire rectus muscle, which is divided with electrocautery. The peritoneum is elevated between hemostats and is entered sharply. The opening is enlarged to the extent of the incision. The falciform ligament usually requires ligation and division to gain adequate exposure.

If acute inflammation or purulent material is encountered, the surgeon should forgo general abdominal exploration. All adhesions between gallbladder and adjacent organs are sharply lysed. Carefully placed abdominal sponges can greatly facilitate exposure and allow the surgeon to work easily through a more conservative length incision. Packing is then performed with a hand inserted, fingertips placed on Gerota's fascia, and the palm retracting the transverse colon inferiorly (Fig. 8.3). Two or three wet surgical sponges are placed between the hand and the gallbladder. With the opposite hand, these sponges are pushed caudally, and a broad deep retractor is inserted to hold them in place.

Similarly, a wet sponge is placed medially between the gallbladder and the duodenum, and a deep narrow retractor can be used to gain exposure (Fig. 8.3). The surgeon may choose to retract the cephalad portion of the incision and liver edge by hand or by using another deep narrow retractor. Mechanical retractors can be used, such as the Balfour, the "upper hand," or the Bookwalter, but all of these may be too cumbersome to use in a smaller subcostal incision.

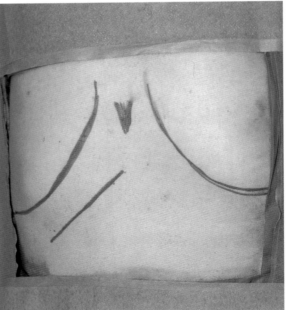

8.1

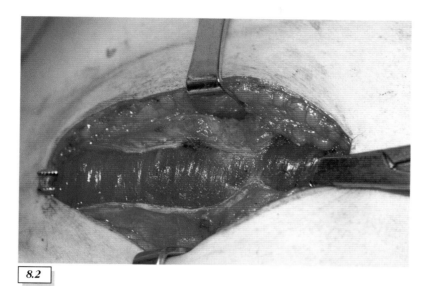

8.2

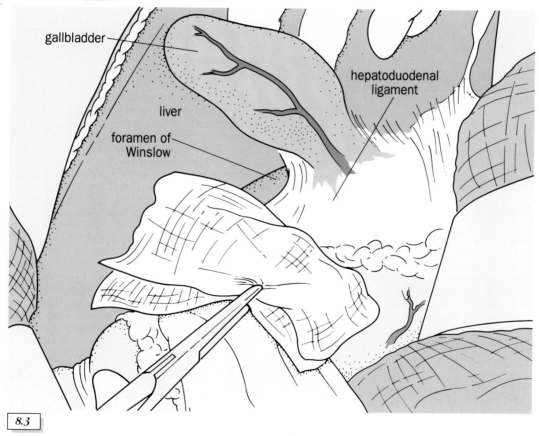

gallblader

liver

foramen of Winslow

hepatoduodenal ligament

8.3

The fundus of the gallbladder is grasped with a Kelly clamp, while a second Kelly clamp is placed more medially. The gallbladder should be retracted inferiorly and laterally (Fig. 8.4). This will splay out the fatty tissues of the hepatoduodenal ligament investing the cystic duct and artery. If the gallbladder is markedly distended such that it obscures the view of the hilar structures, it may be advantageous at this point to drain it with a biliary trocar. A pursestring suture is placed in the gallbladder fundus and the trocar (attached to suction) is inserted (Fig. 8.5).

After adequate exposure is obtained, the peritoneum overlying the area is incised sharply (Fig. 8.6). Using a Kitner dissector (a "pusher"), the fatty tissues are swept medially to expose the cystic artery and duct. Prior to ligation of any structures in the region, the surgeon should be certain that he or she has clearly identified the cystic artery that goes directly to the gallbladder wall (Fig. 8.7). The cystic–common duct junction also must be identified, as this is the most reliable way to prevent common duct injury, since there are many anatomical variations.

A tie or a large clip is now placed on the cystic duct, after it has been palpated for stones, to prevent such stones from entering the common duct during dissection of the gallbladder from its bed. The cystic artery is then ligated and divided (Fig. 8.8). The gallbladder may then be dissected from its bed by division of the duct and by gallbladder removal, from duct to fundus, in a retrograde fashion (Fig. 8.9A). Alternatively, the peritoneum may be incised over the fundus and the gallbladder removed sharply from fundus to duct in an antegrade fashion, in which the duct is only divided as the last maneuver (Fig. 8.9B). We prefer the latter approach.

If the hilar structures are chronically scarred or acutely inflamed, identification of the cystic duct and artery may be difficult or dangerous as an initial maneuver. In that later case, the fundus of the gallbladder is approached first and the gallbladder is removed from its bed, with care taken to stay as close as possible to the gallbladder wall. In this fashion, inadvertent damage to the common bile duct becomes difficult. However, one must accept a potentially higher blood loss. A combination of sharp and blunt dissection is used with electrocautery to remove the gallbladder from its bed and to achieve hemostasis (Fig. 8.10).

If the situation is so difficult that the hilar structures remain unidentifiable in a safe fashion, the gallbladder can be opened and the cystic duct located from inside. In the most extreme situations, the gallbladder can be drained of bile and stones and can be closed over a mushroom catheter (see section on Cholecystostomy). The patient can then be re-explored when the inflammation has subsided and the gallbladder then removed. Partial cholecystectomy also can be done by opening the gallbladder along its long access, removing accessible tissue, cauterizing or stripping the remaining mucosa, and then closing the remnant over a mushroom tube (Fig. 8.11). Subsequent study may show the remnant to be without connection to the biliary tree and free of stones. If that is the case, the tube may be removed 4 to 6 weeks later without the need for additional surgery.

Usually, a cholangiogram is performed. The gallbladder should be opened and its bile cultured. The surgeon should also confirm the presence of gallstones and the absence of mucosal lesions. The gallbladder

bed should be inspected carefully. Electrocautery is commonly used to control small bleeding vessels; suture ligation may be required as well. The surgeon should check carefully for the presence of bile. Small biliary connections can arise directly from the gallbladder bed and, if not ligated, can drain significant amounts of bile during the early postoperative period. These disrupted biliary channels usually heal spontaneously.

In the past, the gallbladder bed was closed routinely by approximation of the peritoneal edges with a running absorbable suture. Most now feel this is unnecessary. We do not close the bed and have not noted any increase in postoperative drainage or complications. Following surgery, the surgeon may or may not want to drain the area. When used, we prefer a closed drainage system and place the tip of the catheter in Morrison's pouch. The drain is then brought out through a separate stab wound inferior and lateral to the incision (Fig. 8.12).

The peritoneum/posterior rectus fascia and the anterior rectus sheath are closed separately with a continuous long-lasting absorbable suture. Subcuticular or interrupted skin closure is utilized as the level of abdominal contamination dictates.

LAPAROSCOPIC CHOLECYSTECTOMY

The gallbladder may be evaluated and removed by a laparoscopic approach in certain patients. At this time that includes those who have not had upper abdominal surgery in the past and those who clearly do not require common bile duct exploration. Other relative contraindications to laparoscopic gallbladder removal include large body habitus, acute cholecystitis, and complicating medical problems necessitating a short anesthetic period. The surgeon with considerable experience in laparoscopic cholecystectomy is able to perform the procedure in more complex settings with significantly shorter operative times than the novice.

Laparoscopic common bile duct explorations are anecdotally reported, but are not the routine at this point. In the patient with a clear indication for possible common bile duct exploration, Endoscopic Retrograde Cholangio Pancreatography (ERCP) is performed preoperatively. The duct is emptied of stones, if necessary, at that time. The use of routine cholangiography during laparoscopic cholecystectomy is the surgeon's preference, as in open cholecystectomy. However, many surgeons feel that routine cholangiography should be performed in laparoscopic cholecystectomy for intraoperative delineation of the anatomy of the biliary tree and prevention of bile duct injury. When asymptomatic common duct stones are found at the time of a routine cholangiogram, many surgeons favor postoperative ERCP to clear the duct of stones rather than converting to an open procedure.

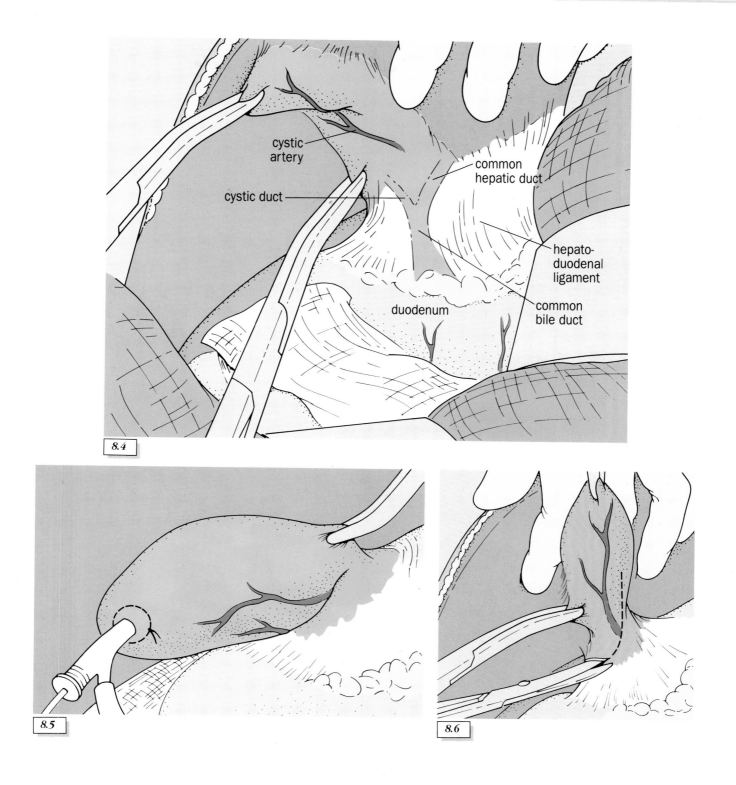

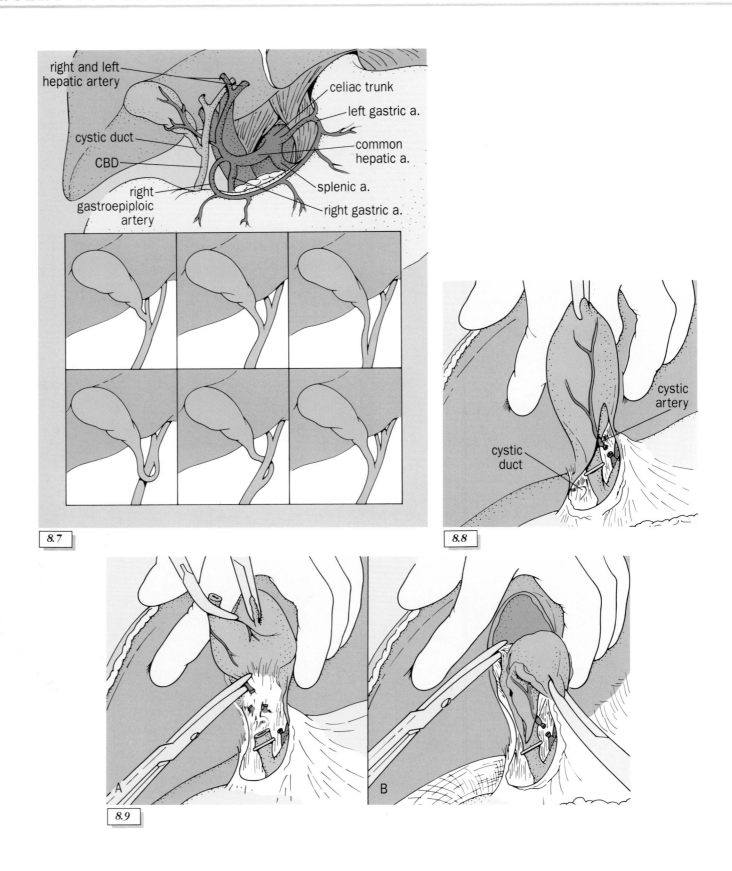

right and left
hepatic artery

celiac trunk

left gastric a.

cystic duct

common
hepatic a.

CBD

right
gastroepiploic
artery

splenic a.

right gastric a.

8.7

8.8

cystic
artery

cystic
duct

A

B

8.9

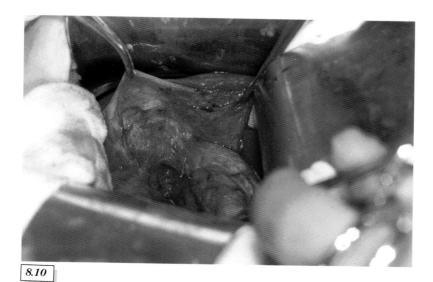

8.10

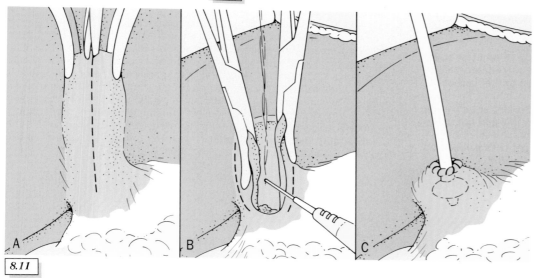

A B C

8.11

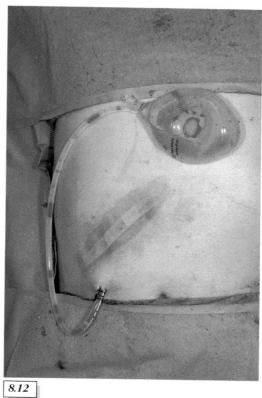

8.12

The rate of conversion to open cholecystectomy is approximately 5%. Those surgeons performing laparoscopic exploration in the patients with acute cholecystitis convert to open cholecystectomy only about 20% to 30% of the time.

The procedure requires a surgeon trained specifically in laparoscopic cholecystectomy, a first assistant with operative experience, a cameraman with anatomic knowledge, scrub and circulating nurses, and laser personnel, if laser use is planned.

LAPAROSCOPIC CHOLECYSTECTOMY

INDICATIONS	• gallstones and biliary colic • acalculous cholecystitis with an otherwise negative workup • acute cholecystitis in certain circumstances
POSITIONING	• supine on an x-ray table
ANESTHESIA	• general with endotracheal tube
INCISION	• vertical intraumbilical incision for laparoscopic examination after placement of a 10- to 11-mm trocar • upper abdominal incision for a 10-mm trocar, at or just to the right of midline, placed under visualization to enter the abdomen to the right of the falciform ligament • two 5-mm trocar sites placed under visualization usually at the anterior axillary line and the right midclavicular line, at a horizontal level determined by the location of the patient's gallbladder with respect to the abdominal wall • an additional 5-mm port may be necessary for retraction or if the surgeon performs a two-handed technique (Fig. 8.13)
PREP	• a Foley catheter and a nasogastric tube should be placed preoperatively • abdomen prepped from nipples to pubis

PROCEDURE

It is wise to be certain all equipment is functional prior to anesthetic induction. This includes the video camcorder, television monitor(s), laser and/or endocoagulator, high flow abdominal CO_2 insufflator, and the irrigation/aspiration system. Ideally, the operating room should be equipped with two video monitors placed to the left and right of the patient's head. This allows both the surgeon and the first assistant to comfortably view the procedure. When only one monitor is available, the table should be turned to the right with the anesthesia equipment moved to the patient's left. The video monitor is then placed at the head of the table. The insufflator should be easily within the surgeon's view for monitoring of the intraabdominal pressure during the case (Fig. 8.14).

The surgeon should clarify the nasogastric tube and Foley catheter have been placed. Using a #11 scalpel blade, a longitudinal intraumbilical incision is made large enough to accommodate a 10- to 11-mm trocar. The Veres needle is inserted at a 45° angle into the peritoneal cavity toward the pelvis (Fig. 8.15). Some surgeons manually lift the abdominal wall dur-

ing this insertion. The Veres needle is aspirated with a 10-cc syringe; there should be no return. Saline should be easily instilled through this syringe (Fig. 8.15). When the syringe is removed from the Veres needle the remaining column of saline should fall rapidly into the abdomen. If these criteria are fulfilled the insufflator is turned on to the lowest setting to provide a slow rate of abdominal insufflation. The intraabdominal pressure should be between 0 and 8 mm during insufflation or consider improper Veres needle placement. There is no exact pressure recommendation to advise for adequacy of insufflation that will provide optimal visualization. The amount of abdominal distension and tympany observed should guide the surgeon as to when he may begin trocar insertion.

A 10- or 11-mm trocar is inserted through the umbilical incision, again using a 45° angle (Fig. 8.16). The blade is removed and the laparoscope with camera attached is inserted. The area below the trocar insertion is carefully inspected. Laparoscopic examination of the abdomen in general is performed. The gallbladder is visualized and an area is chosen for the upper midline trocar which offers a good working angle. Pressure is applied on the skin surface, indenting the anterior abdominal wall, to find an optimal site. This and all subsequent trocars are placed under direct vision. A 10-mm trocar is used in the upper midline position to accommodate the clip applicator and for later laparoscope placement when the gallbladder is extracted through the umbilical port. While using this port with the grasping forceps or scissors a 5-mm reducer is placed over the opening.

The additional trocars are then placed in a similar fashion. These ports are used primarily for gallbladder retraction (Fig. 8.17). In patients who have had previous abdominal surgery, the first trocar can also be placed by an open technique. Through the intraumbilical incision the fascia is reached and exposed sufficiently to place stay sutures on either side of the midline. The fascia is then elevated and opened under direct vision and freed of any underlying adhesions. A phlanged trocar is then bluntly inserted. The stay sutures are used to secure it tightly in place so that the abdomen may then be insufflated (Fig. 8.18). All additional trocars are then placed under direct vision.

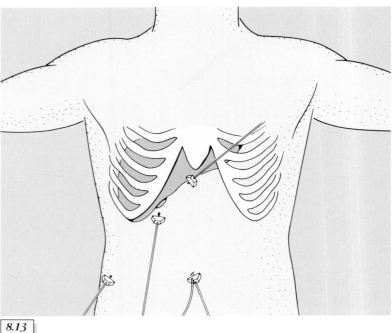

8.13

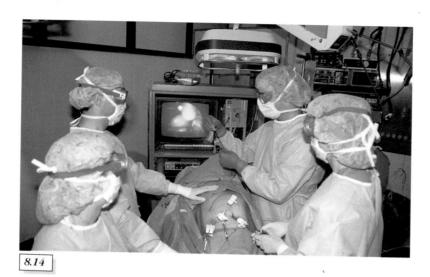

8.14

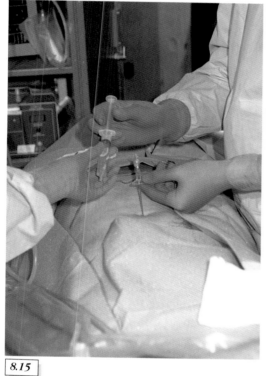

8.15

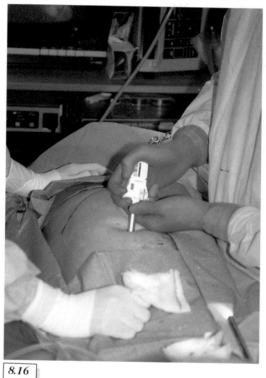

8.16

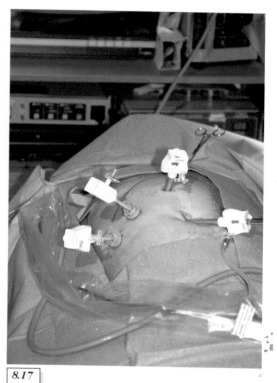

8.17

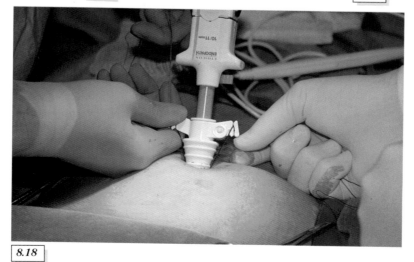

8.18

The gallbladder is then retracted anteriorly and cephalad and the surgeon determines if the procedure is feasible via the laparoscopic approach. The assistant positions one grasper at the fundus and one near the hilum (Fig. 8.19). The midline port is used for surgical dissection. Adhesions are bluntly dissected from the base of the gallbladder to expose the hilar structures (Fig. 8.20). Once the ports are placed and in use the insufflator flow rate should be turned to a higher setting to maintain an adequate pneumoperitoneum.

The cystic duct and artery are cleared of surrounding fibrofatty tissue (FIg. 8.21) and ligated with the application of four clips on each structure, then divided in the middle. The cystic duct is first dissected and clipped proximally and distally, then divided (Fig. 8.22). The cystic artery is then identified, dissected, clipped proximally and distally and divided (Fig. 8.23). It is imperative that the surgeon visualizes completely around both of these structures before clip application. This begins the dissection of the gallbladder from the liver bed (Fig. 8.24).

If a cholangiogram is needed it can be performed in two ways: a cystic duct cholangiogram or a transcholecysto cholangiogram. The cholecysto cholangiogram is performed at the beginning of the procedure, prior to any hilar dissection. Cystic duct cholangiography is performed after the cystic duct has been dissected out.

A cholecysto cholangiogram is performed by needle puncture of the fundus of the gallbladder. Bile is aspirated as thoroughly as possible and full strength contrast is injected. This procedure is best performed under fluoroscopy to determine if the ductal system and duodenum are properly filled with contrast.

When using the cystic duct, only the gallbladder side of the duct is clipped. An incision is made in the cystic duct using the microscissors. The catheter is guided into the duct with a grasping forceps.

Several different systems are available to hold the catheter in place while the x-ray is being taken. As in open cholecystectomy, cholangiocatheter placement takes practice. Static films may be taken or fluoroscopy can be used. After completing the cholangiography, the catheter is withdrawn, and the cystic duct is clipped and then divided.

Either laser or endocoagulation can be used to remove the gallbladder from the liver bed in a retrograde fashion as well as for hemostatic control (Fig. 8.25). The assistant grasps the gallbladder at the hilar end and retracts it cephalad, rotating right and left as necessary to allow the surgeon to separate the gallbladder from its bed. Just before complete separation of the gallbladder from its bed this area should be inspected carefully for bleeding (Fig. 8.26). There are several systems for irrigation and aspiration. A significant amount of the pneumoperitoneum may be lost during aspiration, obscuring the view. Do not proceed until the visualization is adequate. When hemostasis is obtained, the gallbladder is separated from the bed (Fig. 8.26). A drain may be used if necessary by placing it through one of the 5-mm ports, positioning it with a grasper via another port. The trocar port is then slid back over the drain, while the grasping forceps holds the drain in place. A closed system drain should be used, and the end clamped closed to prevent the loss of the pneumoperitoneum during insertion (Fig. 8.27).

The camera is switched along with the insufflating tubing to the upper midline 10-mm port. A large grasping forceps (10–11 mm) is placed through the umbilical port and followed to the liver area where it grasps the gallbladder at the ductal orifice with a large and secure bite (Fig. 8.28).

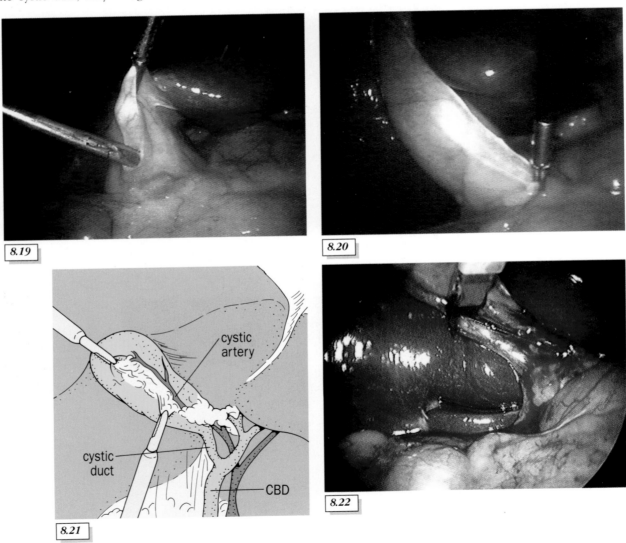

8.19

8.20

cystic
artery

cystic
duct

CBD

8.21

8.22

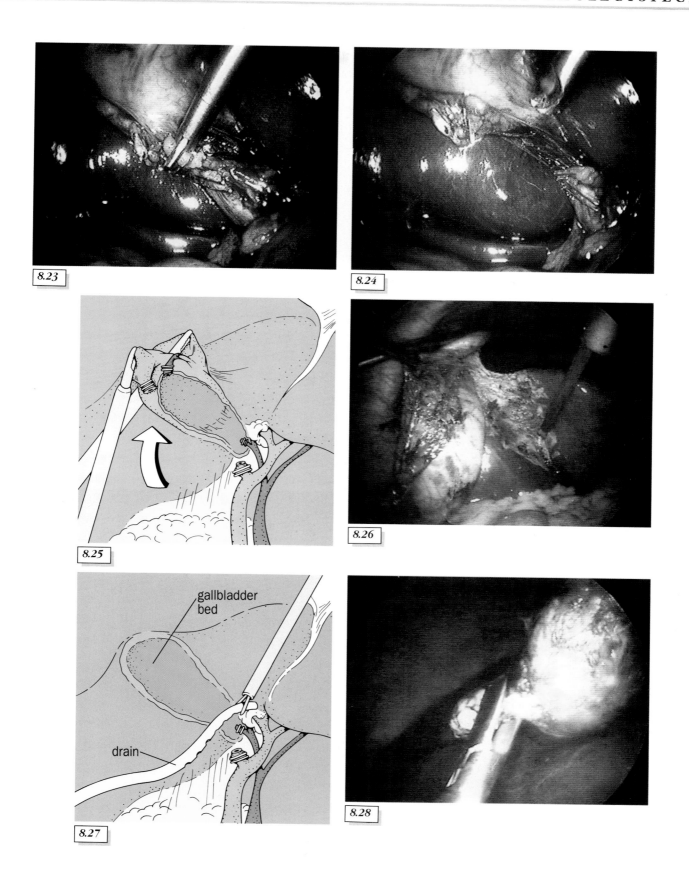

8.23

8.24

8.25

8.26

gallbladder
bed

drain

8.27

8.28

The other graspers may then be removed. The gallbladder is removed through the umbilical trocar site, under direct vision of the camera. The forceps and trocar are pulled back together bringing the clipped cystic duct end of the gallbladder with it. The gallbladder may then be gently manipulated through the umbilical incision. Often stones and bile may need to be emptied before the organ can be totally extracted through the umbilical opening (Fig. 8.29). The umbilical fascial opening may require some enlargement for removal of the gallbladder (Fig. 8.30).

At the completion of the procedure all trocar sites and gallbladder bed are inspected for bleeding. The trocars are removed under direct vision. The remaining CO_2 gas is allowed to escape through the last trocar and it as well is removed under direct vision, slowly pulling the camera back through the abdominal wall.

The umbilical incision is closed with one or two fascial sutures. If an open technique of first trocar placement had been used, the previously placed stay suture may be tied together to get adequate fascial closure. Absorbable sutures are used to close the other skin incisions (Fig. 8.31). Marcaine is infiltrated in all incision sites. Small bandages may be used as dressings. Nasogastric tube and Foley catheter are removed in the operating room. The patient may be started on a house diet after having sufficiently recovered from the anesthetic. The patient may be discharged within 12 to 24 hours in most cases. There are rarely any postoperative activity restrictions. Most patients experience incisional pain as well as right shoulder pain and require narcotic agents for several days.

CYSTIC DUCT CHOLANGIOGRAM

CYSTIC DUCT CHOLANGIOGRAM

INDICATIONS
- multiple small stones
- no stones in resected gallbladder
- single-faceted stone
- enlarged common bile duct (normal size)
- history of jaundice
- history of pancreatitis
- elevated liver enzymes

PROCEDURE

Many surgeons routinely perform a cystic duct cholangiogram with cholecystectomy (see page 8.2). Others use the standard indications listed here. It is easiest to place the cholangiogram catheter into the cystic duct while it is still in continuity with the gallbladder, as the latter can be used for traction (Fig. 8.32). An opening is made in the anterior cystic duct with a #11 knife blade or with Metzenbaum scissors until a lumen is seen clearly. Care is taken to avoid transection. The valves of Heister commonly present obstruction to passage of the catheter. To get beyond the valves, angling of the duct cephalad and the use of firm pressure is necessary.

In many cases, aspiration of bile is possible. A tie or a large clip, carefully applied to avoid catheter occlusion, is used to hold the catheter in place in a watertight fashion. Half-strength contrast medium (final concentration 25%) is introduced in quantities of 5 to 10 mL per injection, with more contrast agent needed if there is obvious dilation of the biliary tree. Full-strength contrast medium is not recommended since small radiolucencies may be obscured as they are heavily coated on both sides by the more radiopaque material. Two films are taken, one supine and one 10°

to 15° right-side down. The second film is used to separate the duodenal–common duct junction from the bony density of the vertebral column. The films should document the presence or absence of common duct stones and free flow of contrast into the duodenum. As abnormal findings may require additional films for delineation, the catheter should not be removed until the surgeon has viewed the original set of films (Fig. 8.33). Figure 8.33A is a normal cholangiogram. An enlarged common bile duct (without stones) is shown in Fig. 8.33B.

The catheter is then removed and the duct is grasped with a right-angle clamp and divided. Absorbable suture or a clip should be used to tie the duct. The surgeon should take care not to leave a long cystic duct remnant, as it has been associated with the formation of common duct stones.

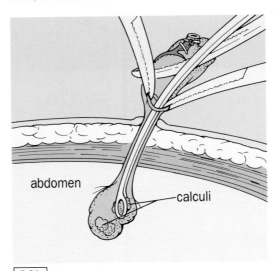

abdomen

calculi

8.29

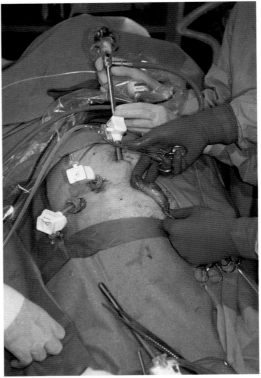

8.30

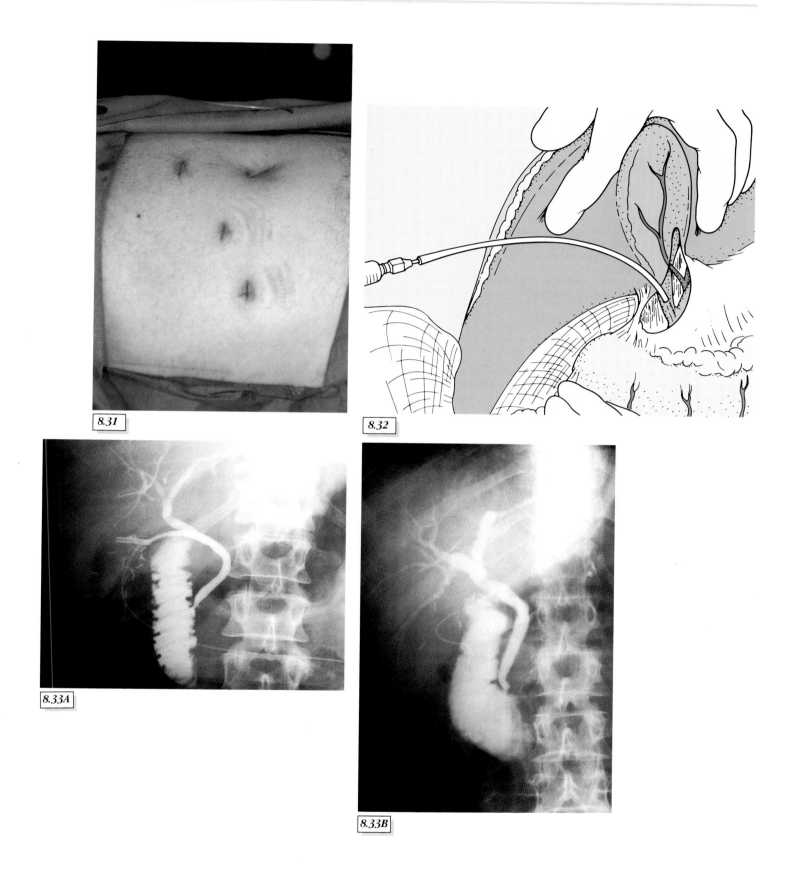

8.31

8.32

8.33A

8.33B

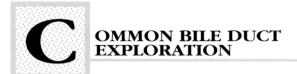

COMMON BILE DUCT EXPLORATION

COMMON BILE DUCT EXPLORATION

INDICATIONS	• obstructive jaundice • cholangitis • palpable stone in the common bile duct • positive cholangiogram showing either filling defects in the common bile duct or no egress of contrast medium into the duodenum (Fig. 8.34) • retained common duct stones postcholecystectomy (not a candidate for, or having failed ERCP)
ANESTHESIA	• general endotracheal
POSITIONING	• supine
PREP	• antibiotic coverage when infection is suspected • vigorous fluid resuscitation in the patient with jaundice and/or cholangitis • correction of coagulation defects • no surgery until patient is hemodynamically stable; if patient is too unstable for general anesthetic, biliary tree drainage rarely may be accomplished by transhepatic or transsphincteric routes

PROCEDURE

Common bile duct (with stones) exploration generally is a part of a cholecystectomy when there is a positive operative cholangiogram (Fig. 8.34). It uses a right subcostal, midline, or right paramedian incision (see Fig. 8.1). The incision and abdominal packing used to expose the gallbladder and the portal area are described in the section on cholecystectomy (see page 8.2).

The patient who is operated on for jaundice or cholangitis should have the etiology of their problem delineated prior to committing to cholecystectomy. With modern imaging techniques, the absence of a relatively firm preoperative diagnosis is unusual. In the case of obstructive jaundice due to bile duct, duodenal, or pancreatic malignancies, the gallbladder may be used to perform the biliary–enteric bypass. It should be carefully preserved until the common bile duct has been inspected and the site for the biliary bypass decided. In this setting, the operative cholangiogram may be obtained using a small, 23- to 25-gauge, butterfly needle inserted into the common bile duct or the common hepatic duct in the direction in which it will lie without impingement of its tip (Fig. 8.35). This is most easily accomplished by placing the needle tip toward the liver. With careful support of the needle within the bile duct, the abdominal packs are removed and the retracted liver surface is allowed to rest gently on the butterfly catheter. The radiographs are obtained as described for operative cholangiogram (see previous section).

Next the bile duct must be carefully exposed, with the surgeon keeping in mind that many anatomic variations of this area are possible. If the cystic duct has not already been identified and followed to the cystic duct–common bile duct junction as part of the cholecystectomy, the peritoneum overlying the ampulla of the gallbladder may now be incised. Then, using blunt dissection, the ductal structures can be delineated without any ligation. The common duct is also identifiable by needle aspiration of bile (Fig. 8.36). The blood supply to the bile duct enters through small vessels along its sides. Therefore, to avoid damage to the supply and the later development of a stricture, dissection in the area should be minimal. Once the duct is identified, two stay sutures approximately 2 mm apart of 4–0 chromic or other fine absorbable suture are placed horizontally on the anterior surface of the duct. The surgeon and the assistant each hold a suture, and a #11 blade is used to make an opening between the two stay sutures in the duct (Fig. 8.37). Potts scissors are then used to enlarge the opening to approximately 1 to 1.5 cm in the longitudinal direction (Fig. 8.38).

The surgeon may perform choledochoscopy at this time to identify the location of the stone or obstructing lesion. Flexible and rigid scopes are available. An 8- or 10-French red rubber catheter is used to irrigate the common bile duct. The catheter is passed gently into the liver and warm irrigation is instilled as it is withdrawn. Irrigation is then repeated in the duodenal direction. Small stones may be flushed out. The tube may pass into the duodenum showing no ductal obstruction. Ballooning of the duodenum may occur from the presence of instilled irrigating solution.

Next, a small biliary Fogarty balloon (#4) catheter is passed into the liver and is gently inflated until some resistance is met to its gentle withdrawal. The surgeon carefully controls the pressure within the balloon to avoid damage to the delicate hepatic ducts. An attempt is made to direct the catheter into the right and left ductal systems. The catheter is then placed in the opposite direction. Often it enters the duodenum easily and the balloon can be palpated within its lumen. The pressure is released enough to pull the balloon back through the ampulla and then it is gently reinflated. Stones can be dislodged and brought back toward the choledochotomy as the balloon is withdrawn in the inflated position (Fig. 8.39).

If these procedures have cleared the bile duct of stones identified by cholangiogram, and if the surgeon is satisfied that the ampulla is adequately patent, the bile duct may be closed over the largest T-tube that it can accommodate. For later possible radiologic manipulation, at least a 14-French T-tube is desirable. The limbs of the T-tube usually are shortened to about 2 to 3 cm and a small wedge is cut from the top of the "T" to allow for easier removal. The duct is then closed using interrupted simple sutures of a fine absorbable material (4–0 chromic or PDS), with very small bites taken on either side of the duct. The last suture is placed at the mid-tube level such that when the suture is tied, the tube is pushed tightly against the hepatic end of the choledochotomy and is secured in a watertight fashion (Fig. 8.40). A completion cholangiogram can be obtained through the T-tube to confirm extraction of all stones and the free flow of contrast medium into the duodenum.

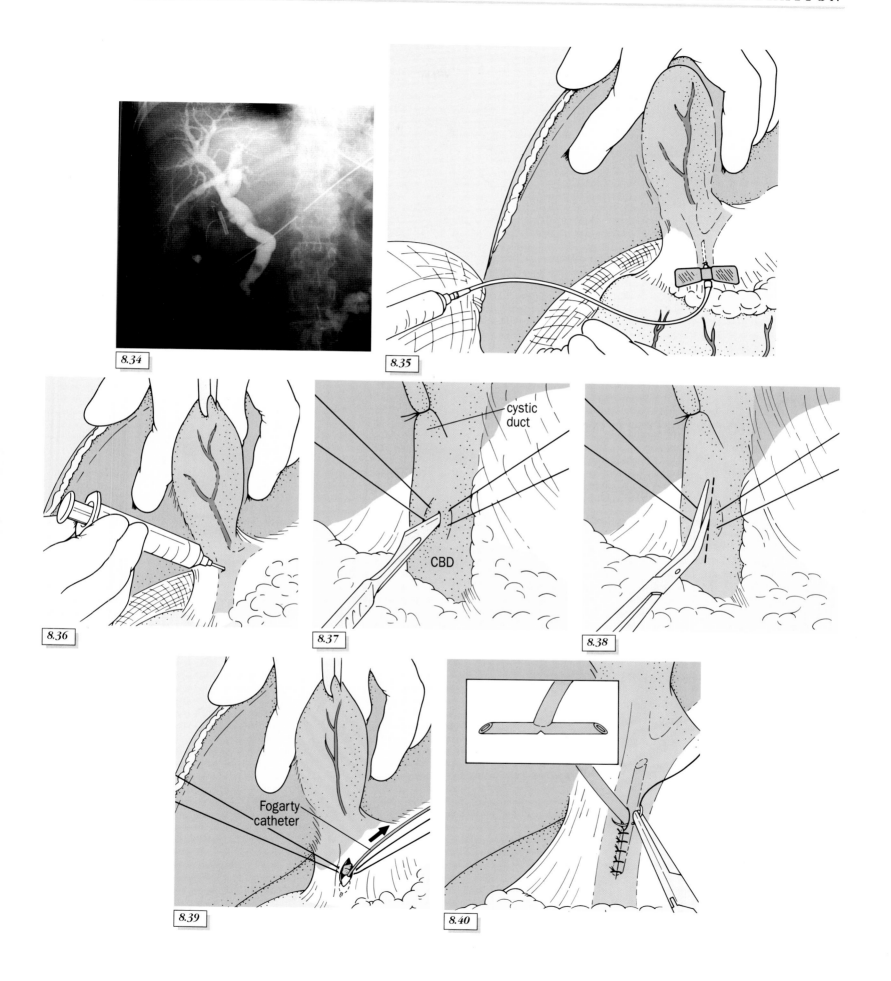

8.34

8.35

8.36

8.37

cystic
duct

CBD

8.38

8.39

Fogarty
catheter

8.40

If the above flushing and Fogarty maneuvers have failed to clear the duct, more rigorous duct exploration becomes necessary using stone forceps and scoops to extract or crush the stone material. In such a case, the duodenum should be freed from its investing peritoneal attachments and it should be elevated and retracted medially so that the surgeon may hold the duodenum and pancreatic head with one hand while manipulating the necessary instruments with the other. This is called the Kocher maneuver (Fig. 8.41), which is mentioned many times throughout this atlas. It is used to gain exposure of the area for a variety of reasons.

The lateral border of the duodenum is now identified and the peritoneum is incised. A right-angle clamp may be used to elevate the tissue and electrocautery used to incise it, thereby gaining exposure of the retroperitoneal duodenum, pancreatic head, and vena cava (Fig. 8.42). Many small blood vessels run in this area and blunt dissection may cause bleeding.

Ampullary patency may be tested with a Bakes dilator, using at most a #4. The passing of larger dilators has been associated with postoperative pancreatitis. When the surgeon is satisfied that the stones have been removed and that the ampulla is open, the duct is closed and T-tube cholangiography is performed as described previously. If duct patency cannot be obtained, consideration can be given to biliary diversions, such as choledochoenterostomy, choledochoduodenostomy (see page 8.22), or sphincteroplasty (see page 6.28).

CHOLECYSTOSTOMY

	CHOLECYSTOSTOMY
INDICATIONS	•same as for cholecystectomy (see page 8.2) with the addition that patient is unable to withstand general anesthesia and/or gallbladder removal upon exploration is too dangerous or difficult due to severe inflammation or abscess, hemorrhage, or intrahepatic location of the gallbladder with or without the above complicating factors
ANESTHESIA	•local infiltration of long-acting anesthetic agent such as bupivacaine hydrochloride, with sedation as tolerated, or general endotracheal
POSITIONING	•supine on an x-ray table
PREP	•preoperative antibiotics •hemodynamic stabilization

PROCEDURE

Cholecystostomy is performed to decompress an acute cholecystitis, extract stones, and provide access to the gallbladder for the future removal of any retained stones. It is occasionally done when cholecystectomy has been abandoned for technical reasons. The preferred surgical incision is a right subcostal one (see Fig. 8.1). Rarely, a paramedian or midline incision is used. If the procedure is performed under local anesthesia, the exposure obtained by the previously described packing technique (see Fig. 8.3) may have to be abandoned if it causes the patient discomfort. As there is no need to expose the hilar structures, if the gallbladder fundus is within easy reach of the incision, the deeper packing and retraction may not be necessary.

Retractors and packs are inserted slowly, with steady tension applied until exposure is achieved. The gallbladder is identified and all adhesions are lysed such that the fundus is mobilized into the midportion of the wound, where possible, by grasping it with a Kelly clamp. Packs are placed around the gallbladder to prevent abdominal contamination. A pursestring suture, 2 cm in diameter, is placed using 0–Vicryl as our preference. With the suture in place, the gallbladder can be drained using a trocar (see Fig. 8.6) or it can be incised and drained with suction. The bile should be sent for Gram's stain and aerobic and anaerobic cultures.

The edges of the cholecystostomy are then grasped with two long Babcock clamps, as stones are extracted with irrigation and suction, forceps, and scoops. Ideally, in acute cholecystitis, the stone obstructing the cystic duct should be removed. However, as it is not always possible, attempts at its removal should be abandoned if they are not quickly successful. A mushroom catheter with the tip cut off is then placed through the cholecystostomy and is secured with the pursestring suture (Fig. 8.43). With the tip removed, easy access to the gallbladder is possible later if necessary. The flange of the catheter is helpful in preventing inadvertent catheter removal in the postoperative period. Demonstration that the closure is watertight is achieved by gentle irrigation of the tube. A cholangiogram can be performed through the tube at the time of surgery or in the postoperative period. Usually with the patient under local anesthesia, additional manipulation at the operating table is not advisable. Additional stones can be extracted at a later date by the interventional radiologist. If communication is demonstrated to the common bile duct, and if unsuspected common bile duct stones are detected, they can be observed or approached by endoscopic retrograde cholangiopancreatography and/or by lithotripsy, if the clinical condition warrants intervention.

The cholecystostomy tube is brought out of the abdominal cavity through a separate stab wound convenient to the gallbladder location. A drain is not necessary in most cases where it was possible to anchor the gallbladder to the peritoneal wall, unless a subhepatic abscess was present. A closed system drain is used if the gallbladder cannot be brought up to the peritoneal surface. Closure is as described with cholecystectomy (see page 8.2).

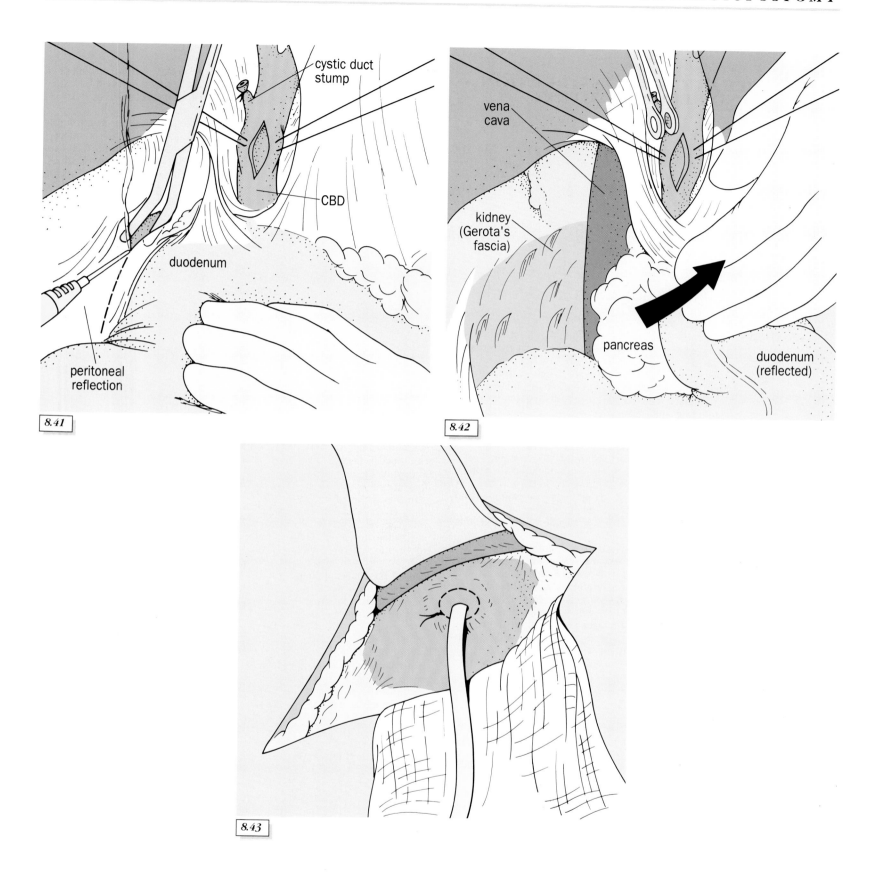

8.41

8.42

8.43

B ILE DUCT RECONSTRUCTION AND RECONSTITUTION

General indications for the procedures discussed in this section—choledo-chocholedochostomy, choledochojejunostomy, choledochoduodenostomy, portoenterostomy, and hepatico-jejunostomy—are presented as a group and reflect significant overlap among certain aspects of the techniques. Specific indications for the procedures are discussed separately, while the operations themselves are discussed individually in the Procedure section. These operations are among the more common ones performed by the general surgeon as well as by the hepatobiliary specialist. Complex hepatobiliary reconstructions are not addressed here.

BILE DUCT RECONSTRUCTION AND RECONSTITUTION

GENERAL INDICATIONS	• bile duct injury • bile duct excision due to choledochocyst, bile duct malignancy, or as part of total or partial pancreatectomy • bile duct stricture due to trauma, surgery, malignancy • bile duct obstruction due to pancreatic, biliary, or duodenal malignancies; chronically impacted gallstones; or ampullar stricture
SPECIFIC INDICATIONS	choledochocholedochostomy (Fig. 8.44) • liver transplantation • immediate bile duct reconstruction in trauma or iatrogenic bile duct injury, although most would favor a choledochojejunostomy in this circumstance, unless the bile duct injury was minimal and there was little if any loss of length choledochojejunostomy (end-to-side anastomosis) (Fig. 8.45) • bile duct excision (see General Indications) • liver transplantation where either insufficient donor or recipient bile duct is available or suitable for choledochocholedochostomy choledochojejunostomy (Roux-en-Y side-to-side anastomosis) (Fig. 8.46) • bile duct stricture (see General Indications) • bile duct obstruction (see General Indications) cholecystojejunostomy (Roux-en-Y side-to-side anastomosis) (Figs. 8.47, 8.48) • same as for choledochojejunostomy (Roux-en-Y side-to-side anastomosis) • choledochoduodenostomy (side-to-side anastomosis) (Fig. 8.49) • bile duct stricture (see General Indications) • bile duct obstruction (see General Indications) portoenterostomy, hepatojejunostomy (Roux-en-Y end-to-side anastomosis) (Figs. 8.50, 8.51) • malignant tumors of the hepatic duct confluence (Klatskin tumor) • restoration of biliary flow following a high bile duct injury with complete obstruction • biliary atresia in neonates
ANESTHESIA	• general endotracheal
POSITIONING	• supine on an x-ray table
PREP	• preoperative intravenous antibiotics

PROCEDURE

A right subcostal, extended subcostal, bilateral subcostal, midline, or right paramedian incision is used. We prefer a right subcostal with the option for extension of the incision as the need for operative exposure dictates (Fig. 8.52; see also Fig. 8.1).

Common bile duct stricture is most often a result of iatrogenic injury during cholecystectomy usually for acute cholecystitis, but also may occur during elective cholecystectomy complicated by intraoperative hemorrhage. Bile duct injury also may occur in procedures performed on the duodenum or pancreas.

If the injury is recognized immediately and if there is little tissue loss, a choledochocholedochostomy may be performed. The incision may have to be extended to obtain adequate exposure. Hemostasis must be obtained. The ends of the bile duct to be anastomosed must be viable and easily approximated, and there can be no tension on this anastomosis. If these requirements are not met, the procedure should be abandoned.

The anastomosis should be performed using 4–0, 5–0, or 6–0 PDS suture depending on the size of the duct. Knots should be placed on the outside. The duct is handled minimally during the anastomosis. A T-tube is then placed through a separate incision, usually distal to the anastomosis if possible. The size of the tube depends on the size of the duct. There should be no tension placed on the inside of the anastomosis.

To place the tube, its proximal limb is guided gently through the anastomosis. The tube can also be placed after the posterior suture line is placed and tied (see Fig. 8.44A), with the anterior line then placed and tied over the tube (see Fig. 8.44B). This latter method is often more cumbersome, however, as the surgeon is then working around the tube in the operative field.

The tube should be left in place as a stent for a minimum of 6 weeks. A closed system drain, such as a Jackson–Pratt, should be left in a dependent position posterior to the anastomosis until the surgeon is sure that there is no bile leakage. A cholangiogram should be obtained on the seventh postoperative day.

An end-to-side choledochojejunostomy may be performed for several reasons (see Specific Indications). When a bile duct injury is recognized immediately and when the remaining bile duct tissue is inadequate for primary anastomosis, this procedure can be employed. Because the common bile duct in this circumstance is of normal caliber (0.5 to 1.0 cm), extreme care must be used in handling of the bile duct to prevent stricture. The anastomosis is stented, where possible, by a T-tube placed proximal to the anastomosis (see Fig. 8.45A). As an alternative, tube stenting through the jejunal limb with an adequately sized red rubber tube (usually 8-French) should be used (see Fig. 8.45B).

For biliary tree reconstruction following resection of a malignancy that caused obstructive jaundice, the duct usually measures from 1.2 to 3.0 cm in diameter and is much easier to handle. It has a thicker wall that holds a large caliber suture with larger bites. There is little chance of stricture in this setting and tube stenting is optional. In either case, a long-lasting but absorbable suture is preferred, such as PDS, whose size is dictated by the size of the common bile duct.

For biliary–enteric anastomoses, a Roux-en-Y jejunal limb is preferred. Where possible, we use a functional Roux-en-Y jejunostomy (see Fig. 8.47) as it is easier to perform with more reliable blood supply. In most cases, it should reach the anastomotic area easily, without tension. If there is any question of inadequate length or tension, a formal or traditional Roux-en-Y should be used (see Fig. 8.48). The method for construction of the traditional Roux-en-Y is described in Chapter 6.

The functional Roux-en-Y is a loop of jejunum that is deemed of adequate length to reach the anastomotic area. An enteroenterostomy is created such that the efferent limb of the biliary–enteric anastomosis will be approximately 40 cm in length. A linear cutting stapler (75 mm) is used to create the enteroenterostomy (Fig. 8.53A). The enterotomy is then closed with a linear stapler (Figs. 8.53B,C), and the afferent limb is closed distal to the enteroenterostomy with a linear stapler (Fig. 8.53D; see also Fig. 8.47).

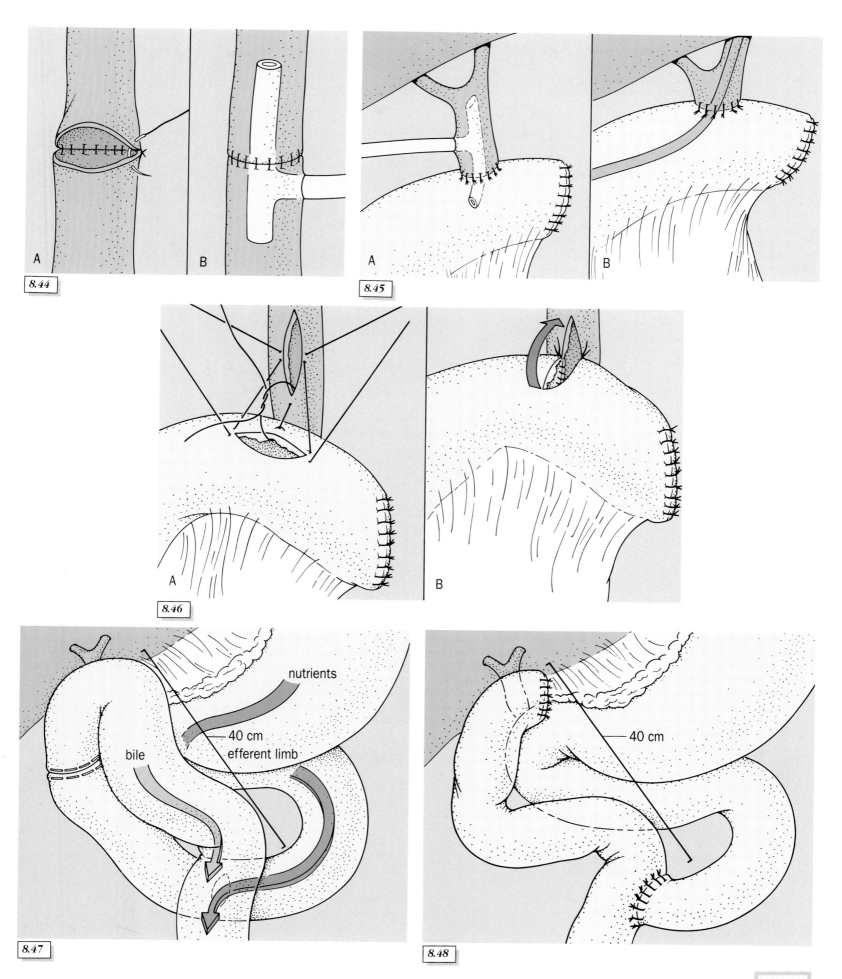

8.44

8.45

8.46

8.47

nutrients

40 cm
efferent limb

bile

8.48

40 cm

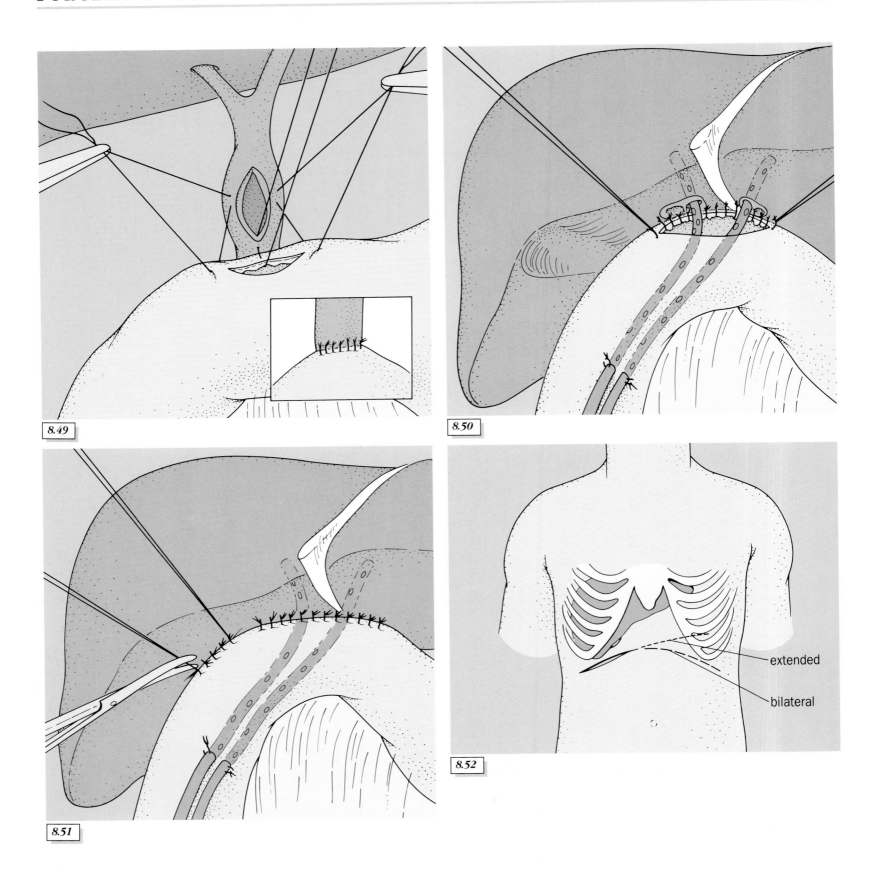

8.49

8.50

8.51

8.52

extended

bilateral

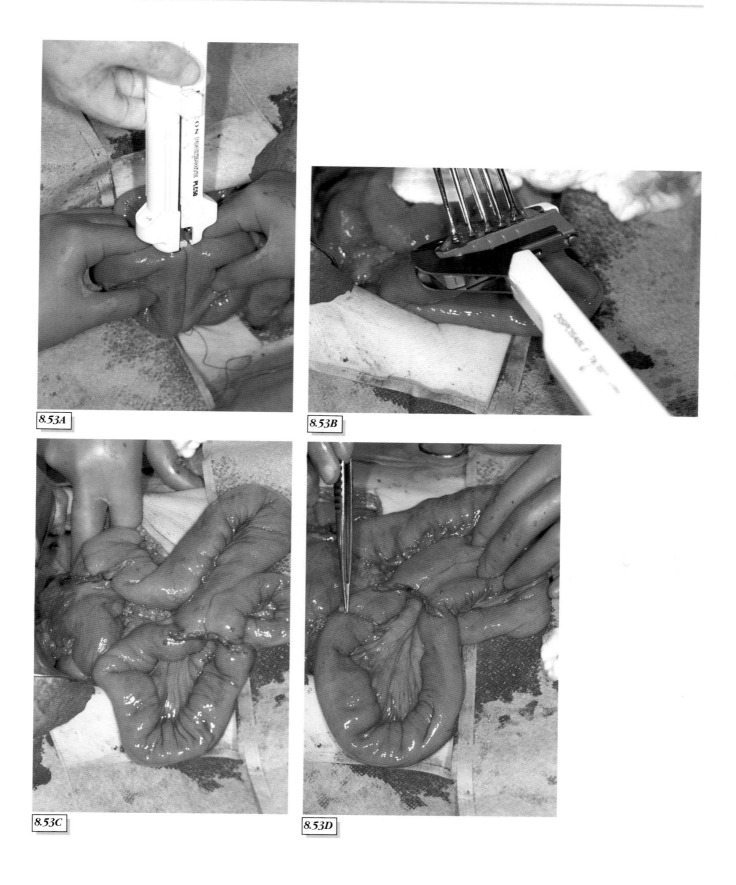

8.53A

8.53B

8.53C

8.53D

The biliary–enteric anastomosis can be performed in a similar fashion regardless of the construction used or the reason for the reconstruction. We routinely perform a seromuscular small bowel to full-thickness bile duct anastomosis using interrupted PDS suture, with caliber dictated by bile duct size. In smaller ducts, the knots should be placed on the outside, while with larger ducts the knots should be located for ease of tying or placement. The small bowel seromuscular layer is incised with cautery on its antimesenteric border for a length appropriate to the bile duct diameter. A hemostat or "mosquito clamp" is then used to spread the layer apart gently. The mucosa is allowed to pout out. Next, a small puncture is made in the mucosal layer, which is then spread to the length of the seromuscular incision (Fig. 8.54A).

Depending on the size of the duct and the ease of suture placement, the surgeon may tie the sutures as they are placed (Fig. 8.54B) or hold them (Fig. 8.54C). In general, it is helpful to place corner sutures first to orient oneself for placement of the remaining sutures in an orderly fashion, without twisting of the duct or creation of disparities. The distance between stitches is dependent on duct size and suture size. The aim is a watertight anastomosis with minimal tissue compromise. We feel that allowing the mucosa to pout out into the bile duct aids in creating a watertight anastomosis with a very low stricture rate. Figure 8.54D shows the placement of the red rubber catheter through the jejunum limb after the first sutures are placed. Figure 8.54E shows the completed choledochojejunostomy. Stent and drain placement has been discussed previously.

When the distal common bile duct requires bypass, several procedures are available. For malignant, nonresectable lesions of the pancreas, duodenum, or common bile duct, we prefer a choledochojejunostomy performed with a Roux-en-Y loop in a side-to-side fashion (see Figs. 8.46–8.48). Due to the insertion of the cystic duct in the lower third of the bile duct, anastomoses to the gallbladder for bypass may be occluded early if the tumor grows. Sometimes, as the massive distension of the biliary tree subsides, the cystic duct may occlude. In a palliative operation the aim should be to achieve the necessary goal of biliary decompression with the safest operation that will allow the best long-term patency. We rely on cholecystojejunostomy only when we are unable to approach the common duct for technical reasons (Fig. 8.55). Similarly, choledochoduodenostomy has been used for bypass in malignant obstruction, as well as in stone or stricture obstruction. We feel that it should not be used in the former case. Since the anastomotic area in choledochoduodenostomy again is closer to the expanding tumor than in a choledochojejunostomy, it could re-obstruct. An alternative to choledochoduodenostomy for benign distal ductal stricture is transduodenal sphincteroplasty, which is described in Chapter 6.

For a choledochojejunostomy and a cholecystojejunostomy, the Roux-en-Y loop is prepared as described previously. The choledochojejunostomy can be performed with or without a cholecystectomy for bypass of the obstructed biliary system, although, in general, the procedure is easier to perform if the markedly dilated gallbladder is removed. The gallbladder should not be removed until the surgeon is sure that the common bile duct is accessible for anastomosis. The bile duct is incised for a distance of approximately 2 to 2.5 cm. The functional diameter of the anastomosis is determined by the cross-sectional diameter of the common bile duct. To enable the loop to lay in the position of least tension, the midportion of the enterotomy is used as the corners with respect to the choledochotomy.

The first sutures of the side-to-side anastomosis are tied after the three distal corner stitches are placed (see Fig. 8.46A). Depending on the exposure, the remaining sutures can be placed, held, and tied later or tied as

they are placed until the proximal corner is reached (see Fig. 8.46B). If the surgeon chooses to hold the sutures, care must be taken to prevent them from tangling and locking. Stenting is optional in the dilated bile duct. We generally use a closed system drain for several days postoperatively.

If the gallbladder is used for anastomosis, a longitudinal incision of a convenient length is made in both the gallbladder and the antimesenteric side of the small bowel, usually at least 3 cm. The anastomosis is carried out using a single layer of interrupted PDS or silk suture, either 4–0 or 3–0 (Fig. 8.56).

A choledochoduodenostomy is also performed in a similar fashion to that described earlier for choledochojejunostomy. A longitudinal choledochotomy is made in the distal common bile duct. The duodenum is freed from its lateral peritoneal attachments (the Kocher maneuver; see Fig. 8.41) and is bluntly displaced anteriorly. The enterotomy is made on the antimesenteric border in a longitudinal fashion, allowing the mucosa to pout up. The midportion of the lateral aspect of the enterotomy is then sutured to the distal common bile duct corner (see Fig. 8.49). Interrupted 3–0 silk or 4–0 PDS suture is used. The anastomosis is then completed as described for choledochojejunostomy.

With very high bile duct strictures or with obstructing tumors of the bile duct, reconstruction often must be performed at the level of the right and left hepatic ducts (Fig. 8.57). We have also coupled resection of tumors of the bifurcation of the bile ducts (Klatskin tumor) with partial hepatectomy to excise a more extensively involved unilateral duct, where indicated.

Resection of these tumors is very tedious and should only be attempted by those who are intimately familiar with this anatomy. Details of the portal dissection are described later in this chapter. In the case of tumor or postoperative scarring, the natural planes between duct, artery, and portal vein may be obscured. Careful blunt dissection is used with incontinuity ligation of all small vessels and lymphatics running between the structures. It is imperative that the surgeon work in a bloodless field. Strictures that are usually the result of previous biliary surgery also are quite difficult to dissect proximally due to heavy scarring. In both of these situations, a previously placed percutaneous transhepatic catheter can prove useful in guiding the operative exploration (Fig. 8.58A). Where resection of a Klatskin tumor is not possible, the tube can serve as postoperative drainage. Later, it can be used as a transtumor route for placement of interstitial radiation. Subsequently, we have our interventional radiologists convert the tube to an internal drainage system through the tumor (Fig. 8.58B). Other tube drainage systems, such as the U-tube, have been described. They are placed operatively and can be changed as needed. However, with advances in interventional radiology, these devices are increasingly outmoded and therefore rarely employed. We believe that they have no advantage over the percutaneously placed devices.

Anastomosis to the proximal bile ducts following tumor or stricture resection is performed using a Roux-en-Y loop of jejunum. An attempt is made to suture seromuscular jejunal wall to full-thickness bile duct using 4–0 PDS suture (see Fig. 8.50). The jejunum also must be anchored to the fibrous tissues of the porta hepatis using a second row of suture (see Fig. 8.51), with 3–0 silk preferred. Both ductal systems are stented with red rubber tubes, which we try to maintain in place for at least 3 months. In the case of bile duct malignancies, the tubes also may be used to place interstitial radiation postoperatively. A closed system drain is left in the subhepatic space and the wound is closed in a standard fashion.

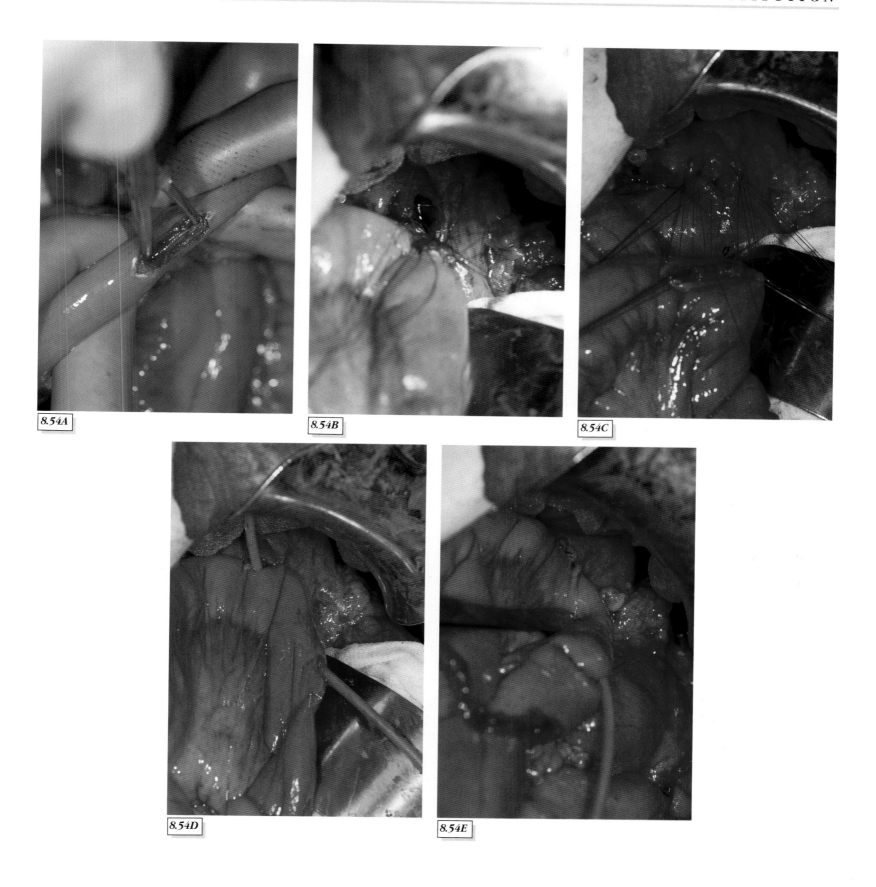

8.54A

8.54B

8.54C

8.54D

8.54E

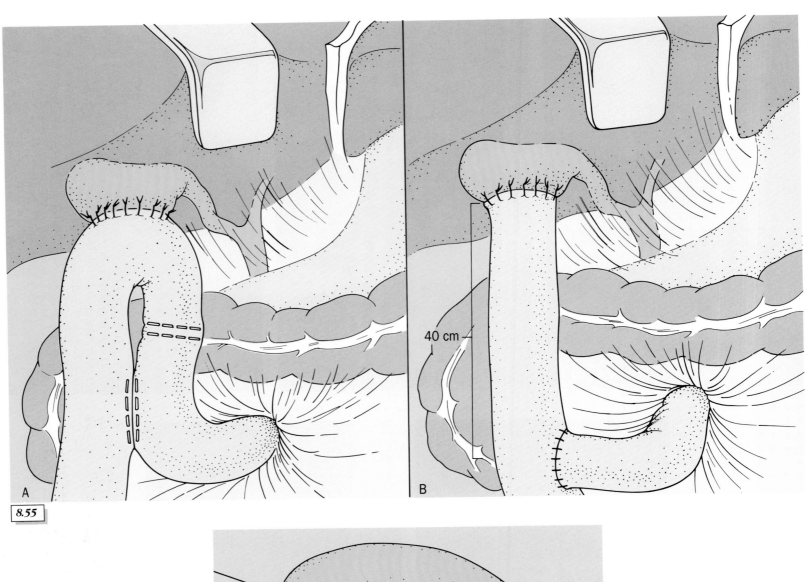

8.55

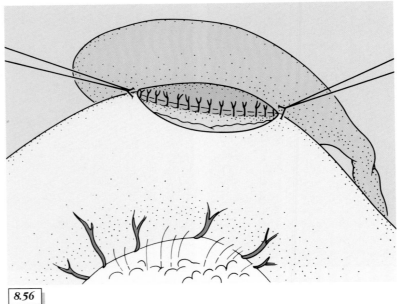

8.56

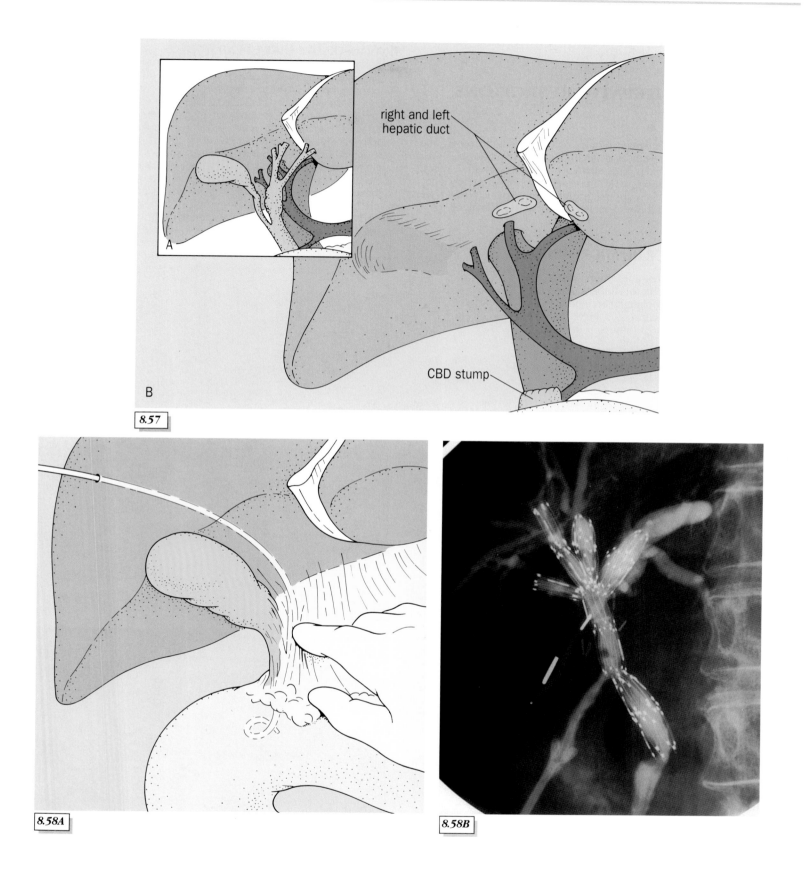

right and left
hepatic duct

A

CBD stump

B

8.57

8.58A

8.58B

MAJOR HEPATIC RESECTIONS

Surgery for benign and malignant tumors of the liver is becoming more commonplace and, with advances in technology and anesthesia, is done with very acceptable morbidity rates. Rather than proceed with a description of each specific operation, we will consider five major components of most liver operations and then approach surgery for specific types of hepatic resections by applying these elements in various combinations.

MAJOR HEPATIC RESECTIONS	

INDICATIONS	• malignant tumors, such as
	  • hepatocellular carcinoma
	  • cholangiocarcinoma
	  • metastatic cancer
	• benign tumors, if there is
	  • bleeding
	  • pain
	• hemangiomas, if associated with
	  • pain
	  • thrombocytopenia
	  • fever

ANESTHESIA	• general endotracheal ✓
POSITIONING	• patient elevated 15° right side up from supine (see below)
PREP	• preoperative CT scan • liver function tests • coagulation tests • angiogram

BASIC SURGICAL TECHNIQUES

THE INCISION

The majority of liver resections can be performed through a subcostal incision, which we prefer. When tumors are very large, when the patient is obese, or when the underlying lesion is malignant, the incision can be extended into the right thorax to afford better access, particularly to the area of the hepatic veins. Preferably, it is extended into the right eighth intercostal space (Fig. 8.59), thereby allowing division of the diaphragm back to the hiatus through which the hepatic veins pass. Extensions of the subcostal incision to the xiphisternum have been found to be of little help in affording extra exposure where it is critically necessary, in the region of the confluence of the vena cava and the hepatic vein. In our hospital, we prefer the Bookwalter retractor system (Fig. 8.60), which is set up after the incision is completed.

MOBILIZATION OF THE LIVER

Once it appears by visualization and palpation that surgery will be possible, mobilization of the liver begins. Division of the left triangular ligament usually is performed first, thus allowing mobilization of the left lobe of the liver. The ligament is divided to the esophageal hiatus with care taken to avoid the phrenic vein, which is often a direct tributary to the vena cava. The round ligament is divided as far superiorly as the peritoneal reflection. The right triangular ligament is then divided back to the bare area, allowing marked downward displacement of the right lobe of the liver. With all three ligaments separated, the liver is adequately mobilized (Fig. 8.61).

INTRAOPERATIVE ULTRASOUND

Following mobilization, the definitive procedure is not undertaken until intraoperative ultrasound of the liver has been performed (Fig. 8.62). The ultrasonographer is present in the operating suite during this portion of the procedure for interpretive guidance. Our experience has shown that, in 25% of cases, the findings of intraoperative ultrasonography have changed the planned operative procedure. In addition, ultrasound can be employed repeatedly without hazard to the patient or to operating room personnel. Using ultrasound guidance, suspicious lesions not previously appreciated, as well as additional unsuspected lesions, can be found, and if necessary, sampled for histologic examination before a major hepatic resection is undertaken. Moreover, lesions that were identified preoperatively but are not palpable at surgery can be localized accurately by ultrasound. We emphasize that intraoperative ultrasonography must be performed after mobilization of the liver to enable access to all areas. Figure 8.63 shows a hepatic adenoma (arrow) found on intraoperative ultrasound. The opposing arrows show the shadowing behind the mass. Figure 8.64 shows a tumor (arrow) just below the liver surface.

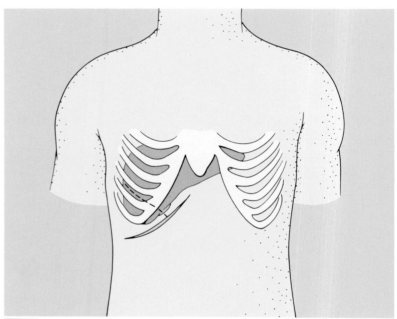

8.59

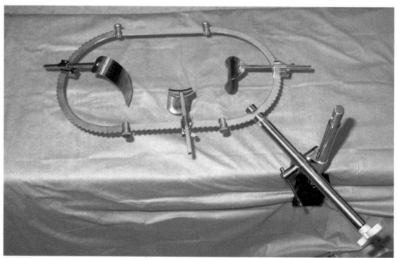

8.60

Bookwalter Retractor

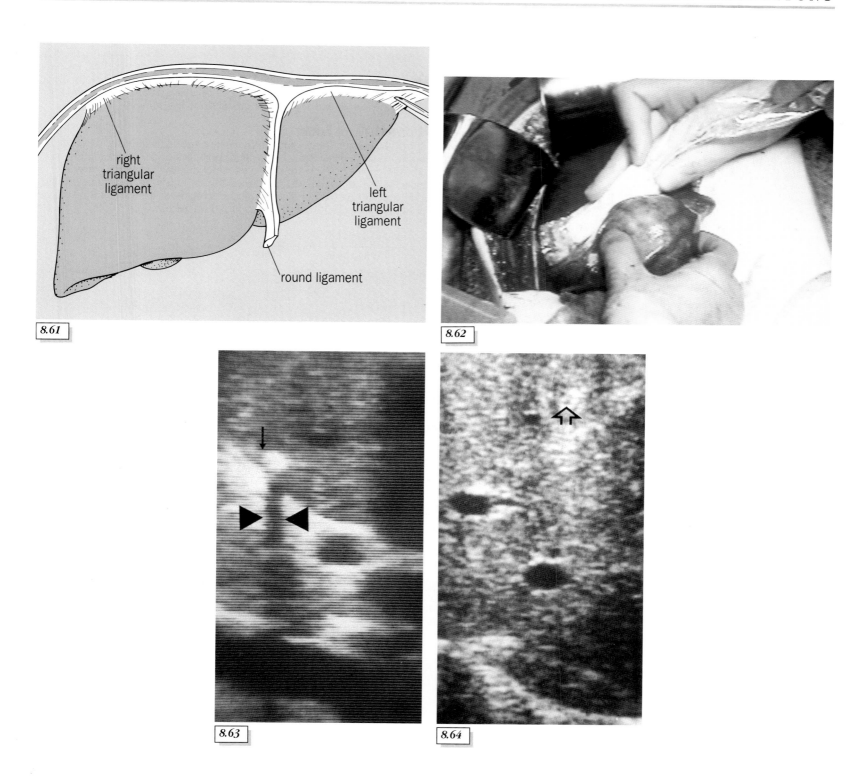

8.61

right triangular ligament

left triangular ligament

round ligament

8.62

8.63

8.64

PORTAL DISSECTION

When it appears that a lobectomy is required, a formal portal dissection is carried out. The usual relationships between the hepatic artery, portal vein, and common bile ducts are well known in the right lateral end of the hepatoduodenal ligament (Fig. 8.65). They represent the anterior lip of the foramen of Winslow, which leads into the lesser peritoneal cavity.

In general, dissection of the artery is done first since it is the most accessible, it is pulsatile, and it lends itself to sharp dissection. An angiogram, which is usually performed preoperatively, is of great help in identifying in advance any anomalies or variations in vascular anatomy. The artery is then traced to its bifurcation into right and left branches and dissected, followed by dissection and division of the portal vein. Because the common hepatic duct bifurcation often occurs just beneath the right branch of the artery, division of the duct is held until last because its dissection is facilitated by the earlier dissection and division of the artery. In addition, because the duct is the most fragile, it is best left until last when there are no other obstructing structures.

For lesser procedures, such as a wedge resection or an enucleation (see below), formal portal dissection is not required. In this instance, the portal vein, hepatic artery, and common bile duct are encircled with a vessel loop and, with the use of tension tubing, are ligated by a controlled Pringle maneuver should there be excessive bleeding (Fig. 8.66). Up to one-half hour of warm ischemia time generally is acceptable.

CAVAL DISSECTION

Caval dissection can be performed either before or after portal triad dissection when the latter is required. One begins with identification of the retroperitoneal cava, which is behind the duodenum. Then, by careful dissection along the anterior surface of the cava and with a lifting pressure on the previously mobilized liver, paired branches passing directly from the liver can be seen entering the anterior surface of the cava. These branches arise directly from the caudate lobe, and usually comprise three to five pairs. They are ligated by careful passage of 3–0 silk sutures using right-angle carriers, with the additional application of clips placed within the space afforded by the two silk ligatures to avoid their migration (Fig. 8.67). As one follows the hepatic branches cephalad, they lead to the hepatic veins. Rarely can the right or left hepatic vein be identified and secured separately in an extrahepatic position since bifurcation of these veins usually occurs intrahepatically. Therefore, we do not dissect the hepatic vein–caval junction extensively. Bleeding in this region is life threatening and we prefer to secure the hepatic veins intrahepatically, distal to their bifurcation.

FRACTURE OF THE LIVER

In major hepatic resections, the final step is a fracture or separation of the liver. With portal and hepatic arterial ligation already achieved, the line of demarcation is easily appreciated and, where possible, liver fracture should occur within the ischemic area. An electrocautery (Bovie) is used to "score" the line of resection and to provide a demonstrable margin to reinforce the plan of the dissection. Using whatever instrument is easiest, the thumb and forefinger are introduced into the liver where they are squeezed together (Fig. 8.68). The hepatic parenchyma thus divides easily. Residual structures persisting after the "squeeze" represent vascular and ductal structures, which are then ligated using 3–0 or 4–0 silk. With a silk suture applied to the residual side, a clip is applied to the side that is to be resected. If the tributaries are large, silk ties are used on both sides.

This portion of the operation is possibly the longest. Referred to as a "finger" fracture, it is really more of a squeezing action. When it is done in a haphazard fashion, considerable bleeding can occur due to liver cross circulation and to the continued availability of blood to the liver through the hepatic venous system. Therefore, it is necessary to "settle in" to the technique, develop a rhythm, and with a thumb and fingerful at a time, proceed in a deliberate fashion with separation of the liver.

SPECIFIC OPERATIVE PROCEDURES

The anatomy of the liver is fairly well demarcated. An imaginary line between the gallbladder fossa and the hepatic vein–caval juncture separates the right and the left lobes while the round ligament divides the left

lobe into lateral and medial segments (Fig. 8.69). With these divisions in mind, one can then speak of right hepatic lobectomy, left hepatic lobectomy, trisegmentectomy (in which the medial segment of the left lobe along with the entire right lobe is resected), and left hepatic segmentectomy (in which only the lateral segment of the left lobe is removed).

RIGHT HEPATIC LOBECTOMY

In a right hepatic lobectomy, all ligaments are divided. Next, a portal dissection is carried out to ligate the right branches of the hepatic artery, portal vein, and common hepatic duct individually. Then the paired caval branches on the right side are likewise ligated and, by finger fracture, the lobectomy is carried out. Finger fracture should occur just within the plane of ischemia that follows ligation of all right branches (Fig. 8.70).

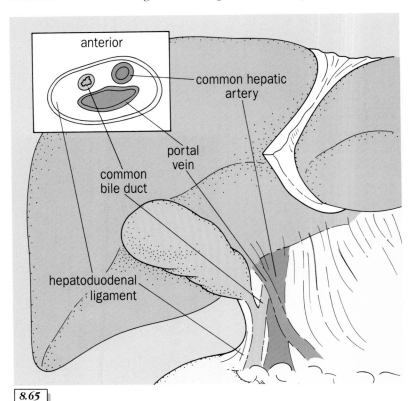

anterior

common hepatic artery

portal vein

common bile duct

hepatoduodenal ligament

8.65

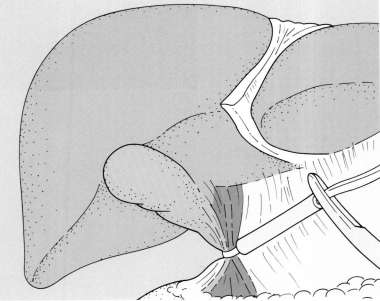

8.66

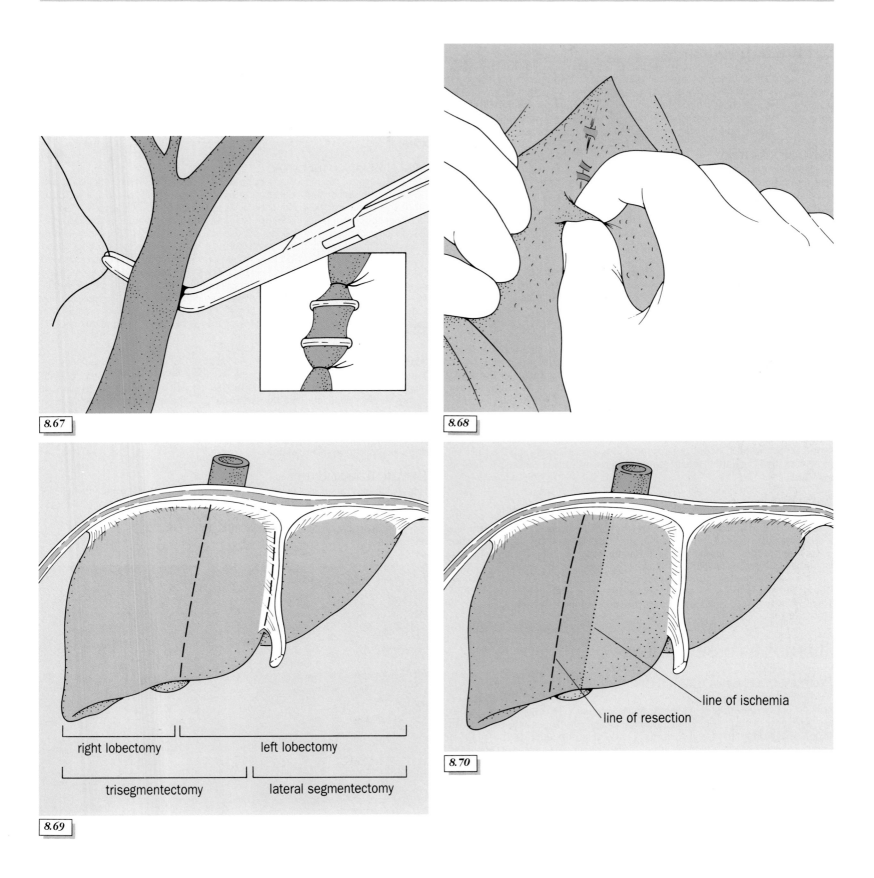

8.67

8.68

right lobectomy   left lobectomy

trisegmentectomy   lateral segmentectomy

8.69

line of ischemia

line of resection

8.70

LEFT HEPATIC LOBECTOMY

Again, division of all suspensory ligaments is performed, followed by portal dissection with securing of the left branches of the hepatic artery, portal vein, and common bile duct. Since the small paired vessels that go directly from the cava are mostly from the caudate lobe, which is mostly within the right lobe, securing of these small branches rarely is necessary in left hepatic lobectomy. Again, finger fracture of the liver occurs within the ischemic area.

TRISEGMENTECTOMY

Trisegmentectomy is the most difficult of the hepatic resections to perform and the most extensive. Great care should be taken to ensure that entirely adequate liver function exists and that there is no evidence of fibrotic change in the left lobe, to ensure adequate hepatic function during the critical phase prior to liver regeneration. The suspensory ligaments are divided, followed by division of both the right and the left paired branches entering the cava. Additional dissection must then be done, up along the left branch of the hepatic artery, portal vein, and left hepatic duct, to identify and secure the major branches going to the medial segment of the left lobe. A preoperative hepatic angiogram often is helpful and an intraoperative cholangiogram may be necessary to perform this additional critical extension of the portal dissection.

LEFT LATERAL SEGMENTECTOMY

Left lateral segmentectomy is probably the simplest of all liver resections. Division of all suspensory ligaments is carried out. A formal portal dissection is seldom necessary since encirclement and compression of the portal triad using a vessel compression loop is usually sufficient, if finger fracture of the lateral segment proves bloody.

WEDGE RESECTIONS AND LIVER BIOPSY

Wedge resections seldom require ligamentary division and since limited in scope do not require portal dissection of any type. Using finger fracture, the liver with the contained small tumor—almost always a surface lesion—is resected.

ENUCLEATION

For hemangiomas requiring resection, a formal wedge resection, in which a margin of normal liver tissue is removed, often is more than necessary. For a clear-cut diagnosis of hemangioma, one can proceed by sharp dissection along the external capsule of the hemangioma, dividing in the course all small vessels feeding into the structure (Fig. 8.71). As enucleation proceeds, the mass of vascular "tumor" undergoes collapse. Often it is possible, through use of a "pusher," to strip away the lining of the hemangioma from adjacent liver tissue, again securing all small feeding vessels in its course.

ADDITIONAL CONSIDERATIONS

POSTRESECTION CHOLANGIOGRAM

We have made it a practice to obtain a cholangiogram after all major resections. It is not done following lesser operations, such as lateral segmentectomy, wedge resection, or hemangioma enucleation. The method following major resection is to use the stump of the resected duct as the point of entry. A small vascular clamp is applied distally, thus ensuring that the injection will proceed into the hepatic radicals. The purpose of the postresectional cholangiogram is less to detect small bile leaks, which are inevitable, than to verify patency and integrity of the ductal system (Fig. 8.72). If, in the course of cholangiography, a major leak is identified, attempted oversewing is carried out. Small leaks are left for spontaneous closure and the resultant bile collections are taken care of adequately by the use of large drains.

DRAINS

We prefer two large Jackson–Pratt drains, one in the lesser sac and one in the right suprarenal fossa (Figs. 8.73, 8.74). The two drains are left in place until the patient has resumed a regular diet and, at that point, advanced. We have had a 7% incidence of large bile and/or blood collections following drain removal. However, in all such cases, there was subsequent drainage percutaneously under ultrasound or CT scan guidance and reoperation was not required.

ARGON BEAM COAGULATOR

The new argon beam electrocoagulation unit differs from the standard Bovie instrument in that it emits a stream of argon gas from the applicator on to the surface to be coagulated and, in the medium of the gas, achieves electrocoagulation (Fig. 8.75). Its two outstanding advantages include the fact that the surface to be coagulated is cleared immediately of blood and fluid, thereby allowing clear visualization. Additionally, because coagulation occurs in the gas medium on the surface of the structure, less tissue damage occurs. Vessels measuring as large as 3 mm in outside diameter can be coagulated by this process, which has greatly facilitated surgery for resection of solid organs such as the liver and spleen. One can also place hemostatic materials such as methyl-cellulose pads or surgical tapes on the surface in question, and by application of the argon beam coagulator "bond" the hemostatic materials to the surface.

STORM LONGMIRE CLAMP

The Storm Longmire clamp (Fig. 8.76) is of help in major resections. Because of gentle compression afforded by its malleable inner jaws, it allows direct visualization of the cut surface of the liver and surface ligation under direct vision. Unfortunately, it cannot always be used when the liver is particularly rounded, in which case it is most likely safer to compress the cut edge of the liver between the hands of an assistant than to risk disruption by application of the clamp.

HEPATIC REGENERATION

Hepatic regeneration is a fortunate accompaniment when sufficient healthy liver tissue is left behind. While the precise mechanisms for hepatic regeneration are unknown, certainly an intact portal venous system is necessary. An insulin or insulin-like protein is thought to be a likely cofactor in liver regeneration.

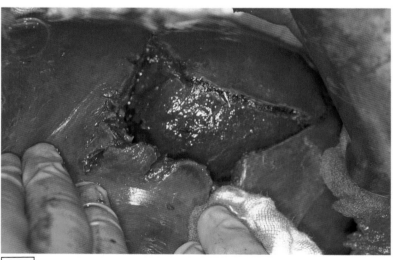

8.71

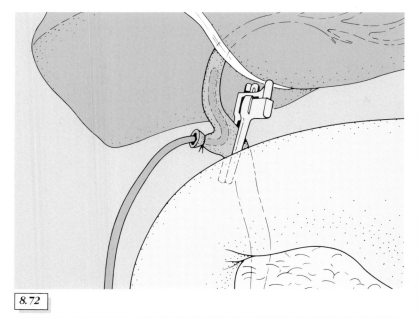

8.72

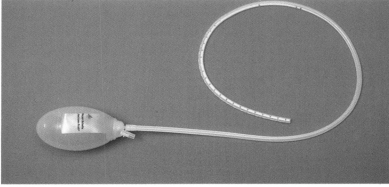

8.73

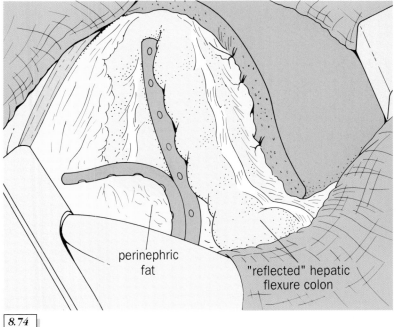

perinephric fat

"reflected" hepatic flexure colon

8.74

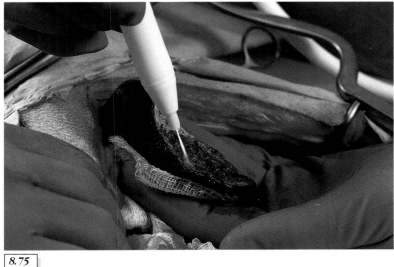

8.75

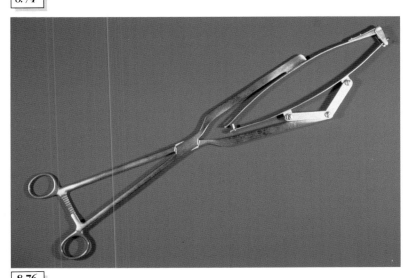

8.76

BIBLIOGRAPHY

Blumgart LH, Kelley CJ. Benign bile duct stricture following cholecystectomy: critical factors in management. *Br J Surg* 1984; 71:836–843.

Broder IW, Dowling JB, Koontz KK, Litwim MS. Early management of operative injuries of the extrahepatic biliary tract. *Ann Surg* 1987; 205:649–658.

Cameron JL. *Atlas of Surgery*, Vol I. Philadelphia, Pa: Decker; 1990.

Longmire WP, Thompkins RK. *Manual of Liver Surgery*. New York: Springer-Verlag; 1981.

McDermott WV, ed. *Surgery of the Liver*. Boston, Ma: Blackwell Scientific Publications; 1989.

Nyhus LM, Baker RJ, eds. *The Mastery of Surgery*. Boston, Ma: Little, Brown & Co; 1984.

O'Neill JA, Templeton JM, Schnaufer L, Bishop HC, Ziegler MM, Ross AG (III). Recent experience with choledochal cyst. *Ann Surg* 1987; 205:533–540.

Ottow RT, August DA, Sugarbaker PH. Treatment of proximal biliary tract carcinoma: an overview of technique and results. *Surgery* 1985; 97(1):251–261.

9

Surgery of the Colon, Rectum, and Anus

Scott D. Goldstein • Maryalice Cheney

ANORECTAL SURGERY
SURGICAL ANATOMY (FIG. 9.1)

ANORECTAL SURGERY

The following are the same for all anorectal procedures discussed, unless otherwise noted.

ANESTHESIA
- spinal used for treatment of abscess or complicated fistula
- general endotracheal rarely necessary
- local with intravenous sedation used in 90% of anorectal surgical procedures (bupivacaine HCl, with epinephrine 1:200,000 to aid in local hemostasis and 2 ampules of hyaluronidase 300 IU to decrease tissue swelling and diffuse local anesthetic into surrounding tissue; bupivacaine is longer acting than lidocaine but more painful on injection)

POSITIONING
- prone jackknife

PREP
- 3- to 4-inch tapes applied to perirectal region to provide lateral traction of buttocks and exposure of anal canal (Fig. 9.2)

DRAINAGE AND EXCISION OF FISTULOUS ABSCESSES

The majority of anorectal fistulous abscesses are cryptoglandular in origin. Almost all originate posteriorly in the region of maximum density of the anorectal glands. All anorectal abscesses require prompt drainage at the time of diagnosis. Delay in treatment (to allow time for "pointing") can only result in further destruction of normal tissue and possibly in incontinence. Two-thirds of all anorectal abscesses treated by simple excision and drainage recur as fistulas in ano. One-third are cured.

DRAINAGE AND EXCISION OF FISTULOUS ABSCESSES

EXAMINATION
- inspection and digital rectal, then Hill-Ferguson retractor (Fig. 9.3 bottom) and Pratt retractor (Fig. 9.3 top) inserted
- Goodsall's Rule is a standard aid during the examination:
  - cutaneous openings posterior to the line dividing the anus in the horizontal plane drain internally to the posterior midline at or distal to the dentate line (Fig. 9.4)
  - cutaneous openings anterior to line dividing anus in horizontal plane drain internally in a radial direction to or distal to the dentate line (Fig. 9.4)

INDICATIONS
- evidence of perianal suppuration or induration
- chronic asymptomatic fistulas

PROCEDURE

Using a 25- to 30-gauge needle, a local anesthetic is injected perianally in a subcutaneous plane (Fig. 9.5). Following this, the anal orifice should become mildly patulous. Next, submucosal injections of local anesthetic are administered to anesthetize the anal canal completely. This is done in four quadrants utilizing approximately 4 to 5 mL in each quadrant (Fig. 9.6).

The following figures illustrate two methods of draining anorectal fistulous abscesses: (1) saucerization (Fig. 9.7) and (2) primary fistulotomy (Fig. 9.8).

Care must be taken to avoid injury to the sphincter mechanism. The distal half of the internal sphincter muscle may be divided safely. Only the most superficial portion of the external sphincter muscle may be divided primarily without compromising the mechanism of continence. When a greater portion of muscle is involved, seton insertion (Fig. 9.9) and secondary fistulotomy is required (Fig. 9.10).

PARTIAL LATERAL INTERNAL SPHINCTEROTOMY

Anal fissure is a linear ulceration commencing at or just below the dentate (pectinate) line and extending distally to the anal verge (Fig. 9.10). One striking feature of this lesion, seen in 90% of cases, is its posterior midline location.

PARTIAL LATERAL INTERNAL SPHINCTEROTOMY

INDICATIONS
- anal fissure with persistent pain, lack of healing, or recurrence
- anal stenosis

PROCEDURE

Following infiltration of local anesthetic, a Pratt bivalve speculum is inserted into the anal canal, placing the sphincter mechanism on slight tension to facilitate identification of the internal and external sphincters. The distal portion of the internal sphincter is then isolated using the following technique. A stab wound incision is made in the intersphincteric groove (Fig. 9.11). Then, a narrow mucosal flap is created to the dentate line, isolating the sphincter medially (Fig. 9.12). The internal sphincter is isolated laterally using minimal dissection within the intersphincteric groove. With the internal sphincter completely isolated, the distal one-third of the internal sphincter is divided (Fig. 9.13). No suture is required. The wound is left open to facilitate drainage.

HEMORRHOIDECTOMY

Tissue commonly referred to as "hemorrhoids" is formed by three radially oriented arteriovenous tufts. There is an internal component covered by mucosa and an external component covered by skin. Internal hemorrhoids, which are normally located within the anal canal, can present with bleeding or prolapse. Operative management of internal hemorrhoids depends on their classification according to degree. External hemorrhoids (covered by perianal skin) can present with painful thrombosis. Without operative management, thrombotic external hemorrhoids resolve spontaneously in 1 to 3 weeks. However, a period of discomfort and a possible residual skin tag may follow.

EVACUATION OF EXTERNAL THROMBOTIC HEMORRHOIDS

EVACUATION OF EXTERNAL THROMBOTIC HEMORRHOIDS

INDICATIONS
- pain, bleeding, prevention of perianal skin tags

ANESTHESIA
- 1% lidocaine with epinephrine 1:200,000 and hyaluronidase 2 to 5 mL

PROCEDURE

This procedure can be performed in an outpatient setting. Following infiltration with local anesthesia into the tissue overlying the thrombosis, a radially placed ellipse of skin is removed (Fig. 9.14A), along with the underlying clot (Fig. 9.14B). The wound is left open to heal by second intention (Fig. 9.14C).

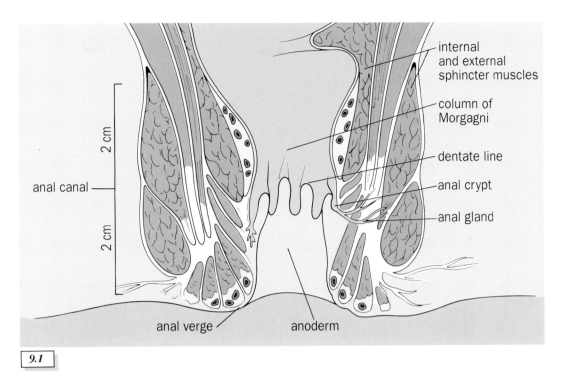

9.1

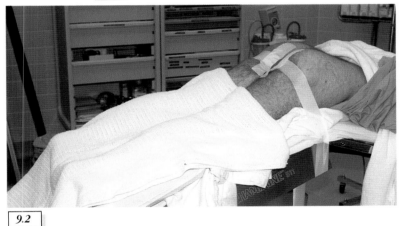

9.2

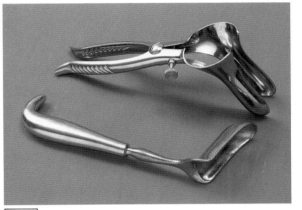

9.3

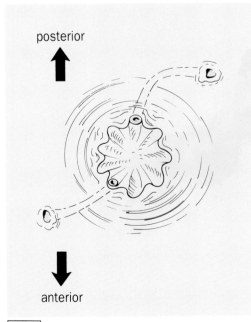

9.4

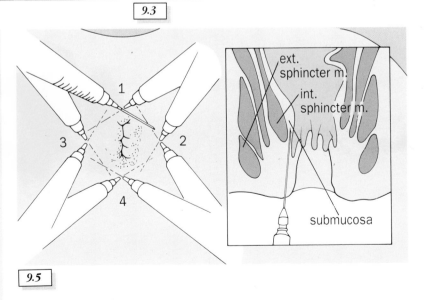

9.5

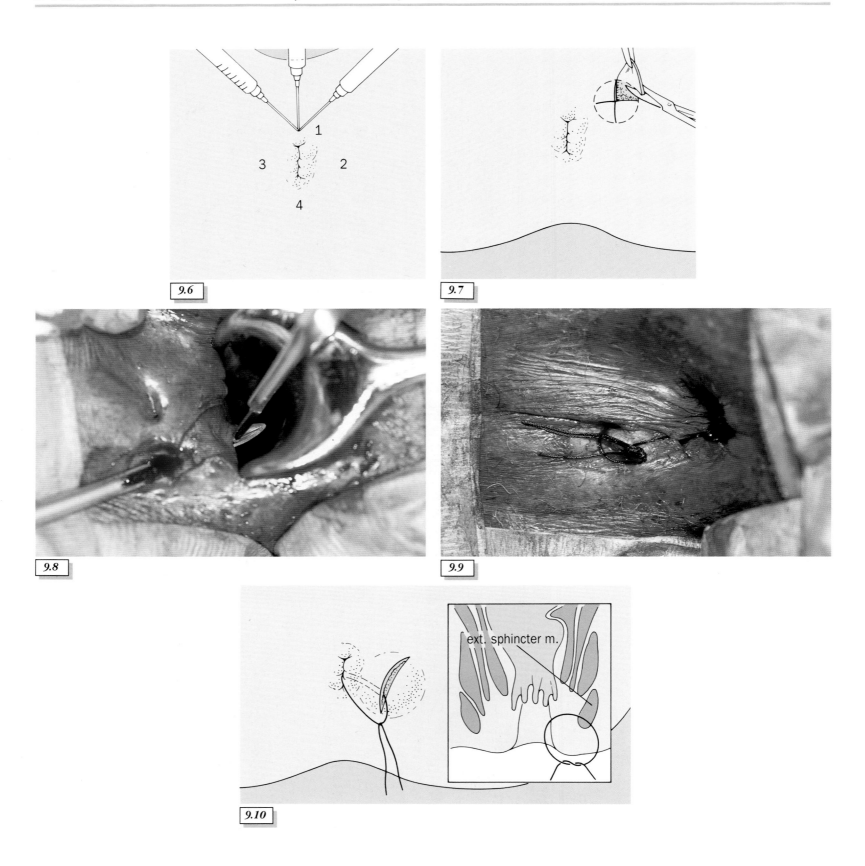

9.6

9.7

9.8

9.9

9.10

ext. sphincter m.

9.4

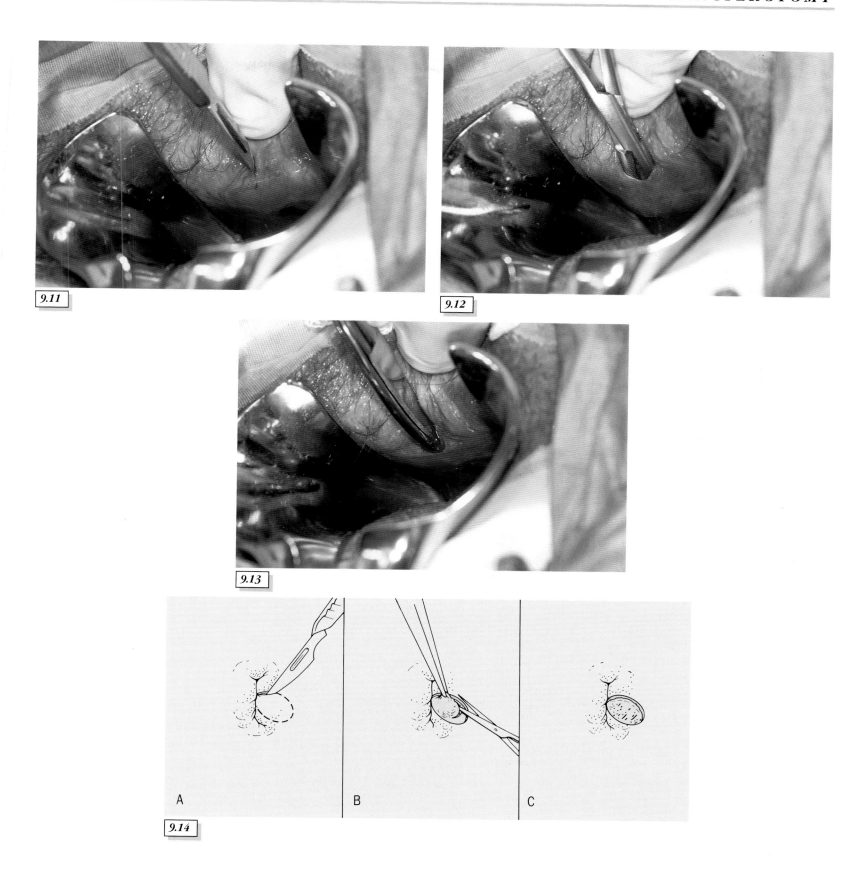

9.11

9.12

9.13

9.14

A   B   C

MANAGEMENT OF INTERNAL HEMORRHOIDS

Internal hemorrhoids are classified into the following four categories:

1st degree: prominent internal hemorrhoidal tissue
2nd degree: internal hemorrhoidal prolapse that reduces spontaneously
3rd degree: internal hemorrhoidal prolapse requiring manual reduction
4th degree: incarcerated internal hemorrhoidal prolapse.

Although many modalities are available for the management of internal hemorrhoidal disease, the most widely used methods are sclerotherapy, rubberband ligation, and operative excision.

SCLEROTHERAPY

SCLEROTHERAPY

INDICATIONS •1st- or 2nd-degree prolapse/bleeding

ANESTHESIA •none

PROCEDURE

With an anoscope in place, 1.5 mL or less of sclerosing solution (5% phenol in cottonseed oil or 2.5% quinine urea) is injected submucosally into the hemorrhoidal plexus just proximal to the dentate line (Fig. 9.15). When performed correctly, the procedure is painless. A properly placed injection results in mucosal blanching. More than one hemorrhoidal bundle can be injected during each session. If symptoms persist, re-injection can be performed in 4 to 6 weeks.

RUBBERBAND LIGATION

RUBBERBAND LIGATION

INDICATIONS •1st-, 2nd-, or 3rd-degree prolapse/bleeding

PROCEDURE

With the anoscope in place, the internal hemorrhoidal tissue is grasped through the barrel of the rubberband applicator and is ligated at its base. One or two bundles can be ligated safely during a single session (Fig. 9.16).

OPERATIVE EXCISION

OPERATIVE EXCISION

INDICATIONS •3rd- or 4th-degree prolapse

PROCEDURE

The distal portion of the hemorrhoidal complex is grasped with a hemostat. A small incision is made at the base of the hemorrhoid (Fig. 9.17). Using a submucosal dissection, the internal hemorrhoidal tissue is separated from the internal sphincter and is excised (Fig. 9.18). The wound is closed using a running 3–0 chromic catgut suture, leaving a small distal opening for drainage (Fig. 9.19). If three major hemorrhoidal groups are excised, mucosal and skin bridges must be preserved.

LOCAL MANAGEMENT OF BENIGN RECTAL TUMORS

LOCAL MANAGEMENT OF BENIGN RECTAL TUMORS

INDICATIONS •benign tumors located within 7 cm of the anal verge

PROCEDURE

Benign rectal tumors located within 7 cm of the anal verge can frequently be removed utilizing a transanal approach under local anesthesia. Local anesthesia containing epinephrine is injected submucosally, raising the tumor away from the muscular layer of the rectum (Figs. 9.20A,B). The lesion is then excised with the rim of normal mucosa (Fig. 9.20C). The resulting defect is closed using interrupted (3–0) absorbable suture material or is left open to heal by second intention.

REPAIR OF RECTOVAGINAL FISTULA

REPAIR OF RECTOVAGINAL FISTULA

INDICATIONS •obstetrical injuries account for the majority of acquired rectovaginal fistulas

PREP •patient should undergo complete mechanical and antibiotic bowel preparation prior to surgery

PROCEDURE

A probe is placed in the rectovaginal fistula to facilitate identification of the tract (Fig. 9.21). A wide rectangular block of tissue consisting of the mucosa, submucosa, and internal sphincter is elevated from the posterior vaginal wall (Fig. 9.22). The flap must be generous enough to allow advancement without tension for approximately 1 to 2 cm distal to the remaining defect in the posterior vaginal wall (Fig. 9.23). The vaginal defect is curetted to remove granulation tissue and ectopic rectal mucosa. The rectal flap is then advanced over the vaginal defect and sutured into place using an absorbable suture (Fig. 9.23). The vaginal defect is left open to facilitate drainage.

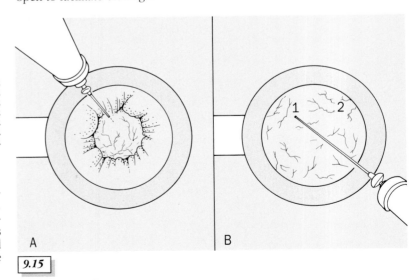

A   B

9.15

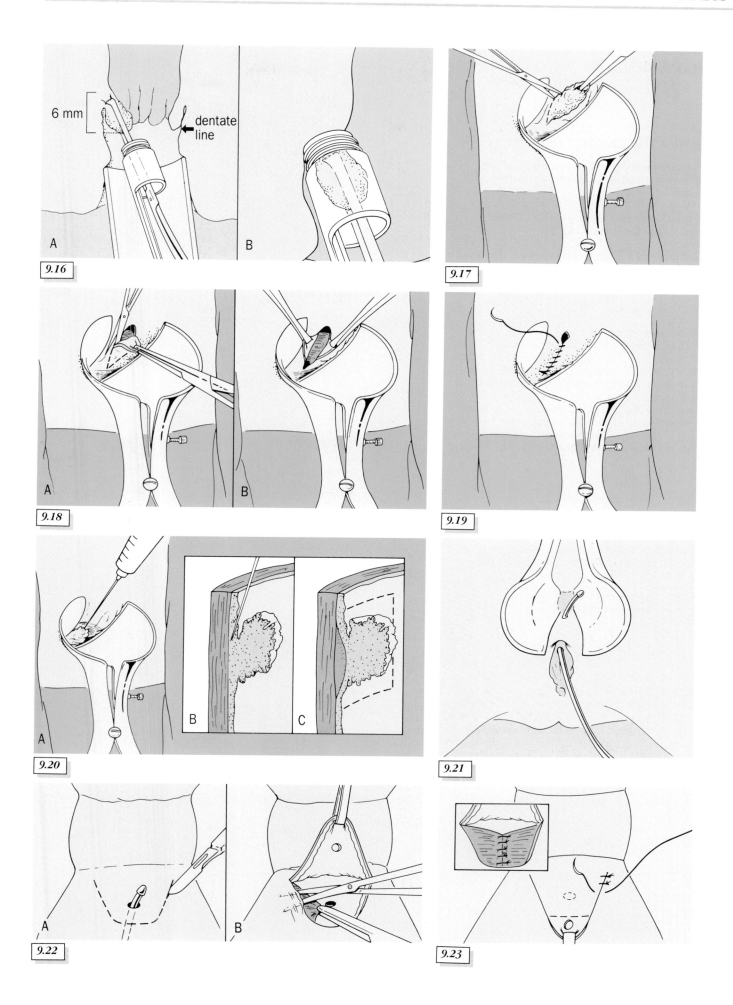

6 mm

dentate line

A

B

9.16

9.17

A

B

9.18

9.19

A

B

C

9.20

9.21

A

B

9.22

9.23

ANAL SPHINCTER RECONSTRUCTION

SPHINCTEROPLASTY

	SPHINCTEROPLASTY
INDICATIONS	•anal incontinence (most commonly resulting from previous anorectal surgery or obstetrical trauma)
POSITIONING	•prone jackknife (see Fig. 9.2), with catheter placed within the urinary bladder
PREP	•bowel prepped with both a mechanical and an antibiotic preparation

PROCEDURE

A curvilinear incision is made approximately 1 cm from the anal verge along the perianal body. The incision is extended approximately 240° around the anal verge and parallels the outer edge of the external sphincter (Fig. 9.24). The perianal skin and anoderm are mobilized from the underlying sphincter mechanism or scar. The sphincter mechanism is dissected widely to enable overlap plication without tension (Fig. 9.25). The cephalad limit of the dissection is the anorectal ring. No scar tissue is removed. Approximately six synthetic absorbable sutures are placed to secure the overlap plication (Fig. 9.26). The wound is partially closed using interrupted absorbable suture. Constipation is avoided in the postoperative period.

POSTANAL REPAIR

	POSTANAL REPAIR
INDICATIONS	•incontinence (usually due to old age or rectal prolapse); anatomically, the sphincter mechanism is intact
POSITIONING	same as for sphincteroplasty
PREP	

PROCEDURE

A posterior incision is made paralleling the course of the external sphincter (Fig. 9.27). The dissection begins in the intersphincteric plane and continues cephalad to the puborectalis muscle. The rectosacral fascia is divided and the levator ani muscle is identified after retraction of the perirectal fat (Fig. 9.28). The levator ani muscle is buttressed but not approximated (Fig. 9.29A). The puborectalis muscle and external sphincter muscles are plicated using interrupted synthetic absorbable suture (Figs. 9.29B,C). The skin is partially closed using interrupted absorbable suture. Constipation is avoided postoperatively.

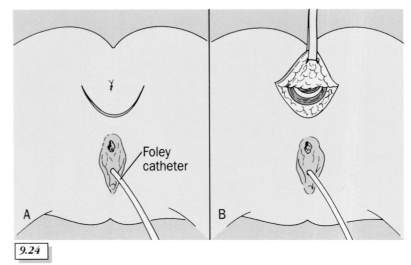

Foley catheter

9.24

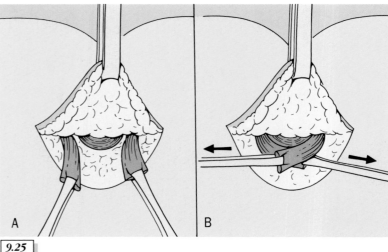

9.25

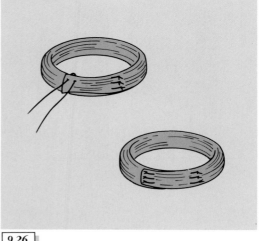

9.26

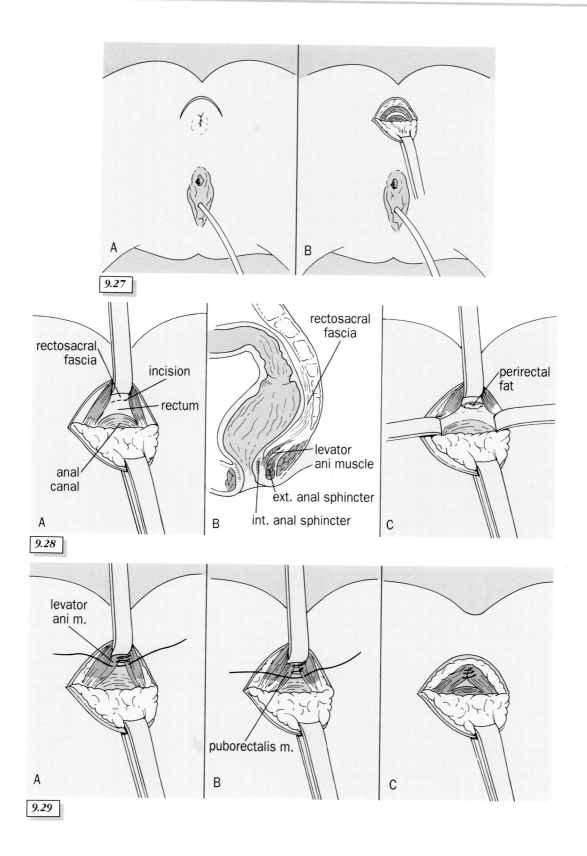

9.27

9.28

rectosacral
fascia

incision

rectum

anal
canal

A

rectosacral
fascia

levator
ani muscle

ext. anal sphincter

int. anal sphincter

B

perirectal
fat

C

9.29

levator
ani m.

A

puborectalis m.

B

C

COLORECTAL SURGERY

COLORECTAL SURGERY

The following are the same for all colorectal
procedures, unless otherwise noted.

ANESTHESIA • general

POSITIONING • supine

APPENDECTOMY

APPENDECTOMY

INDICATIONS • acute appendicitis

PROCEDURE

The McBurney incision is used, an oblique incision extending one-third
above and two-thirds below McBurney's point. McBurney's point
describes a point one-third of the distance along a line drawn from the
right anterior superior iliac spine to the umbilicus (Fig. 9.30). The incision
is deepened by dividing the underlying external oblique, internal oblique,
and transversus abdominus muscles along the course of their fibers (Fig.
9.31). The peritoneum is opened.

Next, the cecum is grasped with the thumb and index finger, and is
"rocked" cephalad and caudad to present the appendix into the operative
field. The appendix is mobilized by dividing the mesoappendix and ligating its vascular supply (Fig. 9.32). The base and proximal portion of the
appendix is "milked" distally prior to clamping (Fig. 9.33). Two
absorbable ties are placed on the base of the appendix prior to amputation (Fig. 9.34). The appendix is amputated (Fig. 9.35) and the exposed
mucosa electrocoagulated. To close the incision, all muscle layers and the
peritoneum are reapproximated (Fig. 9.36).

COLOSTOMY

CREATION OF END COLOSTOMY

CREATION OF END COLOSTOMY

INDICATIONS • usually created as part of Miles' resection or
Hartmann's procedure

PROCEDURE

Creation of the end stoma is the last step of Hartmann's procedure or the
abdominal phase of Miles' resection. The distal descending colon or
proximal sigmoid colon is usually utilized for this purpose. The most
important technical aspect of creating an end stoma pertains to mobilization of the bowel to acquire sufficient length. Adequate length can only
be achieved by mobilizing the bowel at the root of the mesentery and
along the white line of Toldt. The most frequent error leading to stomal
necrosis and retraction involves incorrect mobilization techniques
(Fig. 9.37).

A disk of skin is excised at a predetermined site (preferably preoperatively) in the left lower quadrant (Fig. 9.38). The subcutaneous fat is divided using electrocoagulation. Two army–navy retractors are placed in the
incision to expose the fascia (Fig. 9.39). Traction is placed on the subcutaneous tissue and fascia with Allis clamps (Fig. 9.39). Failure to apply even
traction results in angulation of the defect and potential kinking of the
bowel. The fascia is opened transversely, extending the incision with a
small cruciate cephalad and caudad at the midpoint (Fig. 9.40). The muscle is spread along the course of its fibers exposing the peritoneum (Fig.
9.40). Care is taken to avoid injury to the inferior epigastric vessels. The
army–navy retractors are repositioned to expose the peritoneum, which
is then entered. Two fingers are placed through the defect for sizing
(Fig. 9.41).

Two Babcock clamps are passed through the abdominal wall defect,
grasping the closed end of the colon. The bowel is gently delivered
through the defect, a short distance beyond the skin (Fig. 9.42). The stapled or oversewn colonic end is resected, grasping the edges of the cut
colon with four Allis clamps (Fig. 9.43A). Absorbable sutures are placed to
include the full thickness of the bowel wall and the skin edge (Fig. 9.43B).
Four corner sutures are placed and held. Additional sutures are placed
and tied between the corner sutures. When complete, the four stay sutures
are tied.

CREATION OF LOOP TRANSVERSE COLOSTOMY

CREATION OF LOOP TRANSVERSE COLOSTOMY

INDICATIONS • relief of obstructive lesions of the left colon
• diversion of fecal stream following low pelvic
anastomosis

PROCEDURE

The transverse colon may be approached through a small transverse incision in the right lateral rectus muscle (Fig. 9.44). After the skin incision is
made, the anterior rectus fascia is incised from the middle to the lateral
portion of the rectus muscle, extending laterally for approximately 2 to 3
cm. The muscle is divided using an electrocautery. The abdomen is then
entered by incising the posterior rectus sheath.

The transverse colon is identified by its omental attachments and delivered into the wound. A 2-cm length of omentum is dissected from the
colon, allowing enough room for a rubber supporting tube to be placed
under the colon. An avascular plane in the mesentery is opened with a
cautery and the rubber tubing slipped through this defect (Fig. 9.45).
Immediate maturation is accomplished by making a 3-cm long transverse
incision along the anterior wall of the colon (Fig. 9.46).

Interrupted 3–0 chromic catgut sutures are placed around the entire circumference of the colon. The full thickness of the bowel wall is sutured to
the subcutaneous layer of the skin (Fig. 9.47). A colostomy appliance may
be fashioned and placed at this time.

CLOSURE OF LOOP COLOSTOMY
PROCEDURE

The skin adjacent to the stoma is oversewn in a transverse manner, completely covering the stoma orifice and isolating the abdominal wall from
fecal contamination. The skin is then prepared with a Betadine solution.
An elliptical transverse incision is made encompassing the entire oversewn
area. Once both limbs of the stoma have been liberated from the underlying abdominal wall fascia, the bowel is prepared for anastomosis. The
mesentary is grasped, and is gently retracted to avoid corporating it in the
GIA staple line (Fig. 9.48). Figure 9.49A illustrates the GIA instrument
being inserted into each limb of the stoma. Gentle mesenteric retraction is
maintained, which helps to rotate the lumen of the stoma to an almost
antimesenteric point of opposition without dividing any of the mensen-
tary. The GIA is then mated and fired. The resulting orifice is closed transversely utilizing a TA-55 instrument (Fig. 9.49B), maintaining the GIA staple lines in an opposed position. The abdominal wall fascia is closed
using a running 1–0 PDS suture. The wound is irrigated with kanamycin
solution, and the skin is loosely approximated.

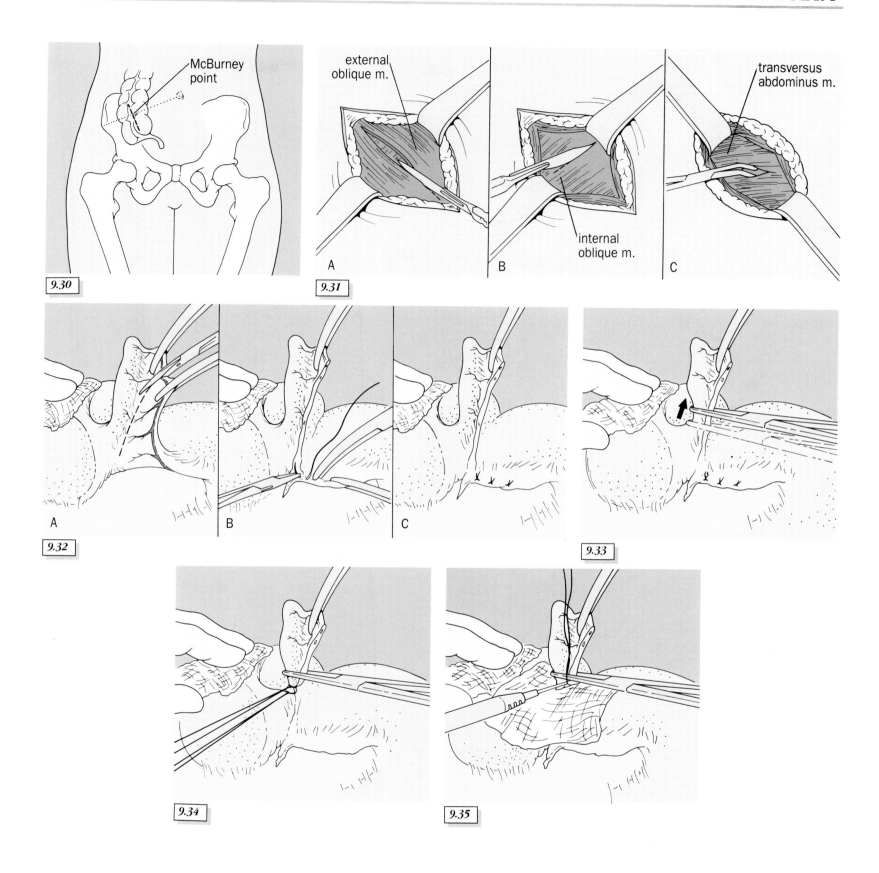

9.30

9.31

external oblique m.

internal oblique m.

transversus abdominus m.

A   B   C

9.32

A   B   C

9.33

9.34

9.35

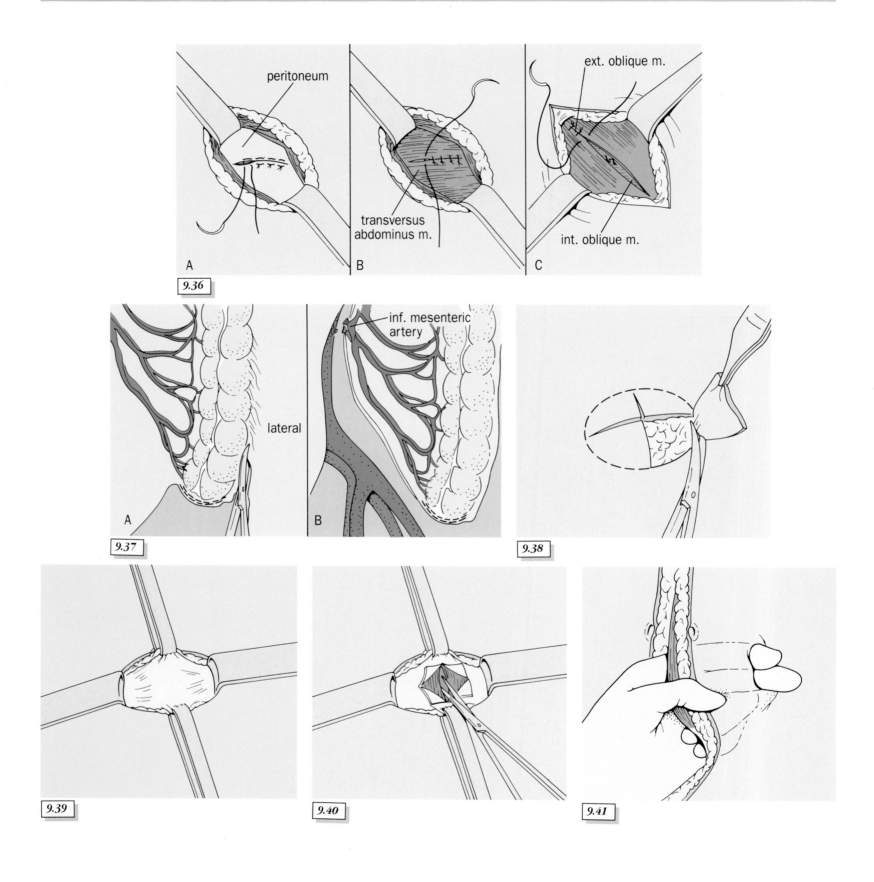

peritoneum

transversus
abdominus m.

ext. oblique m.

int. oblique m.

A

B

C

9.36

lateral

A

inf. mesenteric
artery

B

9.37

9.38

9.39

9.40

9.41

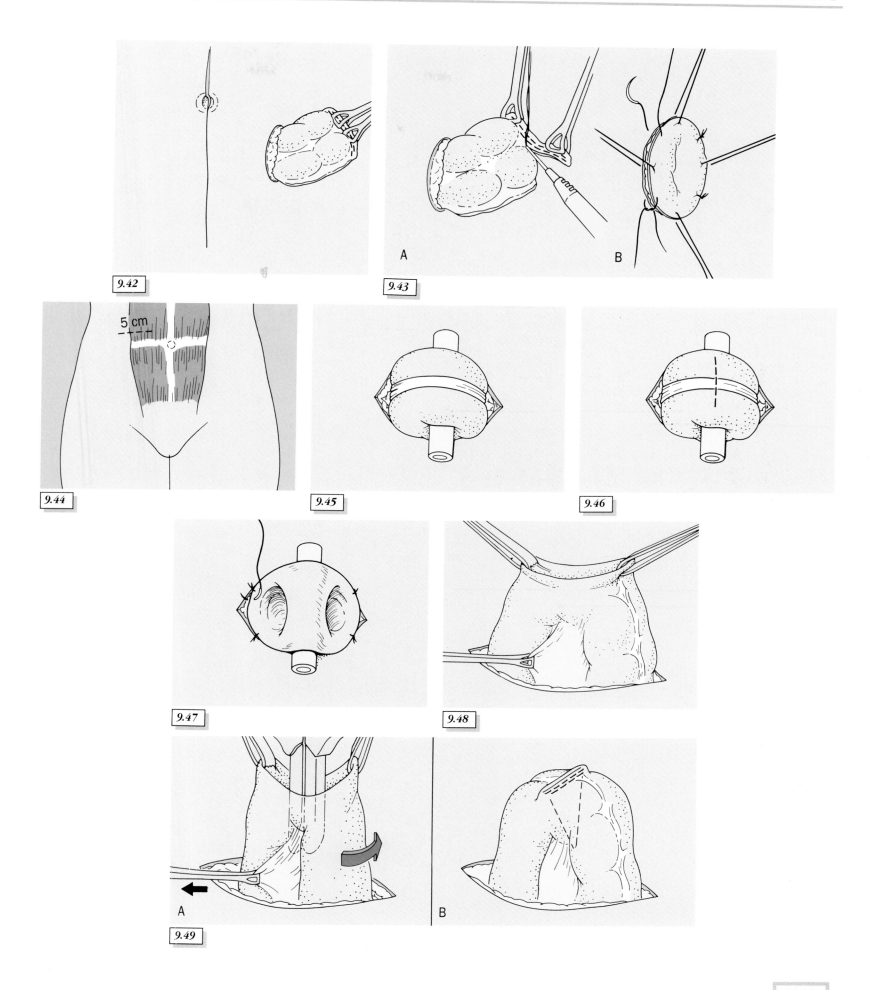

9.42

9.43
A   B

9.44
5 cm

9.45

9.46

9.47

9.48

9.49
A   B

COLECTOMY

RIGHT HEMICOLECTOMY

RIGHT HEMICOLECTOMY	
INDICATIONS	•malignancies occupying the cecum, ascending colon, and hepatic flexure
POSITIONING	•supine

PROCEDURE

A midline incision is made from the mid-epigastrium to a point approximately 8 cm below the umbilicus. Once the abdominal cavity is entered and explored, the tumor is isolated using two bowel tapes. A defect is created in an avascular plane 3 to 5 cm distal to the tumor. A bowel tape is placed through the defect and is tied tightly. Another tape is applied in a similar manner around the distal terminal ileum. The lumen of the bowel proximal and distal to the tumor is then completely isolated. The right paracolic peritoneum is opened along the base of the cecum and the index finger may be inserted deep to this layer (Fig. 9.50). Using an electrocautery, the peritoneum can be incised easily until the hepatic flexure is reached (Fig. 9.51). The duodenum should be gently swept away posteriorly, preventing injury to it. The hepatocolic ligament tends to be vascular and should be clamped and divided.

For tumors of the cecum and ascending colon, the greater omentum can be dissected from the colon using a cautery (Fig. 9.52). For hepatic flexure and proximal transverse colon lesions, the greater omentum should be sacrificed along with the right gastroepiploic arcade. The middle colic artery is ligated near the inferior margin of the pancreas (Fig. 9.53).

The ileocolic trunk is isolated and ligated approximately 1.5 cm distal to its origin with the superior mesenteric artery (Fig. 9.54). An avascular mesenteric "window" is palpated on either side of the ileocolic artery. A Kelly clamp is utilized to open these avascular planes, allowing easy clamping of the main arterial trunks. The mesentery is divided in a similar fashion until the ileal mid-transverse colonic bowel edges are reached, completing the lymphovascular resection.

We use a functional end-to-end anastomotic technique for resecting and anastomosing the ileum to the mid-transverse colon (Fig. 9.55).

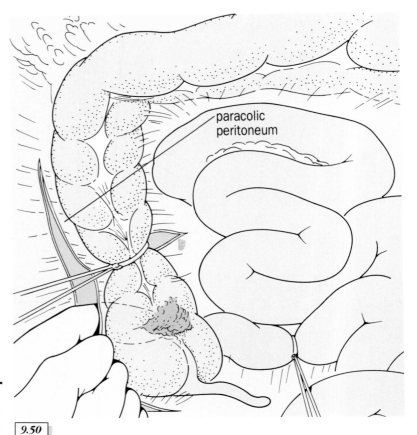

paracolic peritoneum

9.50

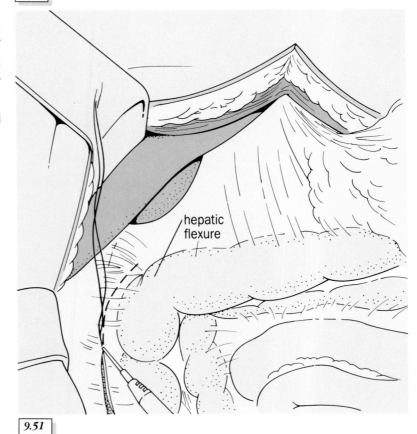

hepatic flexure

9.51

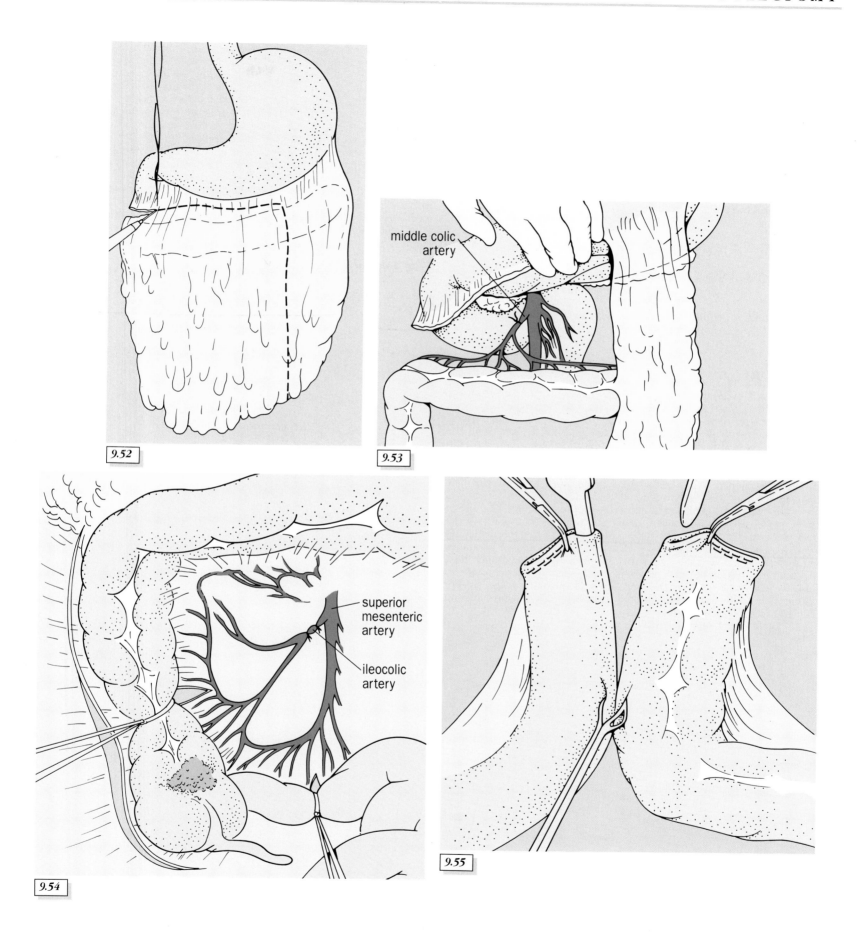

9.52

9.53

middle colic
artery

9.54

superior
mesenteric
artery

ileocolic
artery

9.55

A GIA stapler is used to divide the ileum 7 to 10 cm proximal to the ileocecal valve. The stapler is placed parallel to the mesentery to facilitate an antimesenteric anastomosis. The transverse colon is divided using a TA-55 4.8-mm stapler on the distal side and a Kocher occlusive clamp proximally. The antimesenteric tip of the linear staple lines are removed allowing the GIA stapler to be inserted (Fig. 9.56). An antimesenteric functional end-to-end anastomosis is performed by mating and firing the stapler. The resulting defect is closed using a TA-55 4.8-mm stapler with the GI staple lines held in opposition, ensuring a large, patent lumen (Fig. 9.57). The gaping defect between the ileal and colonic mesentery is closed using several interrupted 3–0 chromic catgut sutures.

LEFT HEMICOLECTOMY

LEFT HEMICOLECTOMY

INDICATIONS	• cancer of the distal transverse colon, splenic flexure, and descending colon
POSITIONING	• lithotomy position, with an irrigating catheter in the rectum

PROCEDURE

The abdomen is entered through a mid-line incision extending from the xyphoid to the pubis (Fig. 9.58). The tumor is then isolated as described previously for right hemicolectomy (see Fig. 9.50). The left colon is mobilized, beginning the dissection in the intersigmoidal fossa, along the white line of Toldt. It is here that early identification of the ureter is possible because of its predictable location (Fig. 9.59). The ureter can be identified easily at the apex of the intersigmoidal fossa, then coursing from lateral to medial, 1 cm below the bifurcation of the common iliac artery (Fig. 9.60).

Dissection continues cephalad along the white line of Toldt. The ureter is swept posterolaterally to prevent injury and to serve as a guide to the correct plane of dissection. Note the lateral location of the spermatic and ovarian vessels relative to the ureter. Mobilization of the colon continues along the white line of Toldt to just below the level of the splenic flexure. A medium-blade retractor is placed in the left upper quadrant to expose the operative field yet minimize the risk of injury to the spleen. An upper-hand retractor provides excellent continued exposure, sparing a fatigued assistant for better purposes.

At this point, the mobilization is continued using a right-angled clamp or blunt finger dissection and the peritoneum is divided using electrocoagulation until complete mobilization of the splenic flexure is achieved (Fig. 9.61). The gastrocolic omentum is separated from the transverse colon along the avascular plane. When the tumor resides in the distal transverse colon or the splenic flexure, the gastrocolic omentum is removed with the specimen along the greater curvature of the stomach, including the arcade of the left gastroepiploic artery. The mesentery is scored along the planned line of resection, including the inferior mesenteric artery (Fig. 9.62). The mesentery is divided and ligated using synthetic absorbable suture. Care must be taken to avoid injury to the ureter when ligating the inferior mesenteric artery. The anastomosis is performed between the mid-transverse and rectosigmoid colon, using mechanical stapling devices or a single layer absorbable suture technique (Fig. 9.63). (Refer to the anterior resection for stapled anastomosis; see Fig. 9.20.)

LOW ANTERIOR RESECTION ✓

In low anterior resection, the appropriate portion of rectum and sigmoid colon are removed. The blood supply nourishing the proximal colon is based on the middle colic artery via the marginal arterial arcade (Fig. 9.64).

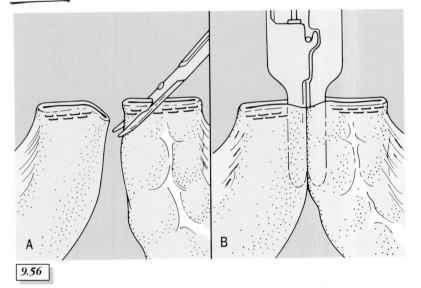

| 9.56 |

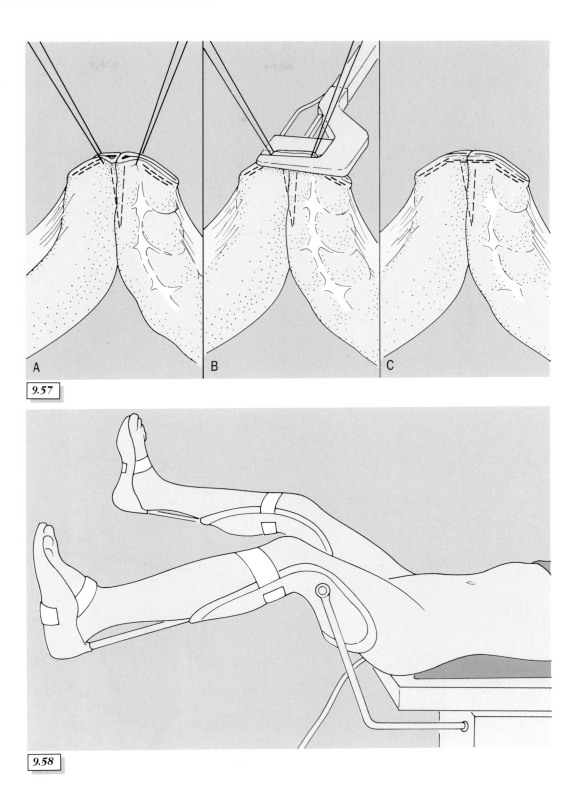

9.57

9.58

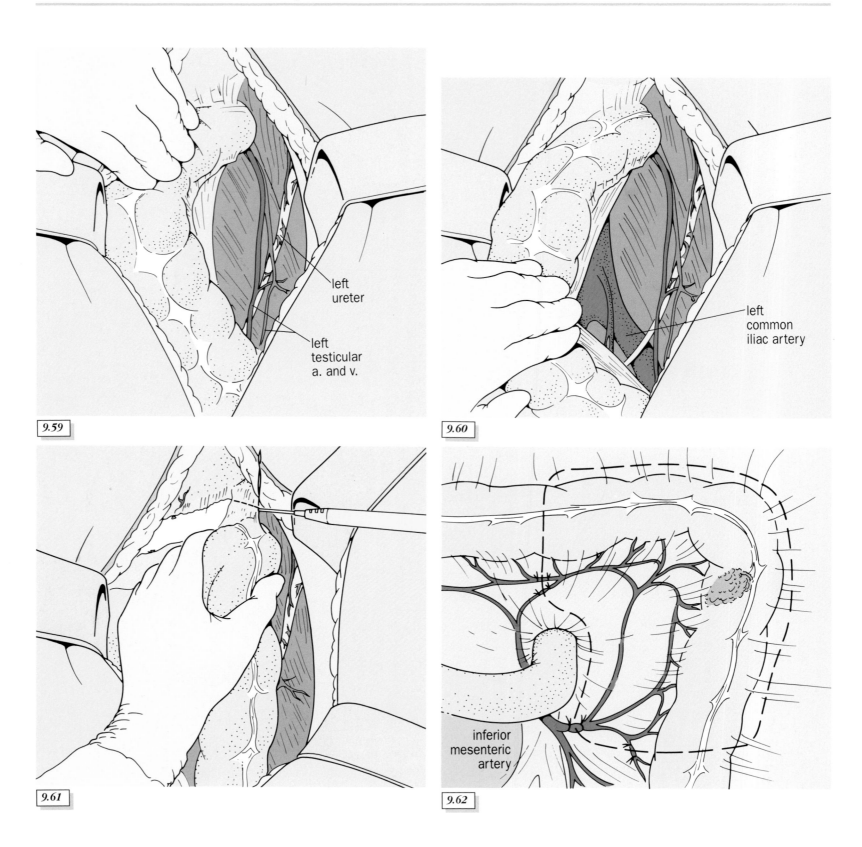

9.59

left
ureter

left
testicular
a. and v.

9.60

left
common
iliac artery

9.61

9.62

inferior
mesenteric
artery

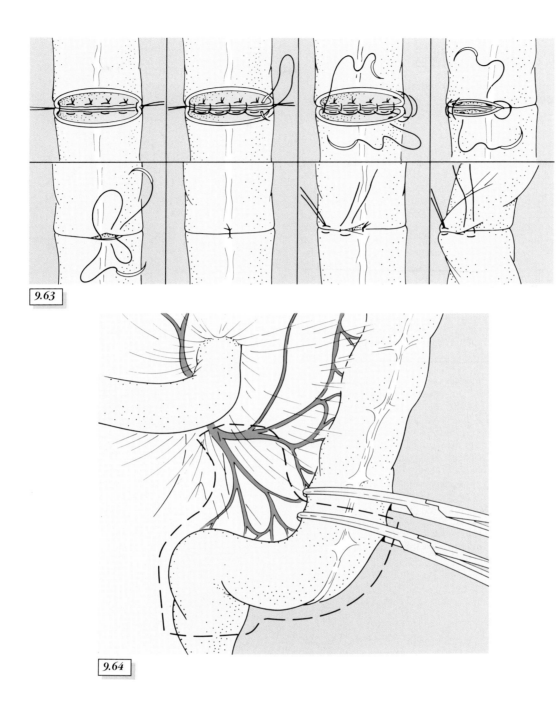

9.63

9.64

LOW ANTERIOR RESECTION

INDICATIONS • tumors of the mid-upper rectal, and distal sigmoid colon

PROCEDURE

A generous mid-line incision is made from the xyphoid to the level of the symphysis pubis. A wound retractor is placed to allow total visualization of the abdomen. The initial step in this procedure is the incision of the lateral peritoneal reflection, referred to as the white line of Toldt (see Fig. 9.59). This will result in total mobilization and straightening of the sigmoid colon (see Fig. 9.60). The mobilization is carried to the level of the splenic flexure proximally and to the anterior peritoneal reflection distally, at which point the mid-line is traversed and the peritoneal dissection is continued on the right side of the colon. The splenic flexure is completely mobilized to allow a tension-free anastomosis. The peritoneal incision is completed on the right side of the sigmoid colon to a level just distal to the duodenal–jejunal angle. At this point, following ligations of the vessels (Fig. 9.65), the pelvic dissection is initiated. The rectosigmoid mesentery is lifted away from the sacral promontory and the presacral space is mobilized utilizing gentle, blunt dissection (Fig. 9.66). The surgeon's hand should be in a plane dissecting the mesorectum anteriorly and leaving the presacral fascia behind. Anteriorly, in the man, Denonvilliers' fascia must be incised, allowing anterior dissection to the level of the prostate. Anteriorly, in the woman, the cul-de-sac has been divided, and careful dissection of the bladder and vagina off of the rectum is performed.

At this point, a margin of 2 to 5 cm is allowed distal to the tumor as a safe point for transection of the bowel (Fig. 9.67). A bowel clamp is then placed beyond the tumor to prevent intraluminal seeding of malignant cells, and the distal rectum is washed out with a hypotonic saline solution (Fig. 9.68). It is our custom to perform a double-stapled anastomosis utilizing a circular stapling device and an EEA instrument at this time. A staple line is placed beyond the clamp on a segment of rectum that has been thoroughly irrigated (Fig. 9.69). The staple line may be performed utilizing a reticulating stapling device. It is then fired and the bowel is transected prior to removal of a clamp. An EEA stapling device is then placed via the anal orifice and the central shaft is poked through the midpoint of the TA staple line (Fig. 9.70).

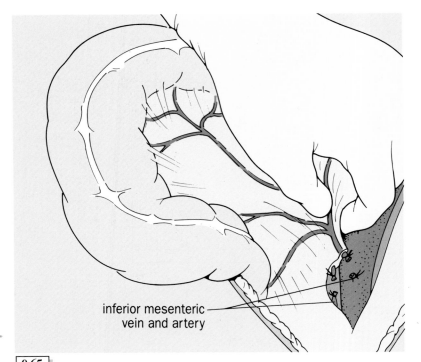

inferior mesenteric vein and artery

9.65

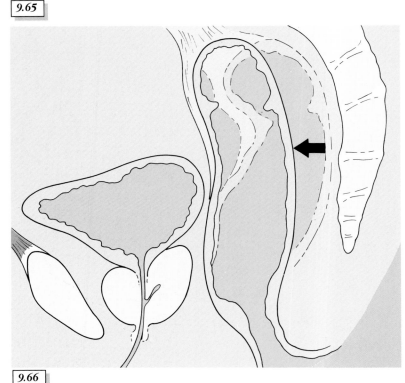

9.66

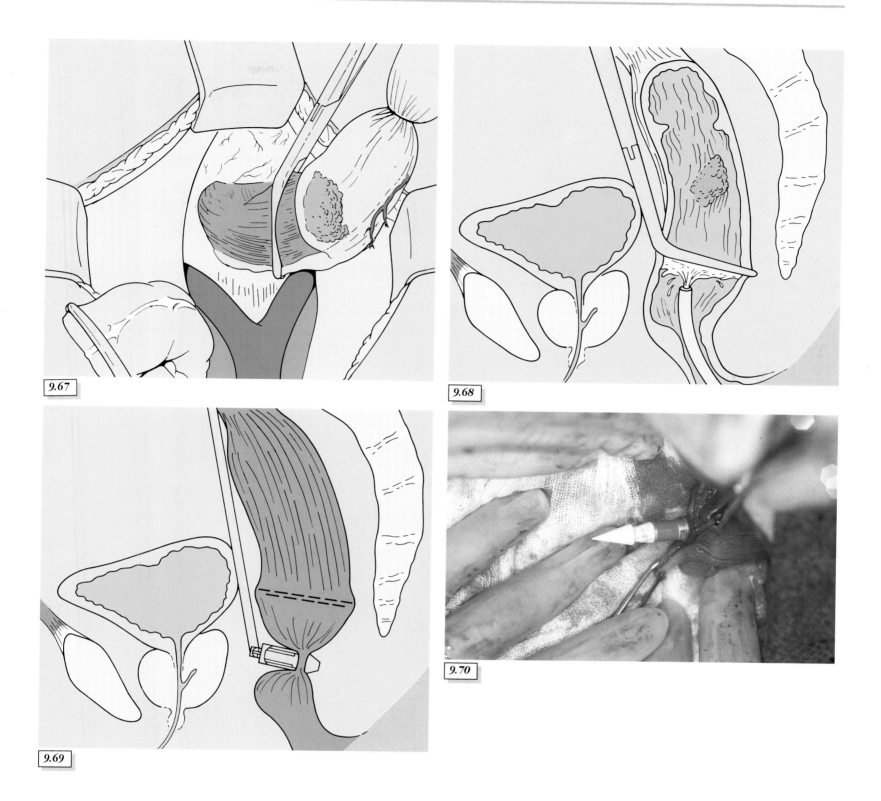

9.67

9.68

9.69

9.70

The proximal colon is prepared utilizing a pursestring clamp. After the clamp is applied, the specimen can be completely removed. The head of the EEA stapling device is then placed into the proximal bowel lumen and the pursestring suture is tied tightly (Fig. 9.71). The proximal colon is then fed gently into the sacral hollow and mated with the EEA stapling device (Fig. 9.72). At the completion of the anastomosis, the integrity of the anastomosis is tested by irrigation of the rectum with a Betadine solution. The abdomen is then closed.

MILES' (ABDOMINOPERINEAL) RESECTION

MILES' (ABDOMINOPERINEAL) RESECTION

INDICATIONS	• currently used for treatment of rectal carcinomas residing within the distal third of the rectum (higher lesions generally can be removed safely utilizing a low anterior resection)

PROCEDURE

Miles' resection is a continuation of the technique described for low anterior resection. Instead of dividing the bowel distally, the dissection is continued to include the sphincter mechanism and perianal tissue. Once the rectum is completely mobilized, the perineal phase of the operation is addressed (Fig. 9.72). The anal orifice is closed using a subcutaneous running pursestring suture to avoid fecal soilage. A generous circumferential incision is made around the anal orifice to include large margins of the perianal skin (Fig. 9.73). The excision extends from the coccyx posteriorly to the urethral bulb anteriorly. The incision is performed in a circumferential manner. The middle hemorrhoidal artery and vein are encountered laterally, and should be clamped and divided (Fig. 9.74). At this point, the perineal and abdominal phases of the operation meet. The specimen can be removed. A left lower quadrant end sigmoid colostomy is fashioned (see Fig. 9.43). The perineal wound must be closed at this time. If a wide pelvic dissection has been performed, the levator ani muscles usually cannot be approximated. The subcutaneous tissue is closed using interrupted 3–0 Vicryl sutures and the skin is closed using metallic skin clips. A drain is left in the pelvis for several days.

ABDOMINAL RECTOPEXY (WITH OR WITHOUT SIGMOID RESECTION)

The decision of whether to perform a sigmoid resection with abdominal rectopexy is based on the patient's bowel history as well as barium enema evaluation. Patients with a long history of severe constipation and a markedly redundant sigmoid colon may well benefit from sigmoid resection (Fig. 9.75A). If a sigmoid resection is to be performed, it should be done following posterior rectopexy, so as not to place any traction on the anastomosis.

ABDOMINAL RECTOPEXY (WITH OR WITHOUT SIGMOID RESECTION)

INDICATIONS	• currently favored for management of rectal prolapse in otherwise healthy patients

PROCEDURE

The rectum is mobilized posteriorly only, making sure to define any bowel redundancy. The rectum is fixed to the presacral fascia utilizing three to four sutures placed in the mid-line, just below the sacral promontory (Fig. 9.75B). If sigmoid resection is indicated, it is performed at this time.

ILEOANAL ANASTOMOSIS WITH J-POUCH CONSTRUCTION

ILEOANAL ANASTOMOSIS WITH J-POUCH CONSTRUCTION

INDICATIONS	• chronic ulcerative colitis ✓ • familial polyposis ✓
ANESTHESIA	• local with epinephrine, injected submucosally to raise the mucosa away from the internal sphincter; patient later given general endotracheal for routine colon resection
POSITIONING	• patient first placed in prone jackknife position, with tape applied to buttocks for traction; patient later placed in supine position

PROCEDURE

A circumferential incision is started at the dentate line with a scalpel (Fig. 9.76). Following this, a mosquito clamp is placed submucosally dissecting the mucosa from the internal sphincter to the level of the anorectal ring. At this point, the cut edge of the mucosa is oversewn with 3–0 chromic catgut to prevent fecal contamination. The patient is then placed in a supine position and general endotracheal anesthesia is administered. The purpose of starting the procedure in the prone jackknife position is to facilitate the rectal mucosectomy, which is tedious and requires excellent exposure.

The patient is then prepared for a routine colon resection, with legs in the Lloyd-Davies stirrups (see Fig. 9.58). The colon is removed to the level of the levators as described in the previous sections on colon excision. The entire colon, including the mobilized distal mucosa, is excised at this time and the terminal ileum is prepared for J-Pouch construction. This is performed by making a J-loop approximately 15 to 20 cm in length (Fig. 9.77A). The two limbs of the terminal ileum are approximated using two or three stay sutures. An incision is made in the apex of the limb and a GIA instrument is inserted into the limbs of the J (Fig. 9.77B). The instrument is then fired creating a common lumen between the two limbs of bowel. When this is completed, the apex of the J-loop is utilized for anastomosis at the level of the dentate line (Fig. 9.77). The anastomosis itself utilizes a 3–0 absorbable suture taking generous bites of the internal sphincter and dentate line region circumferentially (Fig. 9.78). At the conclusion of the anastomosis, a loop diverting ileostomy is constructed to protect the anastomosis for a period of 8 weeks (Fig. 9.79). A water-soluble study is obtained via the distal limb of the loop ileostomy to visualize any imperfections in healing of the anastomosis before the ileostomy is taken down.

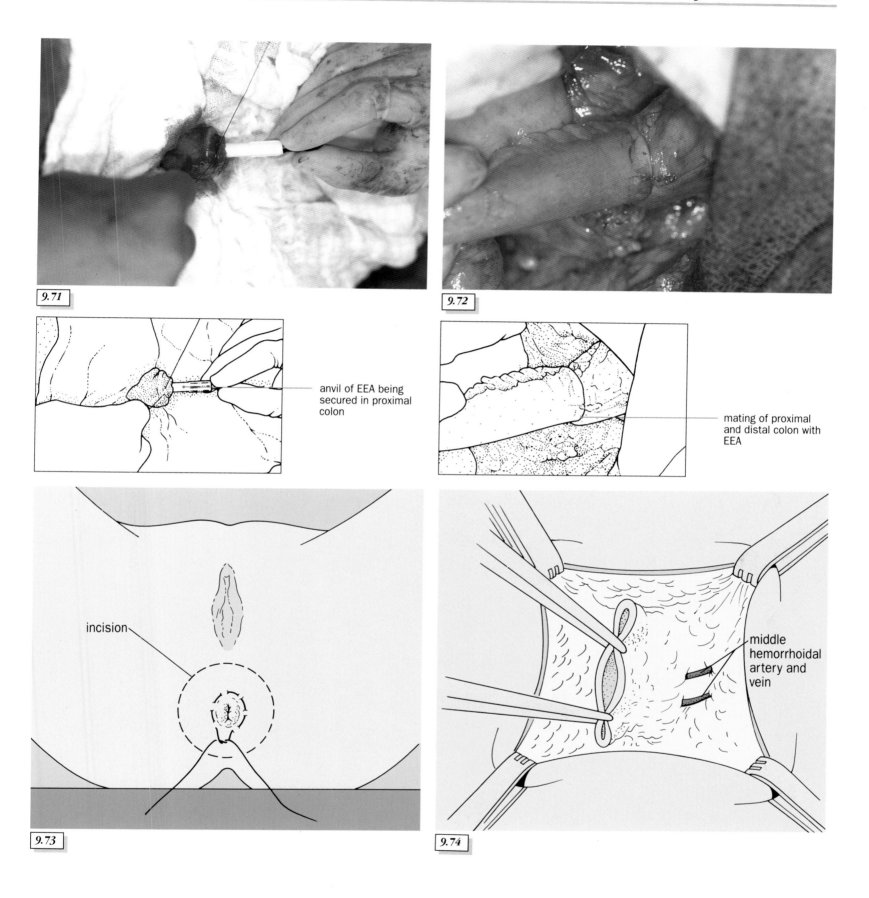

9.71

9.72

anvil of EEA being
secured in proximal
colon

mating of proximal
and distal colon with
EEA

incision

middle
hemorrhoidal
artery and
vein

9.73

9.74

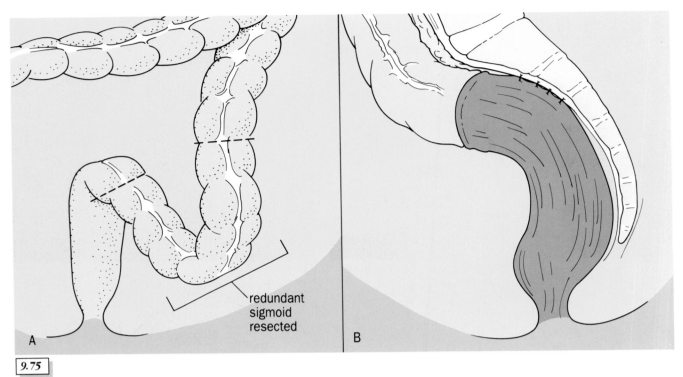

redundant
sigmoid
resected

A

B

9.75

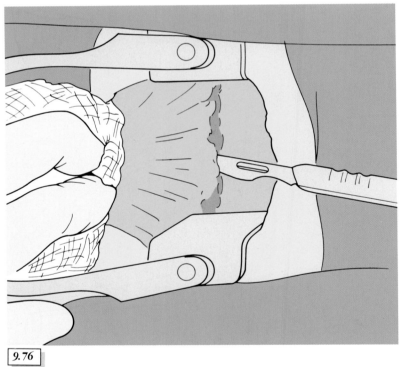

9.76

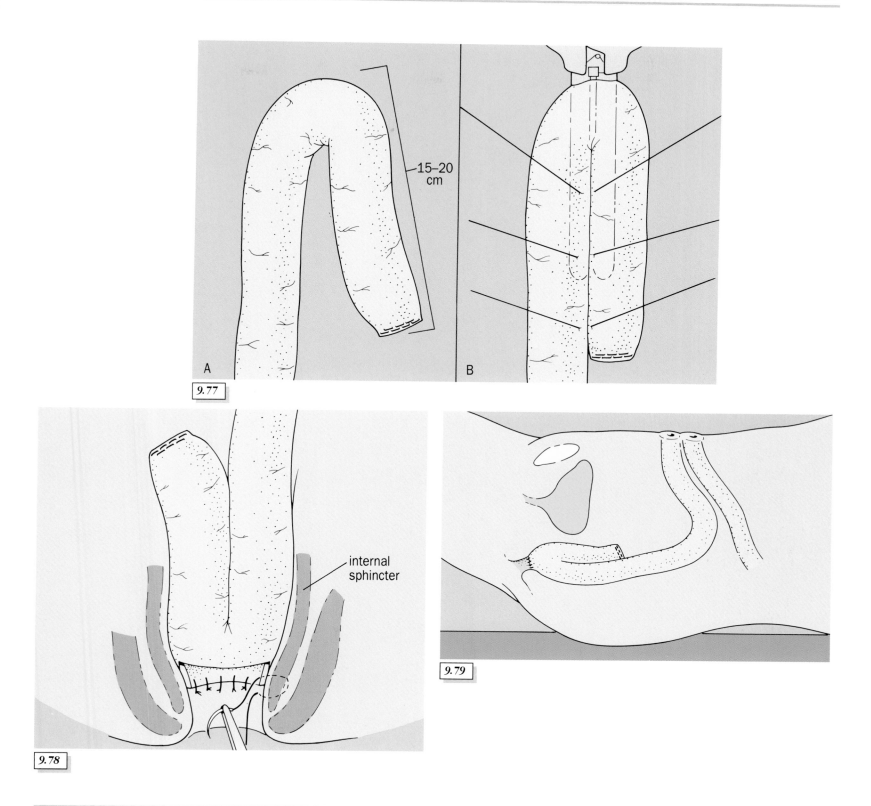

15–20 cm

9.77

A

B

internal sphincter

9.78

9.79

BIBLIOGRAPHY

Chassin J. *Operation Strategy in General Surgery*. New York: Springer-Verlag; 1980.

Goldberg S, Gordon PH, Nivatvongs S. *Essentials of Anorectal Surgery*. Philadelphia, Pa: JB Lippincott; 1980.

Goligher J. *Surgery of the Anus, Rectum, and Colon*. London: Bailliere Tindall; 1984.

Rob CG, Smith L. *Operative Surgery*. St. Louis, Mo: Mosby; 1983.

10

Hernia Surgery

Donna J. Barbot • James E. Colberg

INGUINAL HERNIORRAPHY

Repair of inguinal hernias is usually elective. Emergent repairs are rarely necessary. Most hernias are repaired in the outpatient setting using local anesthesia, with or without intravenous sedation. The use of local anesthesia and early ambulation of these patients has greatly reduced the morbidity of this procedure. Repair is therefore advisable in all symptomatic hernias unless the risk outweighs the benefit in view of the patient's overall medical condition. In the more complex repair or in the patient with a medical problem warranting postoperative monitoring, admission may be scheduled for the day of surgery.

INGUINAL HERNIORRAPHY

INDICATIONS	•symptomatic hernia—indirect, direct, or femoral •enlarging hernia •acute incarceration, strangulation •bowel obstruction due to an inguinal hernia
ANESTHESIA	•local (1% lidocaine or 1/4% bupivacaine without epinephrine) •local anesthesia with intravenous sedation (the anesthetic of choice for the patient's comfort and to decrease anxiety level) •field block (can be given by the surgeon or by the anesthesiologist) •spinal •general (reserved for the more difficult recurrent hernia or the complications of inguinal hernia where a laparotomy may be necessary)
POSITIONING	•supine
PREP	•patient should be shaved in the area of the incision immediately before the procedure
INCISION	•transverse or oblique

PROCEDURE

The line of the incision is infiltrated with the local anesthesia (Figs. 10.1, 10.2). This can be coupled with placement of a field block at the beginning of the procedure or the surgeon may elect to add local anesthesia to the deeper levels as the case progresses (Figs. 10.3–10.5).

The incision is made sharply through skin and subcutaneous tissue (Camper's and Scarpa's fascia) to the external oblique aponeurosis. This area is exposed by bluntly sweeping the subcutaneous tissue in both cephalad and caudad directions until the external oblique aponeurosis is well visualized down to the external inguinal ring. The external oblique aponeurosis is incised laterally, for approximately 1 cm, along its fibers in line with the external ring. The two leaves are elevated and the underside of the fascia is separated from underlying structures by bluntly passing the closed scissors toward the external ring before incising the remaining fascia (Fig. 10.6). Care must be taken to avoid damaging the ilioinguinal nerve, which may lie directly beneath the fascia, particularly close to the external ring.

Both upper and lower flaps of the external oblique fascia are elevated bluntly. When the lower one is elevated, the entire inguinal ligament and the floor of the inguinal canal can be visualized. The ilioinguinal nerve is carefully dissected from its surrounding tissues and protected by placing it on the outside of the external oblique aponeurosis (Figs. 10.7, 10.8), supported by one or two hemostatic clamps attached to the edge of the fascia.

One or two self-retaining rake retractors may be used at this point. Additional local anesthetic should be placed around the lateral aspect of the pubic tubercle and into the spermatic cord before any dissection or mobilization of the cord occurs. The spermatic cord can be bluntly dissected at the level of the pubic tubercle and the lacunar ligament, and then encircled with a Penrose drain. This method may lead to postoperative cord swelling and ecchymosis. Alternatively, in situ dissection of the spermatic cord, as described in the Shouldice method, can be used (Fig. 10.9). The cremasteric fibers are bluntly separated off the anterior surface of the cord, dissected medially and laterally, ligated, and removed (skeletonizing the cord).

This is done sequentially around the cord until only vessels and vas deferens remain with a direct hernia. In the course of this dissection, the hernia sac is uncovered and separated from the cord structures in the indirect hernia (Fig. 10.10). The indirect hernia sac lies anteromedially to the cord structures and is usually a distinct white tissue.

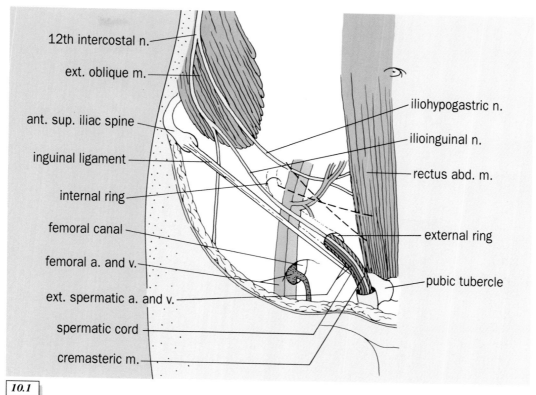

12th intercostal n.
ext. oblique m.
ant. sup. iliac spine
inguinal ligament
internal ring
femoral canal
femoral a. and v.
ext. spermatic a. and v.
spermatic cord
cremasteric m.

iliohypogastric n.
ilioinguinal n.
rectus abd. m.
external ring
pubic tubercle

10.1

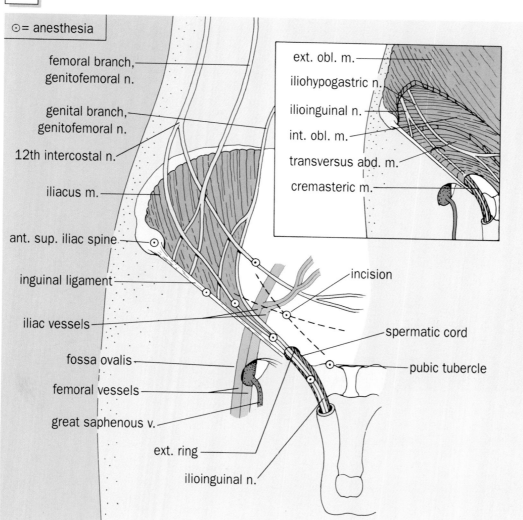

⊙ = anesthesia

femoral branch, genitofemoral n.
genital branch, genitofemoral n.
12th intercostal n.
iliacus m.
ant. sup. iliac spine
inguinal ligament
iliac vessels
fossa ovalis
femoral vessels
great saphenous v.
ext. ring
ilioinguinal n.

incision
spermatic cord
pubic tubercle

ext. obl. m.
iliohypogastric n.
ilioinguinal n.
int. obl. m.
transversus abd. m.
cremasteric m.

10.2

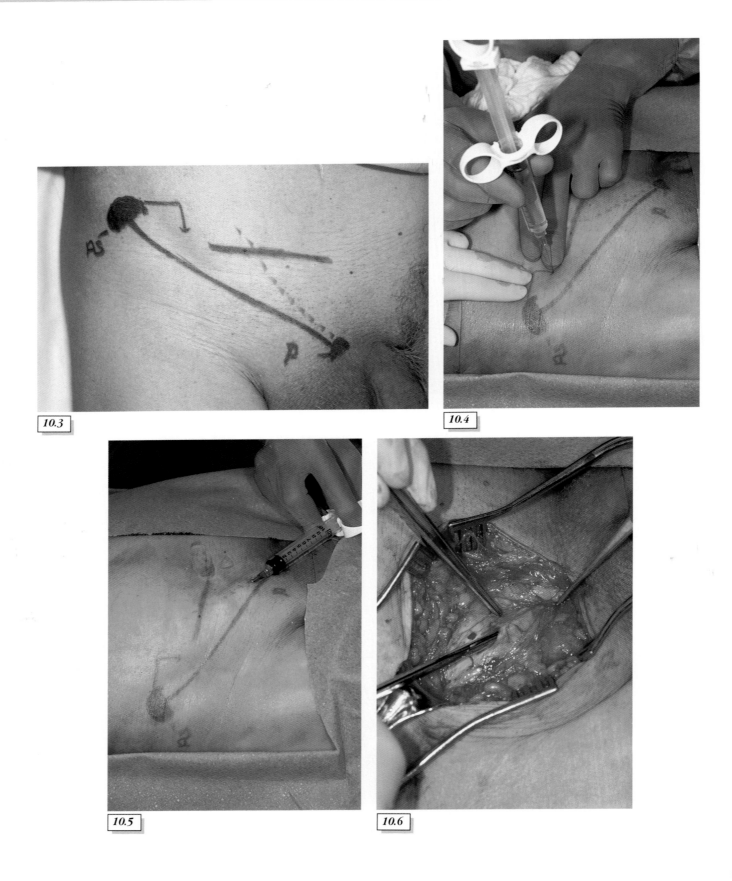

10.3

10.4

10.5

10.6

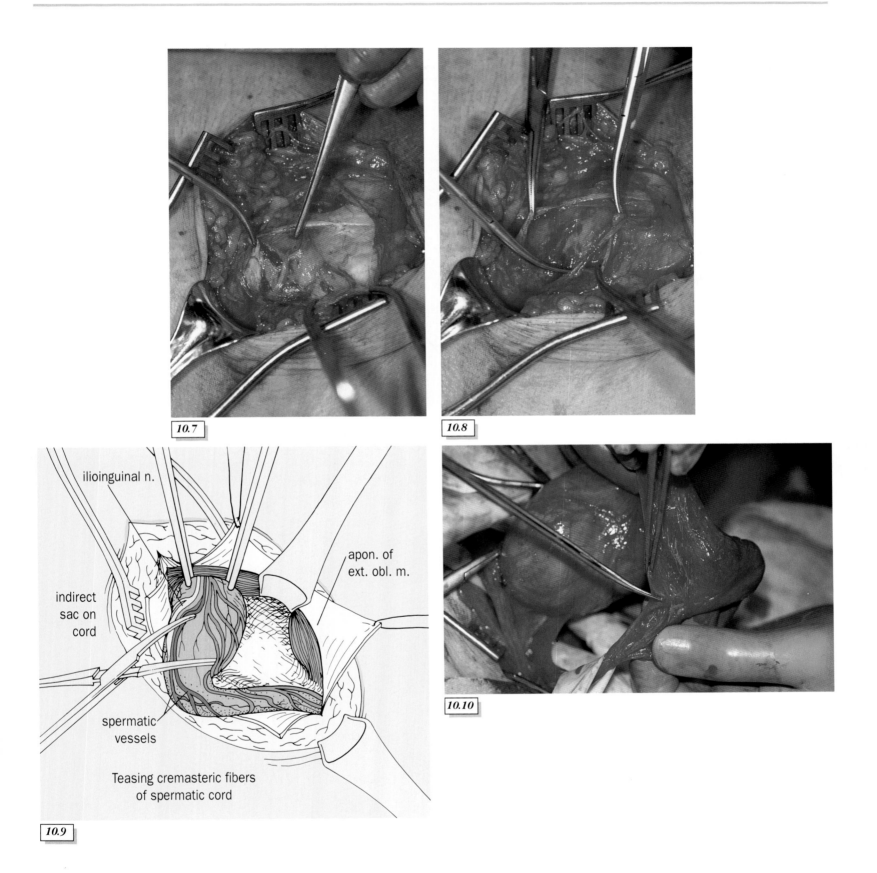

10.7

10.8

ilioinguinal n.

apon. of
ext. obl. m.

indirect
sac on
cord

spermatic
vessels

Teasing cremasteric fibers
of spermatic cord

10.9

10.10

The cord structures are then encircled with the Penrose drain for their protection and manipulation during the repair (Fig. 10.11). Hemostasis is essential and manipulation of the cord should be kept at a minimum to prevent postoperative discomfort.

If the hernia sac is very large, extending into the scrotum (a so-called complete hernia), it may be divided, with care taken to gain hemostatic control of the edges. Often even the large sacs can be brought up easily and separated from the surrounding structures dissecting bluntly and using cautery to cut the more fibrous bands. Regardless of the method used, these patients have significant cord and scrotal swelling postoperatively, which may take several months to resolve. A hernia of this magnitude does not preclude the use of local anesthesia, but good sedation is essential.

The indirect sac is then dissected to the internal ring, carefully separating any remaining cremasteric fibers (Figs. 10.12, 10.13). Care is taken to avoid opening the sac near its neck. If that does occur, it should be closed by placing the ligature below the opening. Dissection superiorly is aided by opening the sac, reducing any contents and placing a finger within the sac (Fig. 10.14). When the neck of the sac is skeletonized and the internal ring is clearly delineated, the sac is suture ligated at or just outside the internal ring. The excess sac is divided and the stump is allowed to retract beneath the internal oblique muscle (Fig. 10.15).

In longstanding hernia sacs, adherent omentum, bowel, or bladder can be found. Often they can be dissected free when there are secondary adhesions to the wall of the hernia sac. When these structures compose the wall of the hernia sac, it is called a sliding indirect inguinal hernia (Fig. 10.16). The viscus forms a portion of the wall of the sac. The sac should be mobilized and opened high and anteriorly; the viscus should not be dissected away from the wall of the sac. Excess anterior sac wall may be trimmed to facilitate suture closure of the sac (Figs. 10.17, 10.18, 10.19).

This form of indirect hernia often causes marked stretching of the internal ring, as well as laxity of the floor of the inguinal canal. Before sac closure, the floor should be inspected. The presence of both an indirect and a direct or femoral hernia constitutes a "pantaloon" hernia. These other sac(s) can be transposed to the indirect position for closure or ligated in the usual manner if the inguinal floor is not opened.

The essential problem in the small indirect inguinal hernia is the presence of the sac and an enlarged internal ring. The important elements of repair in this situation are sac removal and closure of the ring. In the large indirect hernia, the greatly enlarged ring will have weakened the floor of the inguinal canal as well. In this circumstance, repair of the inguinal canal floor is as essential as it would be in the case of the direct inguinal hernia.

Many methods have been described to close or reinforce the floor of the inguinal canal and tighten the internal ring. The essential elements of any good repair should include:
• anatomic closure of the defect
• approximation of strong tissue to strong tissue
• no undue tension
• use of nonabsorbable, nonreactive suture
• use of a relaxing incision or fabric interposition when indicated to reduce tension on the repair.

The surgeon should have several methods available to him so that he can individualize the treatment based on the patient's anatomic situation at the time of surgery.

In the direct inguinal hernia, the floor of the inguinal canal, which is the transversus abdominus aponeurosis together with transversalis fascia, is usually diffusely attenuated but may occasionally have a very distinct defect or sac, which can be closed with a pursestring suture (Figs. 10.20, 10.21).

In the Shouldice hernia repair, the floor is opened from internal ring to the tubercle, taking care to avoid injury to the inferior epigastric vessels (Fig. 10.22). The medial superior flap is elevated (Fig. 10.23) and then sewn to the free lateral inferior edge starting at the pubic tubercle in a continuous fashion (Fig. 10.24). Our preference is 3–0 Prolene suture. At the internal ring the suture is reversed and run back, sewing the free medial superior edge to the base of the shelving edge of the inguinal ligament and tied to itself at the pubic tubercle.

The Shouldice repair is then continued with a second continuous double row of sutures joining the medial arch of the internal oblique and conjoined tendon to the inguinal ligament (Fig. 10.25). The principle of this repair is well-distributed tension along the suture line and imbrication of layer upon layer to remove tension from the deepest layer.

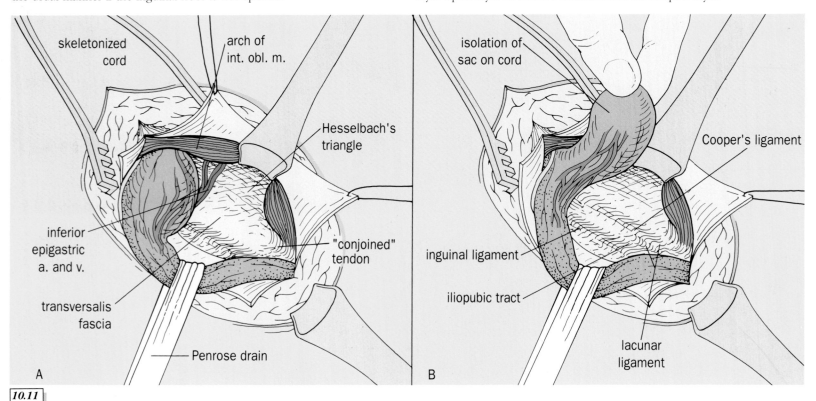

A

skeletonized cord

arch of int. obl. m.

Hesselbach's triangle

inferior epigastric a. and v.

"conjoined" tendon

transversalis fascia

Penrose drain

B

isolation of sac on cord

Cooper's ligament

inguinal ligament

iliopubic tract

lacunar ligament

10.11

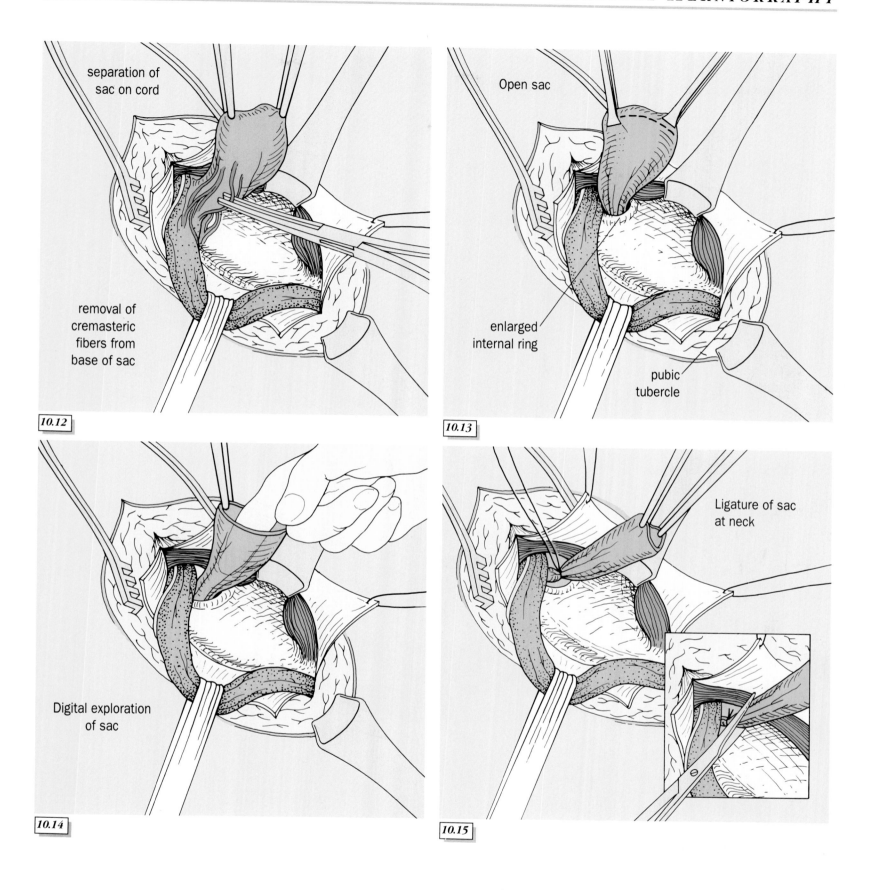

separation of
sac on cord

removal of
cremasteric
fibers from
base of sac

10.12

Open sac

enlarged
internal ring

pubic
tubercle

10.13

Digital exploration
of sac

10.14

Ligature of sac
at neck

10.15

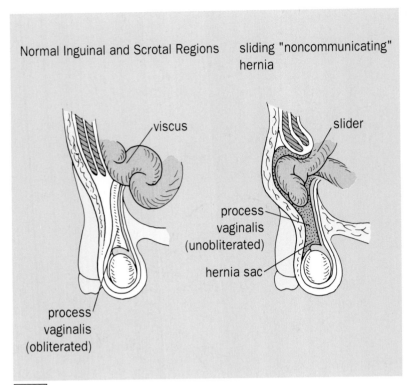

Normal Inguinal and Scrotal Regions   sliding "noncommunicating" hernia

viscus

slider

process vaginalis (unobliterated)

hernia sac

process vaginalis (obliterated)

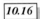

10.16

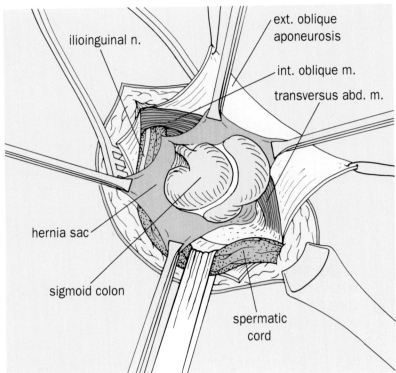

ilioinguinal n.

ext. oblique aponeurosis

int. oblique m.

transversus abd. m.

hernia sac

sigmoid colon

spermatic cord

10.17

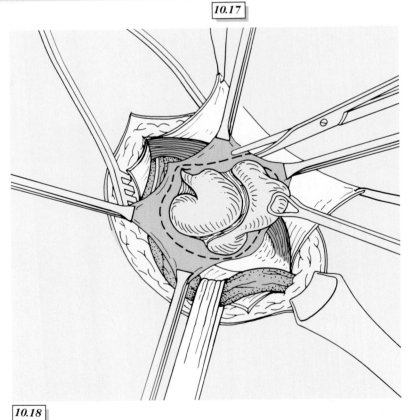

10.18

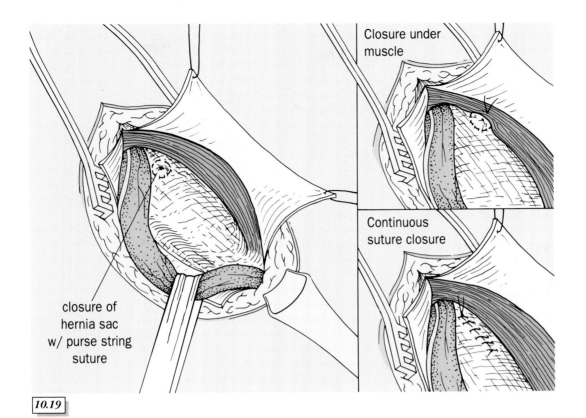

Closure under muscle

Continuous suture closure

closure of hernia sac w/ purse string suture

10.19

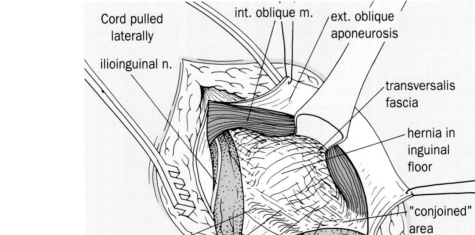

Cord pulled laterally

ilioinguinal n.

int. oblique m.

ext. oblique aponeurosis

transversalis fascia

hernia in inguinal floor

"conjoined" area

inguinal lig.

iliopubic tract

Cooper's lig.

lacunar lig.

pubic tubercle

10.20

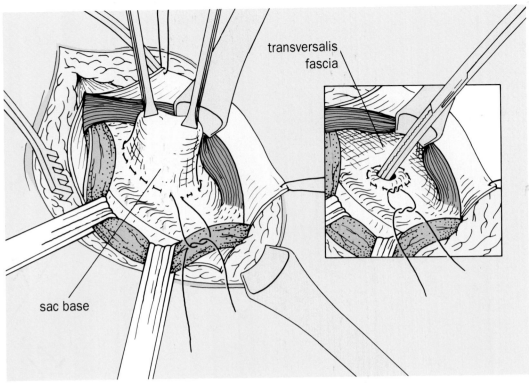

transversalis
fascia

sac base

10.21

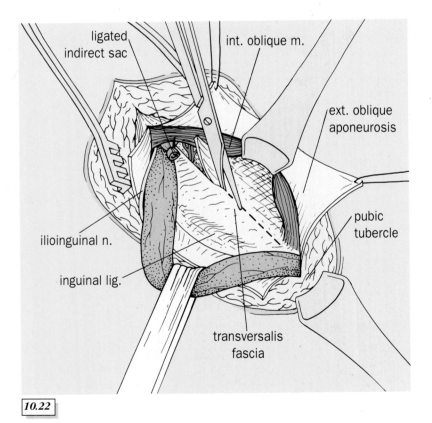

ligated
indirect sac

int. oblique m.

ext. oblique
aponeurosis

ilioinguinal n.

inguinal lig.

pubic
tubercle

transversalis
fascia

10.22

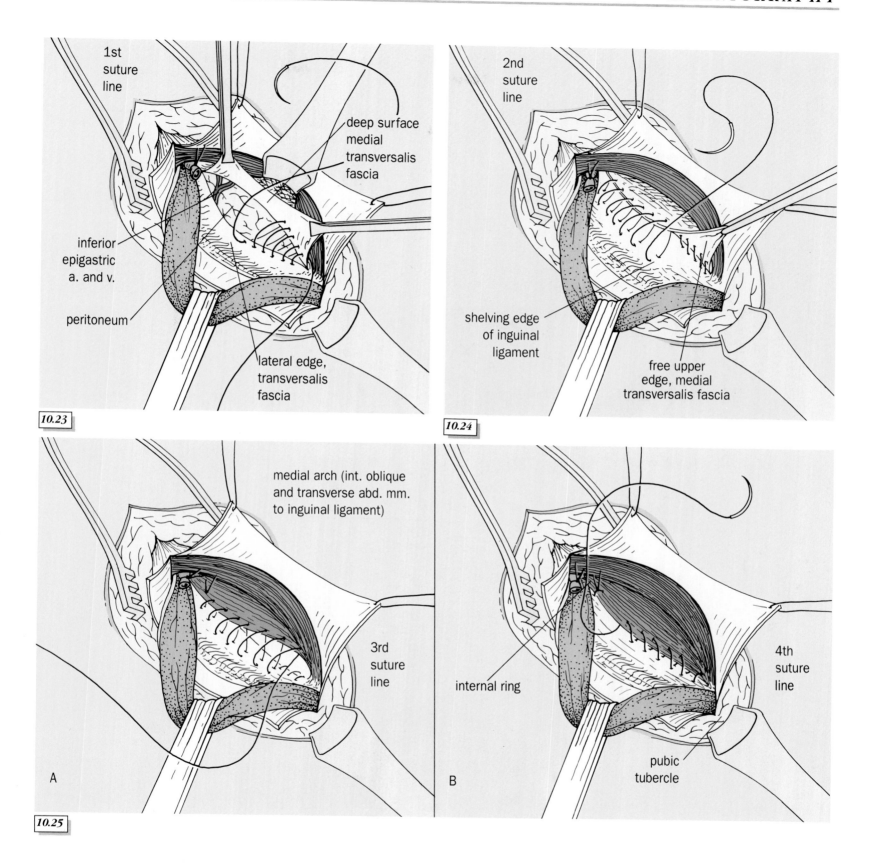

1st suture line

deep surface medial transversalis fascia

inferior epigastric a. and v.

peritoneum

lateral edge, transversalis fascia

10.23

2nd suture line

shelving edge of inguinal ligament

free upper edge, medial transversalis fascia

10.24

medial arch (int. oblique and transverse abd. mm. to inguinal ligament)

3rd suture line

A

internal ring

pubic tubercle

4th suture line

B

10.25

In the Bassini type of repair, the floor of the inguinal canal is reinforced by an interrupted row of nonabsorbable 0 sutures. This line begins at the pubic tubercle between the firm medial component ("conjoined tendon"), which is made up of transversalis and internal oblique fascias, and the shelving portion of Poupart's (inguinal) ligament, extending laterally to a closure of the internal ring (Fig. 10.26). A true conjoined tendon exists in only 5% of patients.

The repair uses the firm edge of tissue palpated medially, which is the edge of the transversus abdominus alone or conjoined with the internal oblique (Fig. 10.27).

The internal ring in either repair described is closed sufficiently so that it admits the tip of the fifth finger beside the cord. Slightly more room is better than less.

In larger direct hernias or in the femoral hernia, it is often desirable to assure that the femoral canal is tightened, in addition to repairing and reinforcing the floor of the inguinal canal. A Cooper's ligament or McVay repair is used in this circumstance. After reduction of the hernia sac, Cooper's ligament (pectinate ligament), the deepest structure just lateral to the pubic tubercle, is then cleared and exposed. Interrupted nonab-

sorbable sutures are placed between the transversus abdominus arch above and starting at Cooper's ligament below, moving laterally along the iliopubic tract, and then transitioning to the shelving edge of the inguinal ligament, closing the floor of the canal to the internal ring (Fig. 10.28). Care is taken not to compress the femoral vein. Placing sutures in Cooper's ligament may be difficult; different needle positions can be tried until the operator is satisfied. This repair may also require deeper sedation for the patient's comfort. In all interrupted suture repairs, all the sutures are placed and then tied.

If the transversus abdominus aponeurosis will not come down to Cooper's ligament without undue tension, a relaxing incision can be made (Fig. 10.29). The other alternative is the interposition of a prosthetic mesh material (Marlex or Goretex) to bridge the gap between the transversus abdominus arch and Cooper's ligament and/or the inguinal ligament. The relaxing incision is made at the base of the reflected external oblique, exposing the rectus abdominus muscle, starting in the midline and extending for 6 to 10 cm as needed. The deeper, inferior component of the anterior rectus sheath may then slide down to effect a tension-free closure.

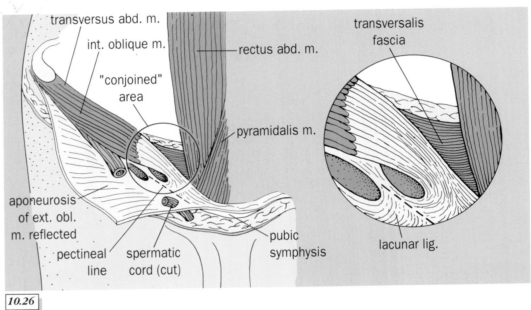

10.26

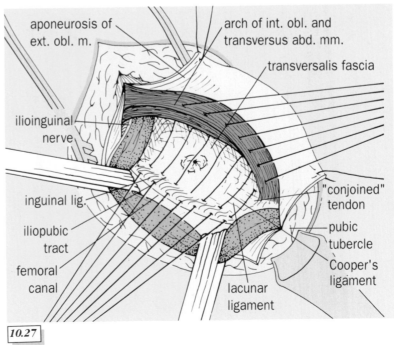

10.27

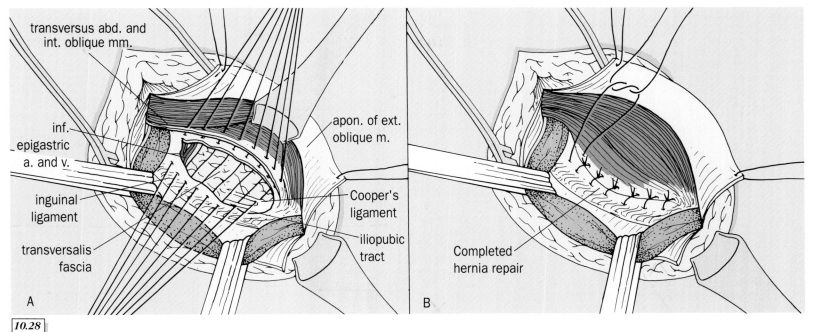

transversus abd. and
int. oblique mm.

inf.
epigastric
a. and v.

inguinal
ligament

transversalis
fascia

apon. of ext.
oblique m.

Cooper's
ligament

iliopubic
tract

A

B

Completed
hernia repair

10.28

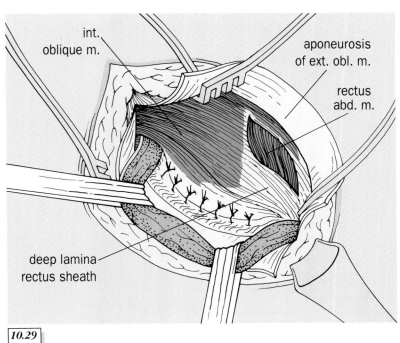

int.
oblique m.

aponeurosis
of ext. obl. m.

rectus
abd. m.

deep lamina
rectus sheath

10.29

A more recent innovation described by Lichtenstein is the "plug" technique of hernia repair. This was initially described in a large series of recurrent herniorrhaphies. This method can produce a tension-free repair by suturing a plug of prosthetic material into the defect.

After repair of the floor of the inguinal canal, the cord and nervous structures are allowed to fall back into place. The area must be inspected and hemostasis must be meticulous. The external oblique is closed with a running suture starting laterally and reconstituting the external ring medially. Care is taken to avoid catching the ilioinguinal nerve in this layer. Scarpa's fascia is closed with either running or interrupted suture. Both of these layers can be closed with a 3–0 absorbable suture. The skin is usually closed with absorbable suture in either a continuous or interrupted fascia and steri-strips. This is more comfortable for the patient and saves an extra office visit for suture or staple removal. At the completion of the procedure, gentle traction is placed on the testicle to straighten the cord structures within the canal.

There are many variations on the basics of inguinal hernia repair that the surgeon experiments with during his career. All surgeons will employ personal variations as needed. If the basic principles of tension-free repair are followed, the recurrence rate should be low. The rate of recurrence of inguinal hernias generally reported is between 1% and 9%. This figure may be grossly inaccurate, as it is unlikely that the patient will return to his original surgeon for a recurrence operation. The repair of the recurrent hernia should take into account all of the principles previously mentioned. The surgeon should review the previous operative report. All structures must be carefully identified in these challenging dissections. The repair must be performed without tension, with any technique that restores the floor of the inguinal canal most satisfactorily. The use of prosthetic material should be discussed with all patients preoperatively and its use liberally applied.

Occasionally it is difficult to pass the hernia through the femoral canal. Additional room may be obtained by incising either the inguinal ligament (Fig. 10.32) or the lacunar ligament (Fig. 10.33). Care must be taken to avoid injury to the obturator artery when this is performed.

A femoral hernia may be repaired from below the inguinal ligament as well. This does not afford inspection of the floor of the inguinal canal, but may be adequate if the surgeon is sure of his diagnosis, as in the case of a palpable incarcerated femoral hernia. This approach avoids general contamination of the inguinal canal in the instance of the perforated incarcerated femoral hernia.

The incision is made above the femoral swelling (Fig. 10.34A, inset). The sac is located and bluntly dissected free of surrounding tissues (Fig. 10.34A), tracing it back and clearing the femoral canal area. The femoral vein should be identified and cleared as well. The sac is opened and viable contents are returned to the abdomen (Fig. 10.34B). Any fluid present should be cultured.

If the hernia neck requires enlargement for reduction, open the inguinal ligament rather than the lacunar. This is easier to repair or incorporate its repair into the hernia closure. The sac is trimmed and closed and reduced through the hernia neck (Fig. 10.35A). Several interrupted sutures of non-absorbable material are used to close the canal between the base of the inguinal ligament and Cooper's ligament or to the pectineal fascia (Figs. 10.35B,C).

The skin and subcutaneous tissue can be closed with absorbable suture. If there was nonviable tissue within the sac, bowel resection should take place through a separate lower midline incision. Consideration should be given to leaving the skin open in the femoral area in this circumstance. Occasionally a femoral hernia may present as an infrainguinal abscess or fistula. One should be prepared for laparotomy in these more extreme circumstances.

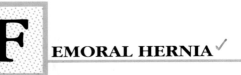

FEMORAL HERNIA

A femoral hernia is a weakness in the transversalis fascia into the femoral ring and canal through which either preperitoneal fat or an intra-abdominal organ may herniate (Fig. 10.30).

PROCEDURE

Two approaches to the femoral hernia are possible. With the first, the inguinal canal is reached and exposed as previously described (Fig. 10.31A). The surgeon, even if highly suspicious of a femoral hernia, should inspect for coexisting hernias (Fig. 10.31B). The neck of the femoral sac can be exposed by opening the transversalis fascia to expose the preperitoneal space, and then bluntly dissected (Fig. 10.31C). Adhesions may be present which require lysis. The end of the sac is then located at the femoral ring and the sac gently reduced back into the preperitoneal space superior to the inguinal ligament (Fig. 10.31D). If there was suspicion of incarceration, the sac is opened and the contents inspected. If not, the contents may be reduced back into the abdomen. The sac is ligated with a pursestring suture. A Cooper's ligament repair is then performed (Fig. 10.31E).

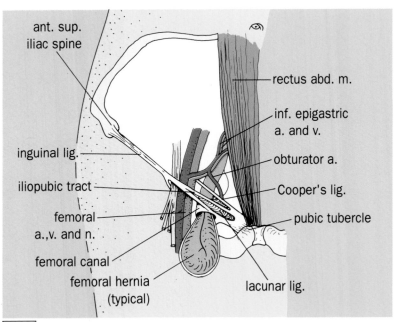

ant. sup. iliac spine

rectus abd. m.

inf. epigastric a. and v.

inguinal lig.

iliopubic tract

obturator a.

Cooper's lig.

femoral a.,v. and n.

pubic tubercle

femoral canal

femoral hernia (typical)

lacunar lig.

10.30

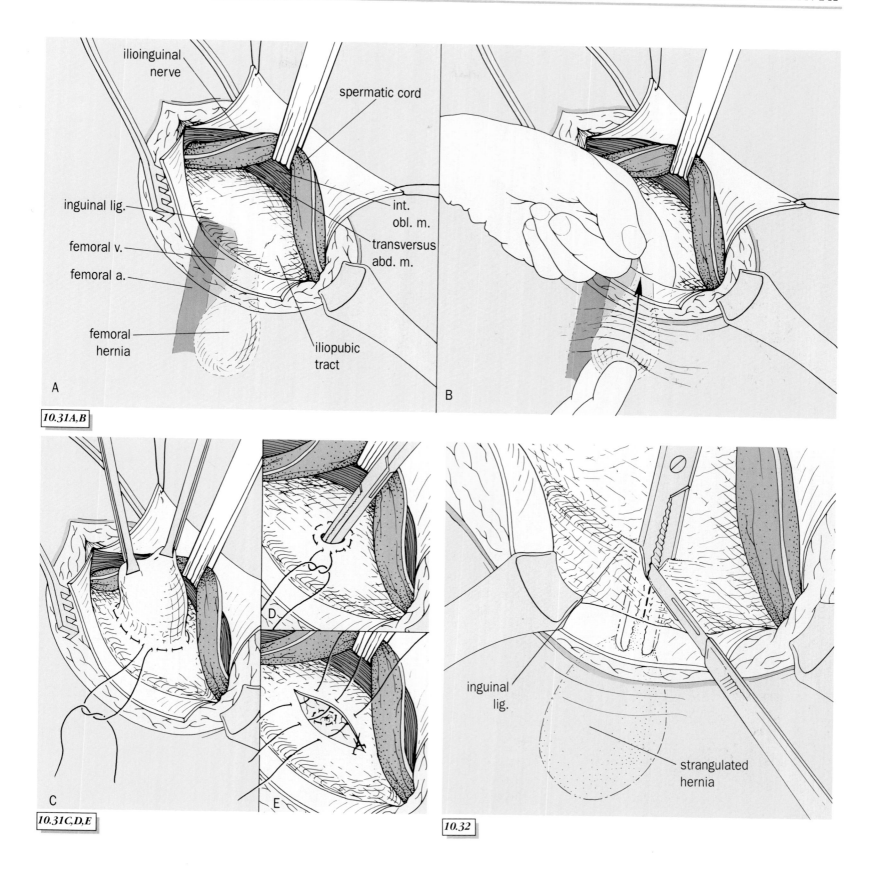

A
- ilioinguinal nerve
- spermatic cord
- inguinal lig.
- femoral v.
- femoral a.
- femoral hernia
- int. obl. m.
- transversus abd. m.
- iliopubic tract

B

10.31A,B

C

D

E

10.31C,D,E

- inguinal lig.
- strangulated hernia

10.32

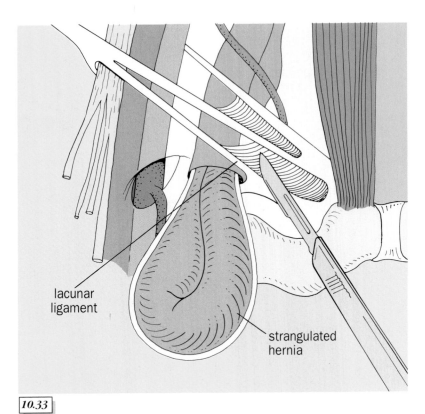

lacunar ligament

strangulated hernia

10.33

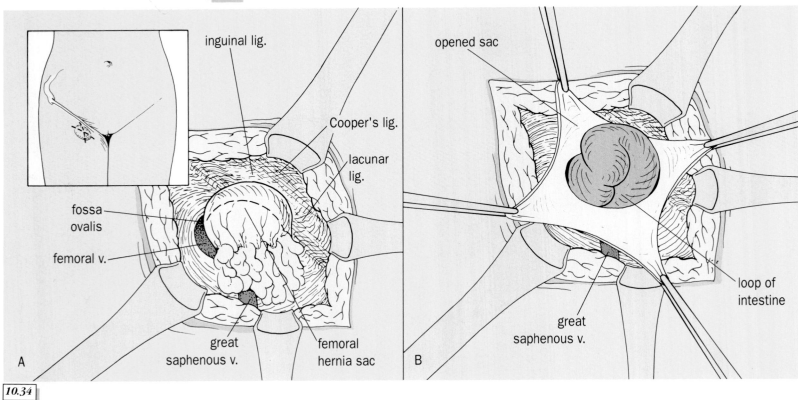

inguinal lig.

Cooper's lig.

lacunar lig.

fossa ovalis

femoral v.

great saphenous v.

femoral hernia sac

A

opened sac

loop of intestine

great saphenous v.

B

10.34

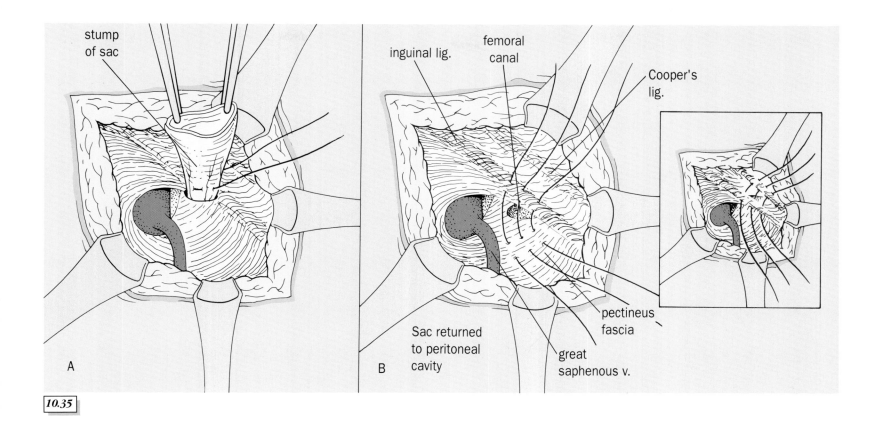

10.35

BIBLIOGRAPHY

Bassini E. *Nuovo metodo per la cura radicale dellernia inguinale.* Padua: Prosperini; 1889.

Halverson K, McVay CB. Inguinal and femoral hernioplasty: a 22-year study of the authors methods. *Arch Surg* 1970; 101:127–135.

Lichtenstein IL, Shulman AG, Amid PK, et al. The tension-free hernioplasty. *Am J Surg* 1989; 157:188–193.

McVay CB. Inguinal hernioplasty—common mistakes and pitfalls. *Surg Clin N Am* 1966; 46:1089–1100.

McVay CB. The normal and pathologic anatomy of the transversus abdominus muscle in inguinal and femoral hernia. *Surg Clin N Am* 1971; 51:1251–1261.

McVay CB, Chapp JD. Inguinal and femoral hernioplasty—evaluation of a basic concept. *Ann Surg* 1958; 148:499–512.

Nyhus LM. Recurrent groin hernia. *World J Surg* 1989; 541–544.

Nyhus LM, Klein MS, Rogers FB. Inguinal hernia. *Curr Prob Surg* 1991; 28(6).

Nyhus LM, Pollak R, Bombeck CT, et al. The preperitoneal approach and prosthetic buttress repair for recurrent hernia: the evolution of a technique. *Ann Surg* 1988; 208:733–737.

Wantz GE. The Canadian repair of inguinal hernia. In Nyhus LM, Condon RE, eds. *Hernia,* 3rd ed. Philadelphia, Pa: JB Lippincott; 1989:236–252.

11

Vascular Surgery

Stanton N. Smullens • John W. Francfort

SURGERY FOR ARTERIAL DISEASE
ABDOMINAL AORTIC ANEURYSM REPAIR

TRANSABDOMINAL APPROACH

Certain preoperative steps are necessary before surgery can be planned for transabdominal repair of abdominal aortic aneurysm. The patient must have no history of recent myocardial infarction (within 3 months), angina, or arrhythmia, and must have a normal electrocardiogram. If any of these factors is present, stress testing should be performed, with a positive test resulting in cardiac catheterization and treatment as indicated. An aortogram should be obtained in the presence of any of the following: hypertension or renal insufficiency; visceral ischemia by history or presence of abdominal or flank bruit; peripheral vascular disease. If none of these is present, computed tomography (CT) scan with dye can be substituted for the aortogram.

In addition, all antiplatelet therapy should be stopped prior to surgery. Autologous donation of blood may be arranged preoperatively, with autotransfusion during the operation. The patient should undergo a preoperative cleansing enema, and should receive prophylactic antibiotics on the morning of, and every 4 hours during, surgery. Antibiotics are continued for 3 to 5 days postoperatively, with a cephalosporin recommended.

TRANSABDOMINAL APPROACH

INDICATIONS	• all symptomatic aortic aneurysms regardless of size • aneurysms greater than 5 cm in width or antero-posterior diameter in good-risk patients (or two times the size of the patient's nondilated suprarenal aorta) • aneurysms enlarging at a rate of 1 cm or greater in 6 months • aneurysms greater than 6 cm in all patients able to withstand surgery
CONTRA-INDICATIONS	• myocardial infarction within 3 months • renal failure with creatinine greater than 3.0 mg/100 dL • intractable congestive heart failure • severe chronic obstructive pulmonary disease
ANESTHESIA	• general endotracheal, with Swan–Ganz pulmonary artery monitoring, indwelling arterial line, and Foley catheter
POSITIONING	• supine, with distal pulses marked
PREP	• abdomen and both groin areas scrubbed with Betadine • Betadine solution used to prep the skin and Betadine-impregnated plastic skin drape used to cover exposed area

PROCEDURE

A long midline incision is made (Fig. 11.1). Following exploration, a self-retracting system, such as the Bookwalter, is set in place (Fig. 11.2). The small bowel is packed to the right of the abdomen and the colon to the left. The peritoneum overlaying the aneurysm is opened with the cautery, with care taken to avoid the mesentery of the left colon. Dissection is then taken superiorly, and the duodenum is lifted from the aneurysm. It is usually helpful to ligate the inferior mesenteric vein after first checking for an accompanying visceral arterial collateral (Fig. 11.3). In addition, the lymphatics draining into the cisterna chyli are ligated carefully to prevent chy-

lous ascites. The incision may then be extended laterally in the transverse mesocolon to increase exposure of the aneurysm neck.

The left renal vein is routinely visualized to make certain of its anterior location, as well as to allow its mobilization for control of the aneurysm neck. In 1% of cases the renal vein is posterior to or encircles the aorta; it is important to determine this prior to the dissection. The plane of dissection about the neck, as well as the plane for visualization of the renal vein, is developed by dividing the multiple lymphatics that are present from the level of the inferior mesenteric artery to the renal vein. It is best to ligate these vessels to prevent leakage of lymph and to reduce bleeding. The renal vein may be divided if necessary, as long as the adrenal, ascending lumbar, and gonadal veins are left intact to ensure venous outflow from the left kidney. An alternative method is to ligate the adrenal or the accessory veins to allow more complete retraction of the renal vein.

Two major approaches are advocated for the neck of the aneurysm. In one, only the anterior and lateral walls are dissected and a vertically placed clamp is used. The alternative approach is to encircle the aorta completely (Fig. 11.4). This allows for a higher mobilization of the aortic neck. When this is done, a plane may be developed in the para-aortic tissues, as described above, which allows a finger to be placed carefully about the neck of the aorta. Frequently, there is a lumbar vessel at this level and the finger can be placed carefully above it in an avascular plane. A #18 red rubber catheter is then passed around the neck of the aorta to facilitate placement of a transverse clamp. The catheter is cut. One jaw of the clamp is inserted in the cut end, and the clamp is pulled around the aorta, without concern for the teeth of the clamp tearing the posterior wall of the vessel.

Minimal dissection of the iliac arteries is then carried out. The iliacs are exposed anteriorly and laterally so that vertically placed clamps can be used. If heavy posterior calcification is present, the vessel can be mobilized in a more lateral plane with passage of the clamps posteriorly. This can be carried out without having to mobilize the area extensively, since the iliac arteries are frequently adherent to the iliac veins. The inferior mesenteric artery is not routinely dissected free, but is controlled within the aorta. Systemic heparinization is used, with 1 mg/kg given intravenously. Since a woven Dacron graft is usually used for replacement of the abdominal aorta, preclotting of the prosthesis is not required. Following heparinization, the distal iliac arteries are first occluded and then the neck of the aneurysm is controlled. This helps prevent distal embolization. The aneurysm is opened with a Bovie cautery along the right side of the aorta to avoid neural tissue on the left anterior wall in an attempt to prevent problems with postoperative impotency in the male patient (Fig. 11.5). After opening the aneurysm, the large amount of thrombotic material is removed. Before the upper and lower ends of the aorta are fashioned, a Weitlander retractor is placed in the aorta—stay sutures of silk may also be used. Control of lumbar artery back bleeding and of the inferior mesenteric artery is carried out using transfixion figure-of-eight sutures of 3–0 Prolene (Fig. 11.6).

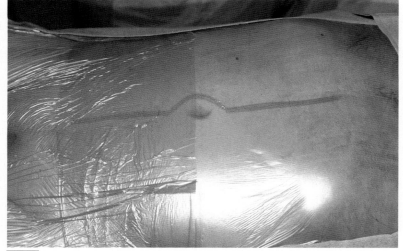

11.1

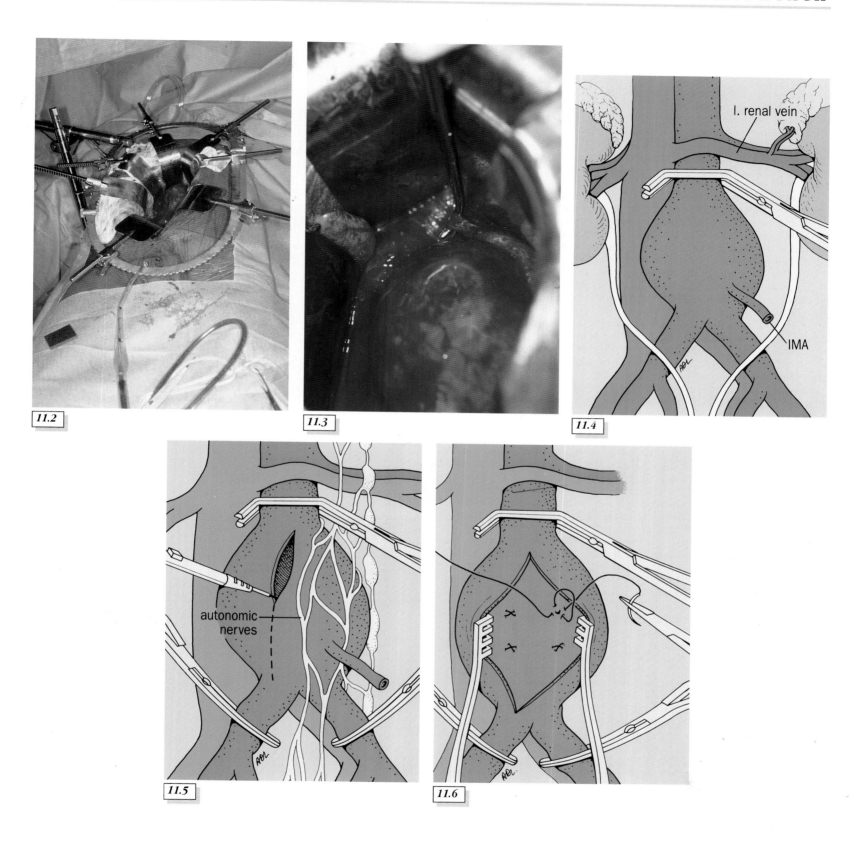

11.2

11.3

11.4

l. renal vein

IMA

11.5

autonomic
nerves

11.6

If a large meandering vessel is seen on the preoperative arteriogram, or if there is a large patent inferior mesenteric artery with poor back bleeding, reimplantation of the inferior mesenteric artery onto the prosthesis may be required. If there is any uncertainty, the inferior mesenteric artery should be excised with a button of aorta and should be controlled with either small vascular clamps or an indwelling, occluding balloon catheter. This will allow assessment of mesenteric blood flow to the left colon at the completion of the aortic portion of the procedure. Assessment for low-lying accessory renal arteries arising from the aneurysm is also made at this time, and if found, they are preserved for reimplantation into the prosthesis.

The neck of the aneurysm is cut in a T-fashion for ease in doing the proximal anastomosis. A decision is usually made at this point as to whether a tube graft or a bifurcated graft to the iliacs or more distal vessels is required. A tube graft can be used in up to 60% of aortic aneurysm resections. Anastomosis of the proximal suture line is constructed in such a way that the sutures posteriorly will encompass a double layer of aortic wall. Using 3–0 Prolene, the first suture is placed as a horizontal mattress in the midline from the inside of the prosthesis. A "parachuting" anastomosis is done and most of the posterior row is placed before the prosthesis is drawn in place (Figs. 11.7, 11.8). The over-and-over suture with a double needle is then brought anteriorly and tied in the midline. Generous bites are required, and the suture line should be placed as close as possible to the renal arteries to avoid the development of an aneurysm in this segment of the aorta. The proximal suture line is then tested by placement of a shod clamp on the prosthesis.

Following this, attention is turned to the distal aorta. This lower area may also be cut in a T-fashion with a shorter lip to the left. The graft is distended and an appropriate length without tension is determined (Fig. 11.9). An end-to-end anastomosis is constructed using 3–0 Prolene, with the initial bite being a horizontal mattress again encompassing a double layer of aortic wall (Fig. 11.10). Frequently, however, there is heavy calcification in the aorta at this point. Although the aneurysm may end at the iliac bifurcation making a tube graft theoretically possible, heavy calcification may necessitate use of the iliac arteries. Occasionally, the calcification in the distal aorta may be removed and the remaining aortic wall can be used if it appears to have sufficient strength. Prior to the completion of the distal anastomosis, both legs are flushed by alternately removing the clamps and compressing the thighs vigorously. The proximal aorta is likewise flushed to remove any clots, and the interior of the graft is washed with heparinized saline to remove any debris. The anastomosis is then completed. The proximal clamp is released and a #20 needle is inserted into the body of the graft in several positions to evacuate air. Each iliac artery is slowly released in turn to avoid postclamp hypotension. Femoral pulses are checked by the surgeon and previously marked distal pulses are checked by the circulating nurse.

If the terminal aorta is not used for the graft, then the anastomoses are performed to the iliac arteries, and the body of the graft is cut short and a bifurcated prosthesis is used. Shortening of the upper graft prevents splaying and kinking of the graft limbs. Dissection of the iliac arteries can be carried out easily once the aorta is decompressed. The arteries are transected. On the right, the end-to-end anastomosis is brought through the open end of the iliac artery, while on the left the prosthesis is best brought through the intact common iliac artery to avoid injuries to the nerve fibers in the area. Occasionally the intima and adherent calcification must be removed to allow a large enough opening for the prosthesis without constricting it. Distal end-to-end anastomoses of the common iliac arteries are carried out with continuous 4–0 Prolene (Fig. 11.11). If com-

mon iliac disease such as heavy calcification or aneurysmal dilatation is present, anastomosis can frequently be carried out to the bifurcation of the internal and external iliac arteries. Occasionally it is necessary to sacrifice an internal iliac artery because of aneurysmal disease and the anastomosis can be carried out end to end to the external iliac. It is imperative that at least one internal iliac artery be preserved, as it will help with left colonic blood flow, particularly if the inferior mesenteric artery is patent and ligated. In addition, it is thought that preserving at least one internal iliac reduces the rare and devastating complication of paraplegia following elective infrarenal abdominal aortic aneurysm repair. Following successful completion of the distal anastomosis (Fig. 11.12), and assurance that distal circulation is intact, heparin may be reversed with protamine sulfate.

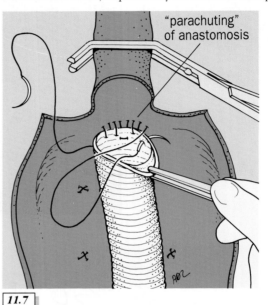

11.7

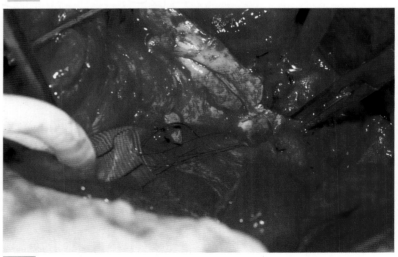

11.8

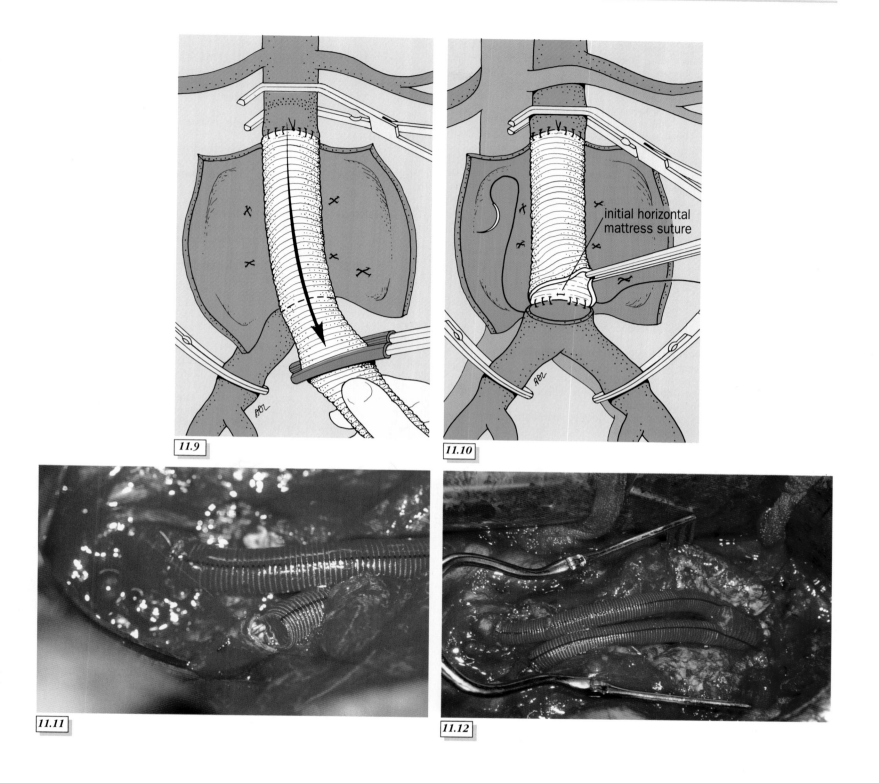

11.9

11.10
initial horizontal
mattress suture

11.11

11.12

Closure is started by controlling bleeding along the wall of the excluded aneurysm. If bleeding is minimal, a Bovie cautery may be used. Usually, however, a continuous locking suture of 0–chromic catgut is required. The aorta is then approximated over the prosthesis with running 0–chromic suture. If the aneurysm is large, the wall is plicated over the aorta to reduce dead space about the prosthesis (Fig. 11.13). The peritoneum is then closed. It is necessary to interpose tissue, usually in the area of the ligated inferior mesenteric vein, under the duodenum. Lymphatic tissue in the area is usually present and the peritoneum can be sutured in this region. The peritoneal closure is completed, with care taken to avoid obstruction of the fourth part of the duodenum. Irrigation with antibiotic solution is carried out prior to the retroperitoneal closure. The abdominal wall is closed with a single layer of continuous 0–Prolene. Metal clips are used to close the skin.

RETROPERITONEAL APPROACH

Preoperative diagnostic and prophylactic procedures are the same as those for transabdominal approach for repair of abdominal aortic aneurysm, except that aortogram is always required.

RETROPERITONEAL APPROACH

INDICATIONS	•aneurysms limited to aorta or proximal iliac arteries •any pararenal aortic aneurysms •obese patients, particularly with cardiac and pulmonary disability •previous abdominal surgery with anticipated multiple adhesions
CONTRA-INDICATIONS	•right iliac artery aneurysm •right renal artery stenosis requiring repair
ANESTHESIA	•same as for abdominal aortic aneurysm (see page 11.2)
POSITIONING	•patient placed supine with the chest slightly elevated approximately 30°, and abdomen flat
PREP	•skin prep and draping same as for routine aneurysm, but extended more posteriorly

PROCEDURE

Incision extends from the tip of the tenth rib on the left across the midline, and below the umbilicus to the region of the right iliac crest (Fig. 11.14). After the abdominal wall has been divided, a retroperitoneal plane is developed laterally with retraction of the abdominal viscera to the right. The spleen and tail of the pancreas are retracted medially. The plane of dissection may be either anterior or posterior to the left kidney. For aneurysms, the plane anterior to the kidney is preferred so that the position of the left renal artery is well visualized. Exposure is not complete until the inferior mesenteric artery is divided. At this juncture, sharp and blunt dissection will expose the aneurysm and the proximal iliac vessels (Fig. 11.15). Self-retaining retractors again are quite helpful (see Fig. 11.2). The remainder of the operative procedure is carried out as for the transabdominal aneurysm resection.

JUXTARENAL ABDOMINAL AORTIC ANEURYSM

Preoperative diagnostic and prophylactic procedures are the same as those for abdominal aortic aneurysm, except aortogram is mandatory.

JUXTARENAL ABDOMINAL AORTIC ANEURYSM

INDICATIONS	•juxtarenal aneurysms that extend to or include the renal arteries
CONTRA-INDICATIONS	•extension of aneurysm above the superior mesenteric artery •obese patients with narrow costal angles
ANESTHESIA	•same as for abdominal aortic aneurysm (see page 11.2)
POSITIONING	•patient placed in supine position for standard midline incision in thin patients; retroperitoneal approach preferred for heavy patients
PREP	•same as for abdominal aortic aneurysm (see page 11.2)

PROCEDURE

The technique of clamping the aorta at the diaphragm should be mastered (Fig. 11.16). It is performed by entering the lesser sac through the avascular portion on the right side of the esophagus. The right crura of the diaphragm, which envelopes the aorta at this level, is freed by blunt finger dissection. A vertical vascular clamp may then be placed (Fig. 11.17). Aneurysms arising just at the renal arteries may be controlled by this method. The aneurysm is opened in the routine fashion (Fig. 11.18) and the proximal suture line is placed just at the level of the renal arteries (Fig. 11.19). Placement above this level will require repair of the visceral vessels.

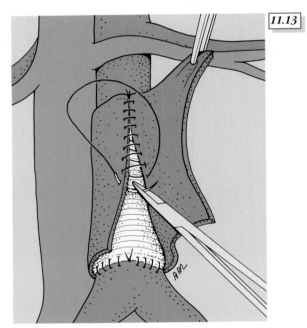

11.13

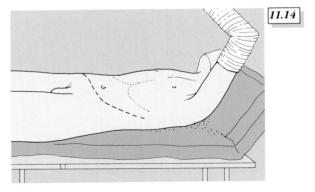

11.14

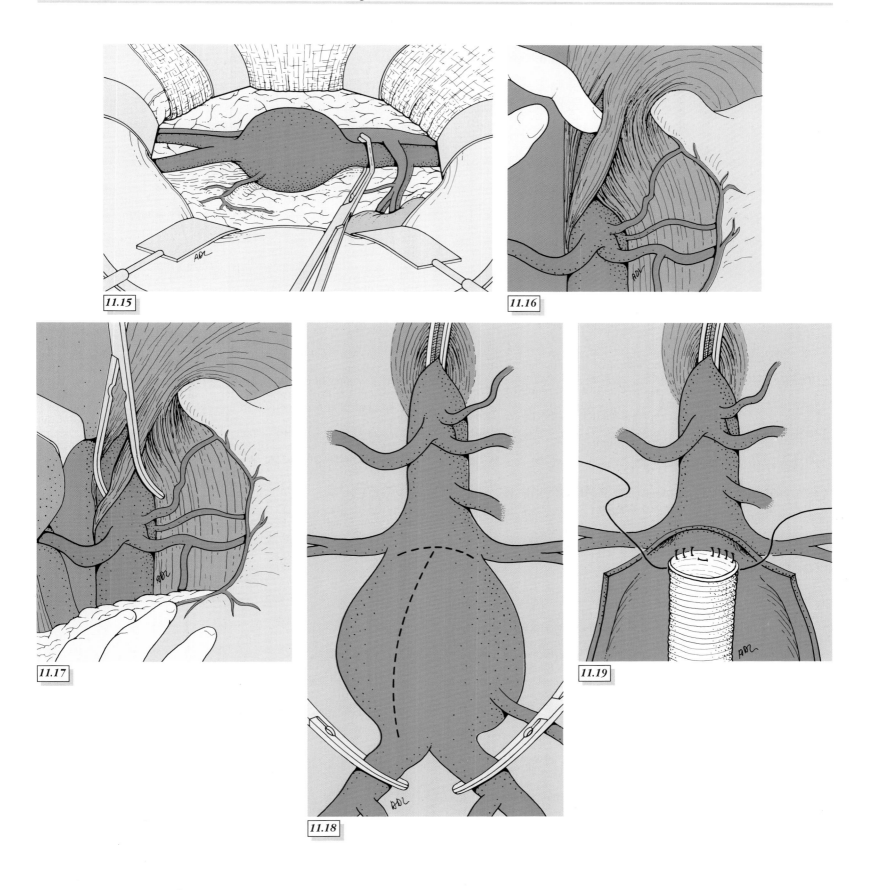

11.15

11.16

11.17

11.18

11.19

SURGERY FOR AORTOILIAC OCCLUSIVE DISEASE

Preoperative diagnostic and prophylactic procedures are the same as those for abdominal aortic aneurysm, except aortogram is mandatory. The decision as to which type of procedure to perform depends on the optimal medical status of the patient.

AORTOFEMORAL BYPASS

This procedure is reserved for good-risk surgical patients, with any of the indications listed below.

AORTOFEMORAL BYPASS

INDICATIONS	• disabling claudication • ischemic rest pain • ischemic ulceration • pregangrenous skin changes • microembolization to feet or toes from aortoiliac source ("blue toe syndrome") • gangrene
CONTRA-INDICATIONS	• same as for abdominal aortic aneurysm (see page 11.2) • gangrene and severe rest pain requiring surgical treatment • vascular repair absolutely medically contraindicated • amputation a possibility
ANESTHESIA **POSITIONING** **PREP**	same as for abdominal aortic aneurysm repair (see page 11.2)

PROCEDURE

A long midline incision is made, with care taken not to place the incision too close to the umbilicus. After abdominal exploration, a self-retaining retractor system is set in place (see Fig. 11.2). The small bowel is packed to the patient's right and the large bowel to the left. The tissue overlying the aorta is opened from the level of the inferior mesenteric artery proximally. The aortic bifurcation is left undisturbed to minimize the chance of injury to neural tissue in the area. The duodenum is lifted from the aorta. It is usually not necessary to divide the inferior mesenteric vein or large lymphatic channels in the area. They may, however, be divided in obese individuals to increase exposure of the infrarenal aorta. The left renal vein is identified in the loose areolar tissue. Occasionally, lymphatics are thick in this area and should be divided to establish a satisfactory plane about the aorta. Identification of the renal vein is important for location of the renal arteries as well as for ascertaining its anterior position. The aorta is mobilized at the level below the renal arteries and is gently encircled. An anterior and lateral exposure may be sufficient if the aorta is to be clamped vertically. If the aorta is occluded to the renal arteries, the arteries should be exposed in order to occlude them temporarily, thus preventing embolization during the thrombectomy of the proximal aorta.

The femoral regions are opened through vertically placed infrainguinal incisions (Fig. 11.20). Great care is essential to avoid undue trauma since the femoral regions are the highest source of infection in aortic surgery. All lymphatic tissue is carefully tied and exposure extends from the inguinal ligament to a level necessary to expose the common femoral artery (CFA), superficial femoral artery (SFA), and profunda femoris artery (PFA). The first 2 to 3 cm of this latter vessel are isolated. The inguinal lig-

ament may be divided to prevent compression of the prosthetic graft limbs. The deep circumflex iliac vein is visualized and usually ligated to prevent tearing of it when the prostheses are placed in the retroperitoneal tunnel (Fig. 11.21). The tunnel can now be started by passing the finger gently, just anterior to the external iliac artery. The wounds are covered with antibiotic-moistened sponges and attention is directed to the abdomen.

The retroperitoneal tunnel is completed by gently dissecting anterior to the iliac vessels on the right, and somewhat more laterally on the left, by placing the graft lateral to the inferior mesenteric artery, again to avoid the neural tissue at the aortic bifurcation and proximal left common iliac artery. The tunnels are always made posterior to the ureters to avoid compression by the prosthesis (Fig. 11.22).

If a knitted Dacron graft is selected, either it is pretreated or it must be preclotted. Its size is determined by the diameter of the aorta and outflow femoral arteries. Frequent sizes are a 16- x 8-mm graft in a man and a 14- x 7-mm graft in a woman.

The patient is systemically heparinized (1 mg/kg). A clamp is first placed distally to prevent embolization, and then the proximal aortic clamp is placed, either vertically or transversely. If an end-to-side anastomosis is to be made, the aorta is cross-clamped to prevent embolization from a side-biting clamp placement. The incision should be placed high on the aorta so that progression of disease will not occlude the graft. A localized endarterectomy or thrombectomy may be necessary in the proximal aorta to make certain of excellent blood flow. The graft is cut at a 45° angle (Fig. 11.23). With both types of anastomoses, the body of the graft is cut short to prevent kinking. Continuous 3–0 Prolene suture is used for the proximal anastomosis. If an end-to-end anastomosis is planned, the aorta is transected 2 to 3 cm below the renal arteries. The distal aorta is cut obliquely and also may require an endarterectomy prior to closure with 3–0 Prolene sutures. In the proximal aorta, the double-armed suture is started posteriorly and is brought anteriorly and tied. Appropriate forward flushing of the anastomosis is performed. If the proximal cuff is not thick, a portion of the prosthesis can be placed around the anastomosis to protect it from the duodenum and for hemostasis (Fig. 11.24). However, if the tissues are heavy, the graft may cause constriction at the anastomotic site. The prosthesis is then carefully placed through the retroperitoneal tunnel, and the limbs passed to the femoral incisions, with care taken to avoid twisting them. The use of long grasping instruments and the markings of the newer grafts help to prevent this.

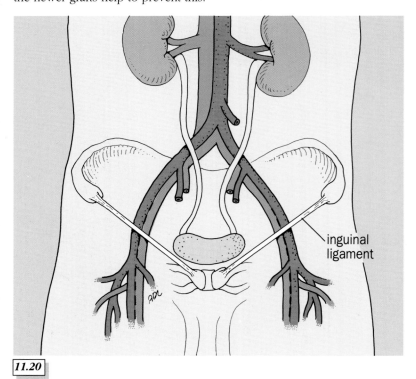

inguinal ligament

11.20

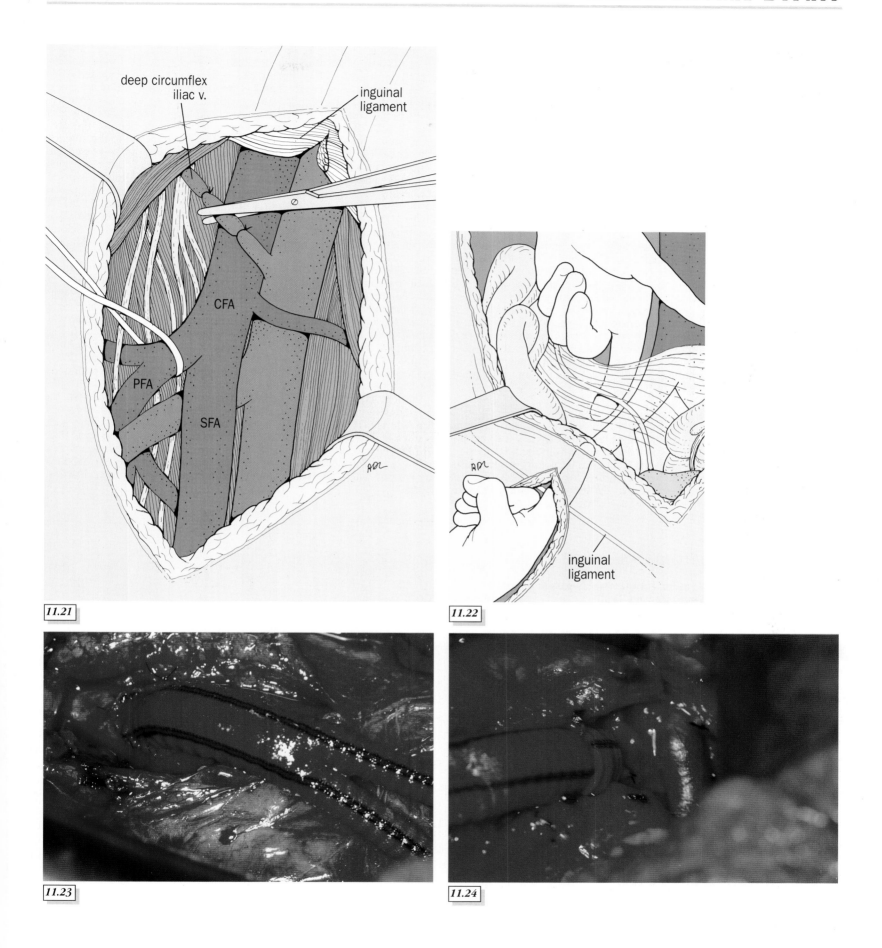

deep circumflex
iliac v.

inguinal
ligament

CFA

PFA

SFA

11.21

inguinal
ligament

11.22

11.23

11.24

At this juncture it is important to appreciate the need for outflow preservation. Significant improvement in long-term patency rates for aortofemoral grafts has been achieved by maintaining flow in the face of disease progression in the SFA. This is achieved by placing the femoral limb of the graft over the PFA orifice to prevent progression of disease at this level, with subsequent loss of the iliac limb (Fig. 11.25). An endar-terectomy or a more extensive profundaplasty may be necessary to maintain outflow. Techniques of profundaplasty have been described elsewhere, and may include extension of the graft limb over the PFA, local endarterectomy with graft covering this, or a long endarterectomy and patch, with the limb of the graft sewn into the patch. With SFA occlusion, a prosthetic graft may be sewn end to end to the PFA. The prosthesis is cut to an appropriate length, and the anastomosis is made without tension using 5–0 Prolene sutures. Forward and back flushing of the anastomosis is always performed.

The heparin is reversed with protamine sulfate, and time is spent in achieving hemostasis. The retroperitoneum is washed with antibiotic-containing solution and is closed with absorbable suture to exclude the aortic suture line from the duodenum. The midline abdominal incision is closed in one layer using 0–Prolene as a continuous suture, interrupted and tied in several locations. The groin is thoroughly irrigated, dried, and closed in at least two layers using absorbable material. Care should be taken to avoid placement of the sutures too deeply and trapping of the femoral nerve, leading to significant postoperative morbidity. All skin incisions are closed with carefully placed metal skin clips. The patient is maintained on prophylactic intravenous antibiotics for 1 to 2 days or until all central intravenous lines are removed.

AXILLOFEMORAL BYPASS

Preoperative diagnostic and prophylactic procedures are the same as those for aortofemoral bypass. Unilateral axillofemoral bypass is to be discouraged since long-term patency is not as good as with the bilateral procedure. In the bilateral procedure, if no difference in blood pressure exists between the two arms, the right arm is chosen for inflow since there is less of a chance of subsequent stenosis in the innominate artery as compared to the left subclavian artery. The use of two surgical teams is optimal with this procedure.

AXILLOFEMORAL BYPASS	
INDICATIONS	•same as for aortofemoral bypass in poor-risk patients (see page 11.8) •retroperitoneal infection
CONTRA-INDICATIONS	•stenoses or occlusions of innominate and subclavian arteries
ANESTHESIA	•same as for aortofemoral bypass (see page 11.8) •epidural for lower half of body and local for upper portion •local anesthesia with sedation
POSITIONING	•supine, with arm extended on the side of the donor axillary artery
PREP	•operative field scrubbed with Betadine soap, skin prepared with Betadine, and covered with Betadine-impregnated plastic drape

PROCEDURE

The axillary artery is exposed in its first portion, medial to the pectoralis minor muscle. An incision is made below the clavicle, on the selected side, for a distance of 5 to 6 cm (Fig. 11.26). The pectoralis major muscle

is split in the direction of its fibers. The pectoralis minor may be divided or preserved as the situation dictates. Nerves to the pectoralis muscle should be preserved, if possible. The artery is palpated and exposed, with careful attention given to the cords of the brachial plexus and nearby axillary vein (Fig. 11.27). Exposure for a distance of 2 to 3 cm is necessary. The femoral vessels are exposed as described for the aortofemoral bypass (see Figs. 11.20–11.22). A subcutaneous tunnel is made deep to the pectoralis minor muscle along the lateral chest wall and medial to the anterior iliac spine. The DeBakey tunneler is useful for this and can be passed the entire length without the need for a counter incision. Counter incisions should be avoided since they have shown poor healing. A tunnel is made connecting the two femoral incisions, and is placed in the hollow superior to the pubic bone, just anterior to the abdominal fascia (Fig. 11.28). A knitted Dacron graft, or an externally supported expanded polytetrafluoroethylene (ePTFE) graft, usually an 8-mm diameter, is used. It is helpful to place the graft in the tunnel prior to the axillary anastomosis, with care taken to avoid twisting it.

In constructing the axillary anastomosis, great care must be taken to avoid tension since kinking of the axillary artery is a frequent source of graft failure. It is also important to bevel the anastomosis so that the graft exits the axillary artery in a gentle, forward curve rather than at a right angle. Placing the anastomosis in the first part of the axillary artery is important for this reason. The patient is systemically heparinized with 1 to 1.5 mg/kg. The axillary vessels are occluded with appropriate vascular clamps and an arteriotomy is made in the inferior–anterior aspect of the axillary artery (see Fig. 11.27). An anastomosis is made with continuous 5–0 Prolene suture.

The femoral anastomosis is constructed similarly to the anastomosis for the aortofemoral bypass, with placement of the graft overlying the PFA orifice (see Fig. 11.25). After this is completed, a side arm of the 8-mm graft is sewn end to side to the graft, proximal to the femoral anastomosis (Fig. 11.29). The second femoral anastomosis is performed in the same manner as the first. The heparin is reversed with protamine sulfate, the wounds are washed with antibiotic-containing solution, and they are then closed in layers.

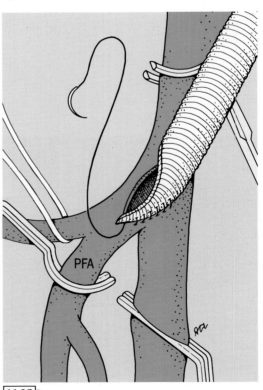

PFA

11.25

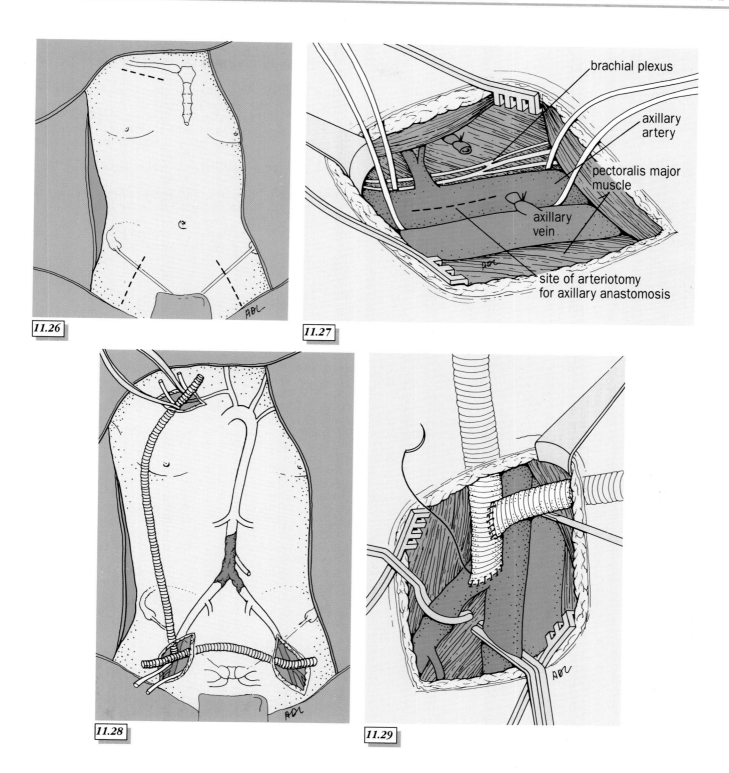

11.26

11.27

brachial plexus

axillary
artery

pectoralis major
muscle

axillary
vein

site of arteriotomy
for axillary anastomosis

11.28

11.29

FEMOROFEMORAL BYPASS

Preoperative diagnostic and prophylactic procedures are the same as those for aortofemoral bypass. This procedure is reserved for patients at poor surgical risk, with any of the indications listed for aortofemoral bypass.

PROCEDURE

The femoral vessels are exposed through vertical incisions, and a suprapubic tunnel connecting them is made by blunt finger dissection, just anterior to the fascia (Fig. 11.30). Although much has been written regarding "S" configuration versus "C" configuration for the donor artery anastomosis, experience has shown no difference in patency rates. In the S configuration, the graft is taken from the external iliac artery and passes retropubically in the space of Retzius. A forward-flowing anastomosis is constructed. With the C arrangement, the graft is taken from the CFA and flow must go retrograde. The C configuration is the technically easier one and is preferred. Usually a 6- or an 8-mm knitted Dacron or ePTFE graft is selected depending on the size of the patient's arteries.

Following preclotting of the Dacron graft, the patient is systemically heparinized. The graft is placed in the tunnel, and the donor artery is occluded with vascular clamps (Fig. 11.31). If the donor artery is large enough, a slightly oblique incision is made in its anterior wall. The graft is cut to an approximate 45° angle, and the end-to-side anastomosis is made with continuous 5–0 Prolene tied at the "toe and heel." The graft is cut without tension, and the second anastomosis is made to include the PFA orifice, as previously described (Fig. 11.32). Flushing of the graft and artery is always standard. The heparin is reversed, the wounds are irrigated, and they are then closed in at least two layers using absorbable suture. If the skin is not unusually thin or fragile, subcutaneous skin closure is recommended. Antibiotics are continued for 1 to 2 days or until all central IV lines are removed.

SURGERY FOR COMMON FEMORAL ARTERY DISEASE

COMMON FEMORAL ENDARTERECTOMY AND BYPASS

Prior to surgery, preoperative noninvasive vascular studies are performed, as well as arteriography to define inflow vessels and distal runoff. Associated cardiovascular risk factors should also be evaluated prior to surgical reconstruction. Prophylactic antibiotics are administered prior to surgery.

PROCEDURE

An infrainguinal longitudinal incision is made over the CFA using a somewhat lateral approach to avoid the lymphatic pad (Fig. 11.34). Vessel loops are placed about the proximal CFA, SFA, and PFA (Fig. 11.35). If the atherosclerotic plaque extends into the SFA or PFA, further mobilization of these vessels may be necessary to perform an endarterectomy. The lateral femoral circumflex vein and other perforating veins must be divided to expose the PFA distal to its origin (Fig. 11.36). The skin incision can be extended along the medial border of the sartorius muscle to enhance PFA exposure for a distance of up to 15 cm.

Endarterectomy is ideal for patients with localized disease of the CFA and more proximal segments to the femoral bifurcation. After heparin administration (1 mg/kg), a soft vascular clamp is placed on the CFA while vessel loops are tightened distally. Most commonly this procedure is performed in the presence of SFA occlusion; thus the arteriotomy is extended from the CFA into the PFA. The endarterectomy plane is begun proximally at the junction of the outer one third and inner two thirds level of the media (Fig. 11.37; see also Fig. 11.75).

Careful endarterectomy of side branches ensures good outflow and patency of the repair. The distal end of the plaque should be entirely removed and the remaining intima visualized to prevent intimal flaps from causing postoperative thrombosis. If the flaps are not adequately adherent, 7–0 Prolene intimal tacking sutures are inserted. Patch angioplasty of the entire arteriotomy site is best performed with vein and 6–0 or 7–0 polypropylene suture. However, if vein is to be preserved for future procedures, either the endarterectomized SFA that was occluded or prosthetic patching material provides good long-term patency (Fig. 11.38).

We prefer to bypass those patients who require a long patch or an extended profundaplasty. Those patients with a patent but extensively diseased SFA and PFA are more likely to develop SFA occlusion after CFA endarterectomy and are also better served with a bypass. In both cases we bypass from the distal external iliac artery or CFA to a relatively disease-free portion of the PFA. The anastomoses are performed in an end-to-side fashion, utilizing 6–0 or 7–0 polypropylene sutures (Fig. 11.39). Vein graft is preferred, but prosthetic grafts are durable with acceptable patency rates.

Groin closure is performed in three layers. Two subcutaneous layers are repaired with absorbable suture prior to skin approximation. Distal pulses (or Doppler signals in the patient with SFA occlusion) should be present prior to awakening of the patient. Ankle–arm pressures are obtained postoperatively.

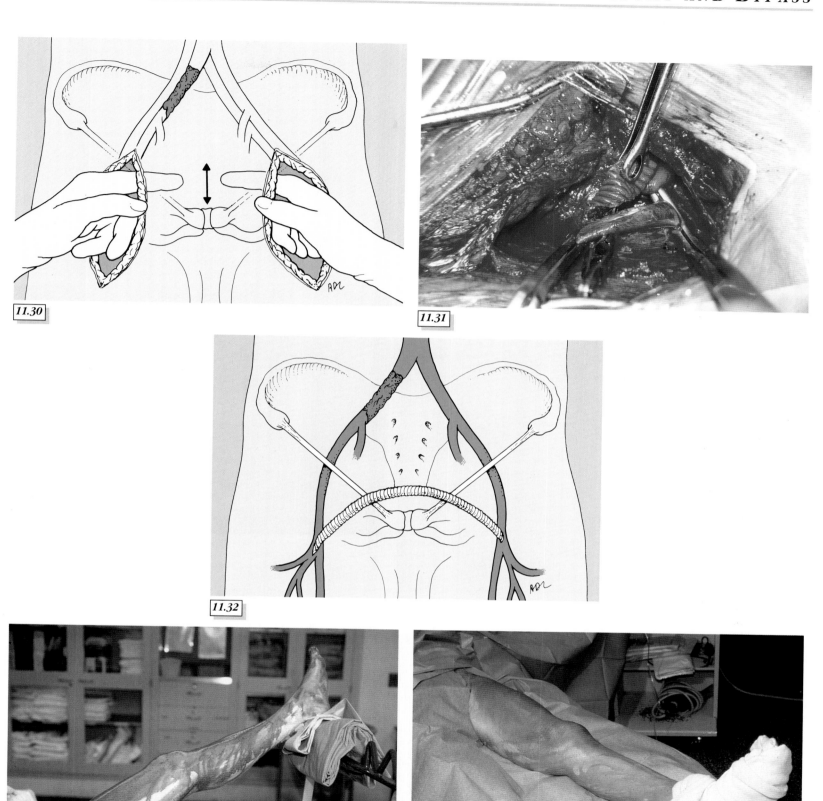

11.30

11.31

11.32

11.33A

11.33B

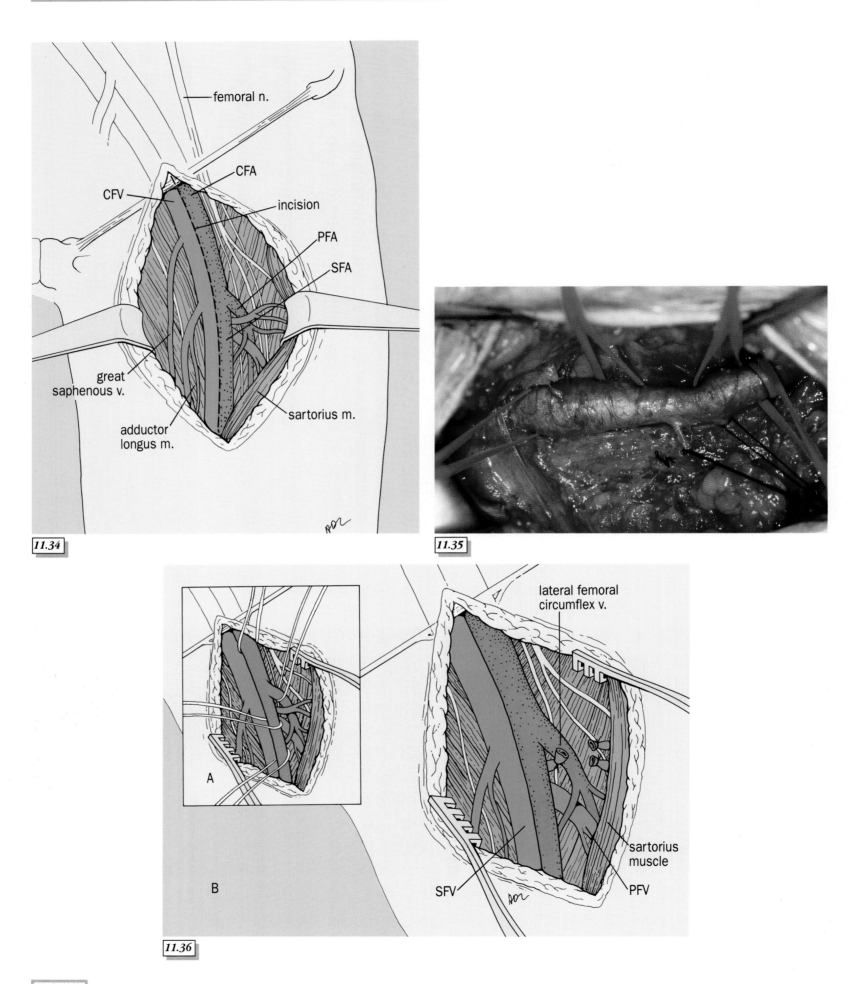

11.34

femoral n.

CFV

CFA

incision

PFA

SFA

great
saphenous v.

adductor
longus m.

sartorius m.

11.35

11.36

A

B

lateral femoral
circumflex v.

sartorius
muscle

SFV

PFV

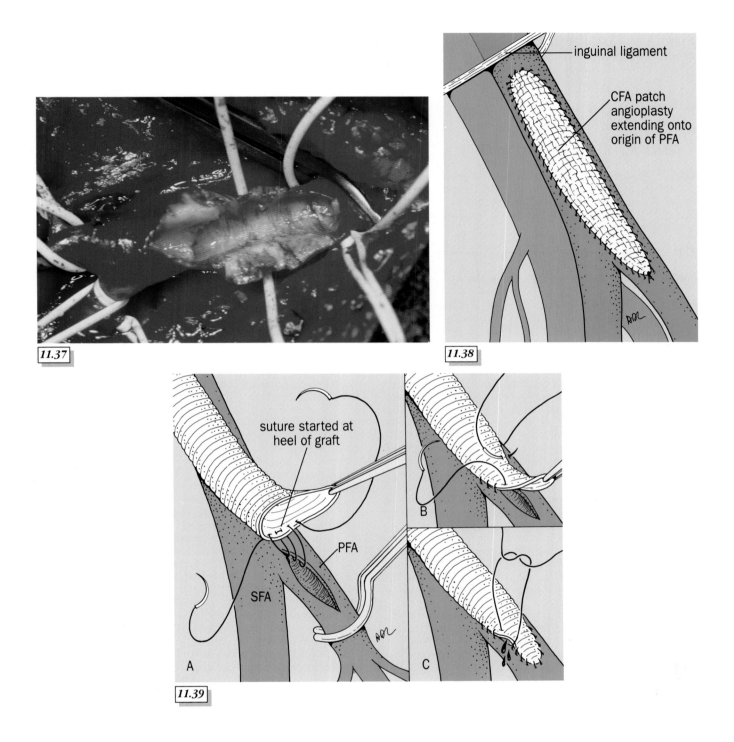

inguinal ligament

CFA patch
angioplasty
extending onto
origin of PFA

11.37

11.38

suture started at
heel of graft

PFA

SFA

A

B

C

11.39

FEMORAL ARTERY ANEURYSM REPAIR

Prior to surgery, Doppler pressure and waveform examinations are performed, along with cardiac evaluation and arteriography, if occlusive disease is present. CT scanning is sufficient to demonstrate the proximal and distal limits of involvement. Concomitant aortic, popliteal, and SFA aneurysms may be detected. Antibiotic prophylaxis should also be given.

FEMORAL ARTERY ANEURYSM REPAIR

INDICATIONS	•aneurysms twice normal femoral vessel size •symptoms due to nerve or vein compression •embolization of luminal thrombus •femoral aneurysm thrombosis requiring emergency repair
ANESTHESIA	•general endotracheal, epidural, or local
POSITIONING	•supine, with Foley catheter in place
PREP	•sterile preparation of abdomen and entire leg (see Fig. 11.33)

PROCEDURE

An infrainguinal longitudinal incision is made over the CFA. Lateral approach to the artery decreases the chance of lymphocele formation. Most aneurysms can be approached from the groin, dividing the inguinal ligament for proximal exposure of the external iliac artery as necessary. Proximal control is first obtained by placing a vessel loop about the CFA (see Figs. 11.35, 11.36A). More distally, loops are placed about the SFA and PFA distal to the femoral bifurcation (Fig. 11.40). After heparinization (1 mg/kg), clamps are applied proximally, while vessel loops are tightened distally.

The aneurysm is opened anteriorly and small bleeding vessels are sewn from within the sac (Fig. 11.41). If the femoral bifurcation is not diseased, a 6- or 8-mm prosthetic graft is sutured with continuous 6–0 polypropylene suture to bridge the aneurysmal defect. In the event that the femoral bifurcation is aneurysmal, the distal anastomosis is performed to the SFA (Fig. 11.42). If there is SFA occlusion, an iliac–PFA bypass is performed (Fig. 11.43). If the SFA is aneurysmal, a femoropopliteal bypass with saphenous vein is necessary, followed by ligation of the intervening SFA (Fig. 11.44).

Groin closure is performed in three layers. Two deep subcutaneous layers are repaired with absorbable suture prior to skin approximation. Distal pulses (or Doppler signals in the patient with SFA occlusion) should be present prior to awakening of the patient. Ankle–arm pressures should be obtained preoperatively and postoperatively.

FEMORAL–POPLITEAL–TIBIAL RECONSTRUCTION
FEMOROPOPLITEAL BYPASS

Noninvasive vascular studies are performed preoperatively, along with arteriography. If proximal iliac stenosis greater than 50% is present, demonstrating a pressure drop of 15% or more across the lesion, preoperative angioplasty or surgical correction is required. Proximal or midpopliteal artery disease (stenosis or aneurysm) necessitates distal popliteal bypass. Ultrasound mapping of the saphenous vein should be performed, if indicated. Cardiac evaluation should be performed prior to all vascular cases. Prophylactic antibiotic therapy should also be instituted.

FEMOROPOPLITEAL BYPASS

INDICATIONS	•atherosclerotic occlusive and aneurysmal disease of the femoral and popliteal vessels •disabling claudication •rest pain •distal gangrene or nonhealing ulcers
ANESTHESIA	•general endotracheal or epidural
POSITIONING	•supine, with Foley catheter in place
PREP	•entire groin and leg prepped and draped in a sterile fashion, with the foot placed in stockinette

---

PROCEDURE

A vertical incision is made in the groin over the CFA with the lower portion extended medially toward the greater saphenous vein (GSV). Care is taken to ligate the lymphatic tributaries to avoid lymphocele formation. Exposure of the CFA and its bifurcation is performed as for CFA occlusive disease (see Figs. 11.35, 11.36). The GSV is identified medial to the artery at the fossa ovalis (Fig. 11.45; see Fig. 11.34). The knee is flexed 30° to 60° by placing a rolled sheet under it to facilitate vein exposure. A continuous or discontinuous incision, thereby leaving skin bridges, is made directly over the vein to a level that obtains sufficient length for the bypass (Fig. 11.46). All tributaries are identified and divided between 4–0 silk ligatures. The vein is left in situ for continuity of flow until the distal artery is dissected and heparin has been administered.

The above-knee popliteal artery is exposed through the same skin incision used to harvest the vein (Fig. 11.47). The remaining subcutaneous tissue and fascia, above the sartorius muscle, is incised exposing the fat pad of the popliteal space (Fig. 11.48). Care is taken to avoid vein and nerve injury while dividing small venous collaterals to expose adequate popliteal artery length. Finger palpation over a right-angle clamp helps to evaluate the extent of disease and to identify a soft area for the arteriotomy. The subsartorial tunnel is bluntly developed either by finger technique or with a long tunneler (Fig. 11.49). A Silastic sling is brought through the tunnel, which is inspected for hemostasis prior to heparin administration. Intravenous heparin (1 mg/kg) is administered prior to vein division. The vein is gently dilated with a heparinized (5 units/mL) solution of saline and papaverine HCl (0.1 mg/mL) or with heparinized blood prior to performing the distal anastomosis (Fig. 11.50). In cases where vein is not available, ePTFE may be utilized.

The popliteal space is held open by a self-retaining retractor. Using magnification loupes, an arteriotomy is made in the vessel after flow is occluded. Outflow patency must be ensured by direct visualization and, in some cases, passage of coronary dilators. Care to avoid plaque dissection is essential. Length of the arteriotomy should be adequate to assure good exposure. The reversed vein wall is split longitudinally for the appropriate length and the toe is trimmed to remove dog-ears. The anastomosis is performed using a 6–0 polypropylene double-armed suture in a continuous fashion beginning at the heel (Fig. 11.51; see Fig. 11.39). Stitching should tack down intimal plaque from inside out to prevent flap formation and also to incorporate at least 2 mm of adventitia (Fig. 11.52). Upon completion of the anastomosis, clamps are released to identify leaks that should be repaired.

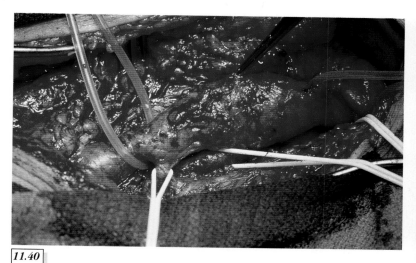

11.40

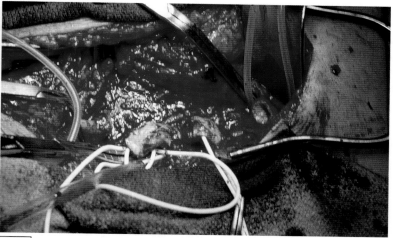

11.41

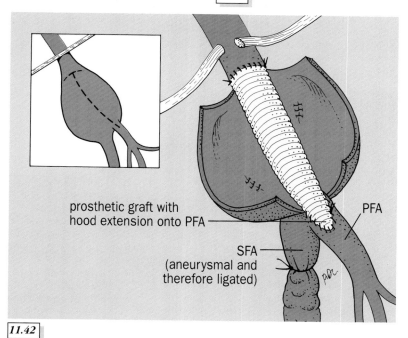

prosthetic graft with
hood extension onto PFA

PFA

SFA
(aneurysmal and
therefore ligated)

11.42

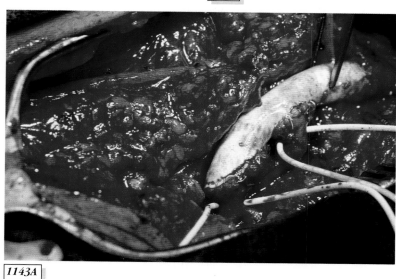

1143A

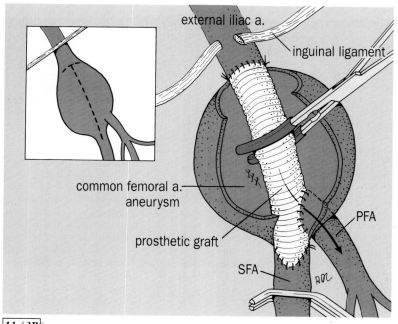

external iliac a.

inguinal ligament

common femoral a.
aneurysm

prosthetic graft

PFA

SFA

11.43B

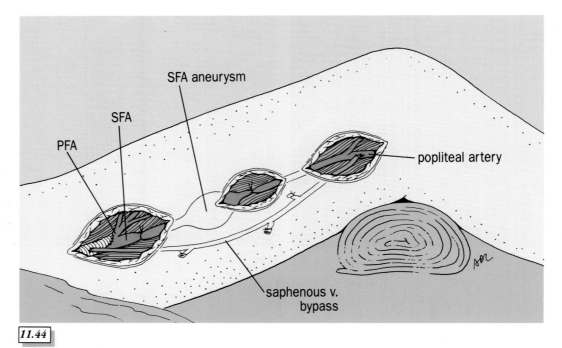

SFA aneurysm

SFA

PFA

popliteal artery

saphenous v. bypass

11.44

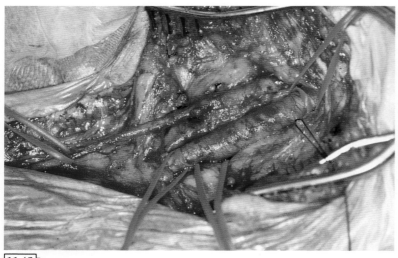

11.45

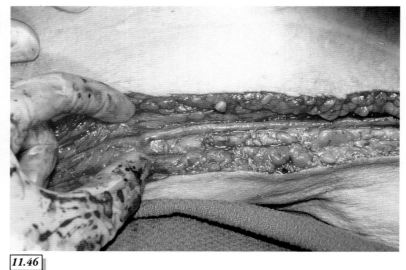

11.46

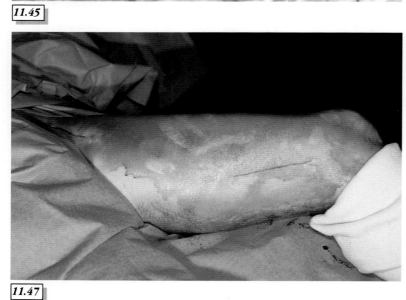

11.47

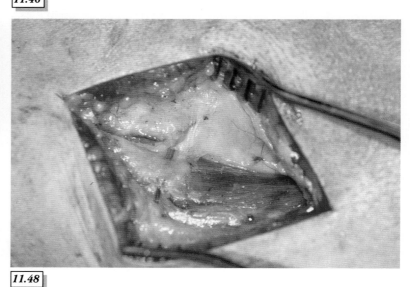

11.48

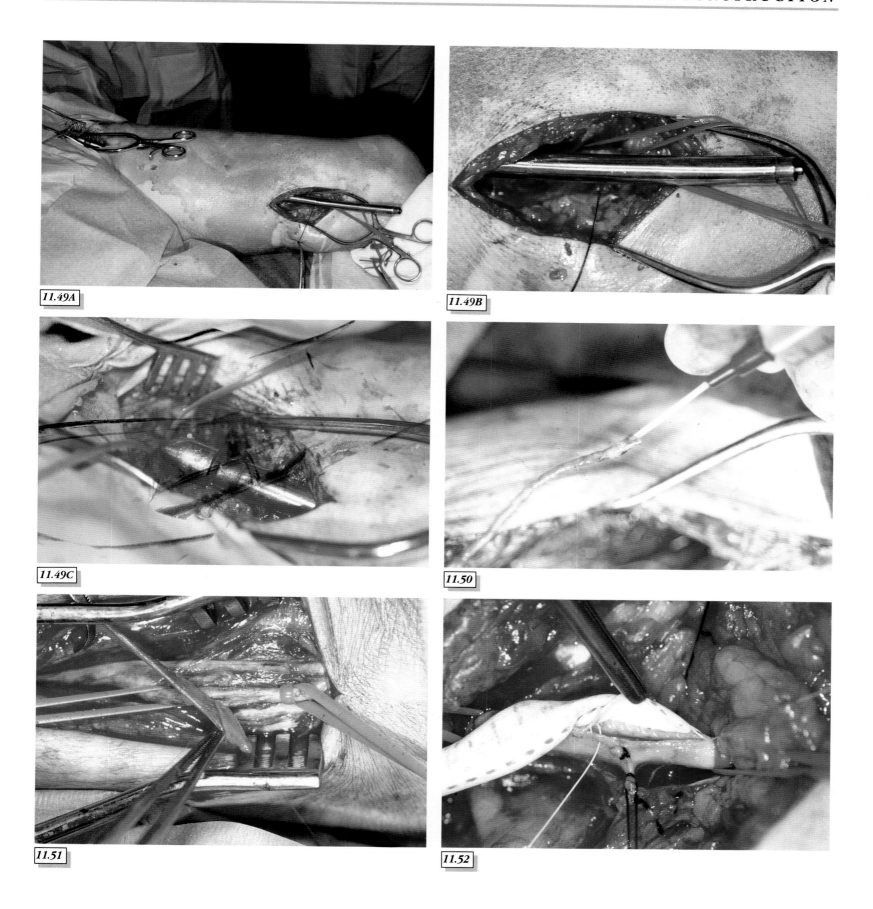

11.49A

11.49B

11.49C

11.50

11.51

11.52

After distention of the vein graft with heparinized solution to ensure proper orientation, it is brought through the subsartorial tunnel (Fig. 11.53). Clamps and vessel loops are tightened on the CFA and its tributaries (see Fig. 11.45). A longitudinal arteriotomy is made in the CFA. The vein is cut and tapered to the appropriate length for the end-to-end anastomosis, which is performed with a continuous 6–0 polypropylene double-armed suture. Careful flushing to assure removal of debris from the CFA should be performed prior to completion of the anastomosis.

A completion arteriogram is essential to identify technical flaws that may lead to early postoperative occlusion. This is performed by placing an 18-gauge butterfly or angiocatheter into the saphenous vein just distal to its origin from the CFA (Fig. 11.54). Full-strength contrast reagent (20 mL) is injected distally while the proximal GSV is occluded. The catheter entry site is repaired with 7–0 Prolene suture. Poor distal outflow, intimal flaps, and twisted grafts may then be identified and corrected.

For below-knee bypass, the infrageniculate popliteal artery is exposed through the saphenous vein–harvesting incision (Fig. 11.55). The subcutaneous tissue and fascia should be opened from the level of the knee joint to just below the origin of the soleus muscle. The knee is flexed 60° and the thigh is abducted and externally rotated. The artery is found in the popliteal fat pad when the medial head of the gastrocnemius is retracted posteriorly. Venous tributaries are divided, allowing arterial mobilization. Venous loops are placed proximally and distally. A popliteal tunnel must be bluntly created between the heads of the gastrocnemius muscles (Fig. 11.56), and is accomplished by finger dissection from the above- and below-knee popliteal space incisions. Silastic slings are placed through this tunnel and the subsartorial tunnel prior to anticoagulation. The techniques used for proper placement of the arteriotomy in a soft area and for assuring adequate outflow are similar to those used for the above-knee anastomosis. Should the distal popliteal bypass be performed for a popliteal aneurysm, the popliteal artery above the anastomosis is suture ligated through both the above- and below-knee incisions, prior to clamp removal, to exclude it from the circulation (see Fig. 11.55). The femoral incision is closed with two absorbable deep layers prior to skin closure. The leg incision is closed in two layers with absorbable 3–0 subcutaneous suture and either 4–0 subcuticular suture or staples.

IN SITU TECHNIQUE FOR FEMORAL–POPLITEAL–TIBIAL BYPASS

IN SITU TECHNIQUE FOR FEMORAL–POPLITEAL–TIBIAL BYPASS

INDICATIONS	•same as for femoral–popliteal–tibial reconstruction (see page 11.16)
ANESTHESIA	•general endotracheal or epidural
POSITIONING	•supine
PREP	•entire groin and leg prepped and draped in a sterile fashion, with the foot placed in a stockinette

PROCEDURE

The major advantage of this technique is that veins 3.0 to 4.0 mm in diameter, previously too small for a reversed bypass, are now acceptable. The CFA and its bifurcation are dissected as described earlier for CFA disease surgery (see Figs. 11.34, 11.36A). The knee is then flexed 60° and the saphenous vein is exposed without skin bridges, until sufficient length is obtained for the bypass. The vein is left in situ without ligation of any tributaries (Fig. 11.57). A moist sponge is placed over the vein to prevent desiccation while the distal artery is exposed.

The posterior tibial artery (PTA) is approached from the same incision that exposes the GSV (Fig. 11.58). With the GSV displaced posteriorly, the muscular fascia is incised (Fig. 11.59). The soleus insertion on the tibia is divided with cautery and then retracted posteriorly (see Fig. 11.58). The PTA is found just behind the tibialis posterior muscle (Fig. 11.60; see also Fig. 11.58). Crossing veins are divided to expose 2 cm of the PTA. Vessel loops are placed proximally and distally.

After heparinization, the first 6 cm of GSV below the fossa ovalis are freed from the surrounding tissue and tributaries. The vein is divided proximally, taking a small piece of common femoral vein for use as the hood of the proximal anastomosis (Fig. 11.61). The femoral vein is repaired with continuous 5–0 polypropylene suture (Fig. 11.62). The vein hood is everted 1 to 1.5 cm to expose the ostial valve, which is excised under direct vision (Fig. 11.63). Rarely, the vein will not reach the CFA. The proximal anastomosis should then be performed to the PFA or SFA. Continuous suture technique with 6–0 polypropylene is performed (Fig. 11.64). After the release of the clamps, arterial blood will distend the vein to the first intact valve. Mills valvulotomes are introduced via the larger side tributaries (Fig. 11.65). To lyse the anterior leaflet, the valvulotome is placed (tip up) 90° to the skin plane. To lyse the posterior leaflet, the blade is turned 180° (tip down). After valvulotomy is completed for that portion of the vein, all tributaries are ligated with 4–0 silk ties. Only three tributary entrance points are needed to lyse all valves. Placement of the valve tip in a side branch should be carefully avoided, thus preventing vein-wall injury.

Prior to division of the vein, the tibial artery is opened and inspected. A coronary dilator (1.5 mm) may be used to determine outflow should there be any question of patency. The vein is then divided. A valvulotome is passed through the end of the cut vein to ensure complete valve disruption (Fig. 11.66). The anastomosis is performed with 7–0 polypropylene suture (Fig. 11.67). Flushing to remove debris resulting from valve lysis should be done prior to completion of the suture line. A completion arteriogram is performed as described.

The peroneal artery is found through the same incision, just lateral to the PTA and the posterior tibial nerve, behind the tibialis posterior muscle and medial to the fibula (see Fig. 11.58). The anterior tibial artery can be found in the anterior compartment just deep to the tibialis anterior muscle (Fig. 11.68; see also Fig. 11.59). When exposed in its proximal two-thirds, the saphenous vein is either directly tunneled through the interosseous membrane near the level of the anastomosis or is brought through the natural perforation, which the anterior tibial artery and vein penetrate. By necessity, this removes the vein from its in situ bed below the knee. Near the ankle the vein is tunneled subcutaneously over the tibia (Fig. 11.69).

Other techniques for in situ bypass exist but are not used as widely as the one described herein. Currently the next most popular method employs a floating valvulotome brought blindly through the GSV after exposure of the vein and arteries at the level of the proposed anastomoses. Vein branches must be identified and ligated through multiple stab sites or arterio–venous fistulas will ultimately cause graft failure. Techniques for arterial exposure and anastomosis are otherwise unchanged.

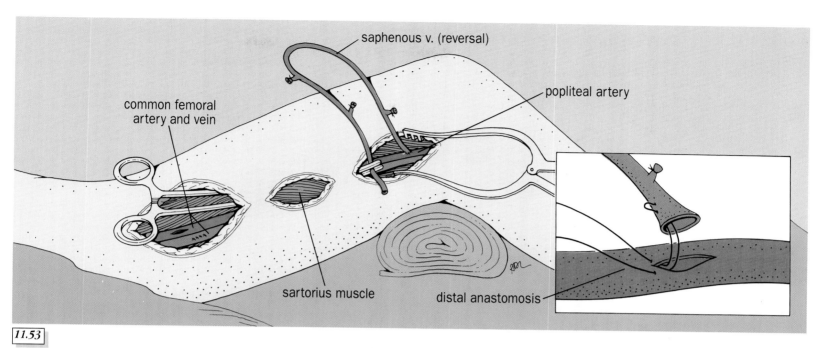

saphenous v. (reversal)

popliteal artery

common femoral
artery and vein

sartorius muscle

distal anastomosis

11.53

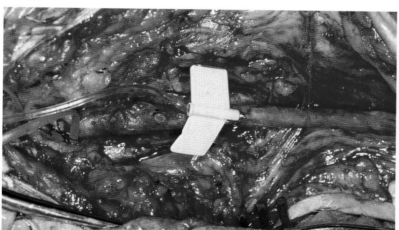

11.54A

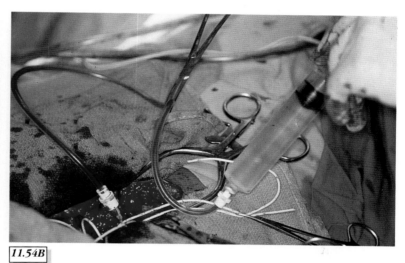

11.54B

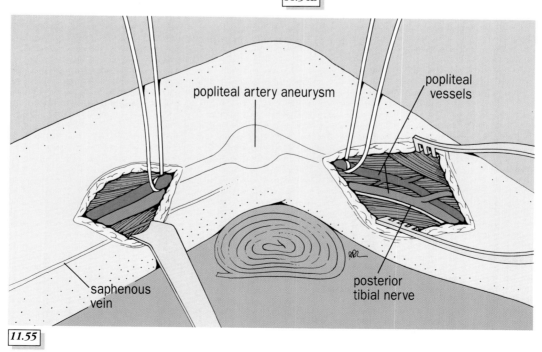

popliteal artery aneurysm

popliteal
vessels

saphenous
vein

posterior
tibial nerve

11.55

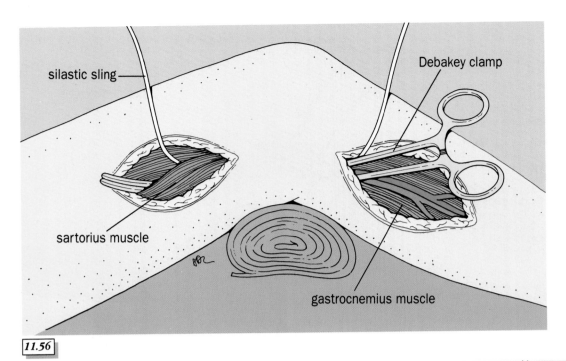

silastic sling

Debakey clamp

sartorius muscle

gastrocnemius muscle

11.56

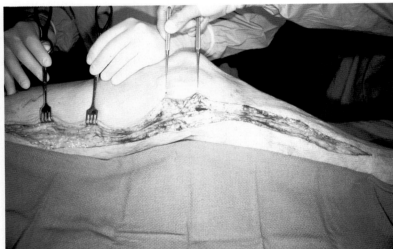

11.57

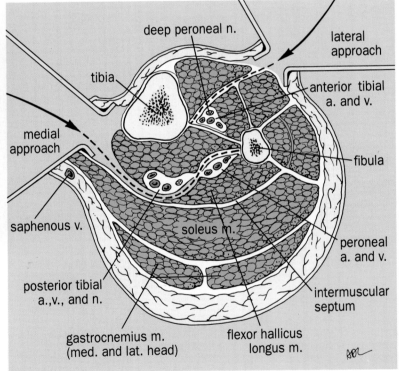

deep peroneal n.

lateral approach

tibia

anterior tibial a. and v.

medial approach

fibula

saphenous v.

soleus m.

peroneal a. and v.

posterior tibial a.,v., and n.

intermuscular septum

gastrocnemius m. (med. and lat. head)

flexor hallicus longus m.

11.58

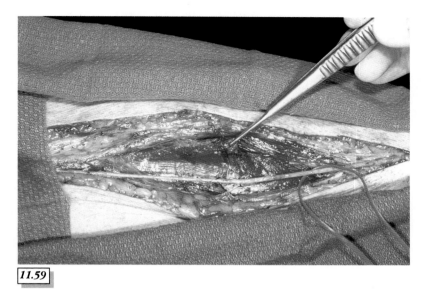

11.59

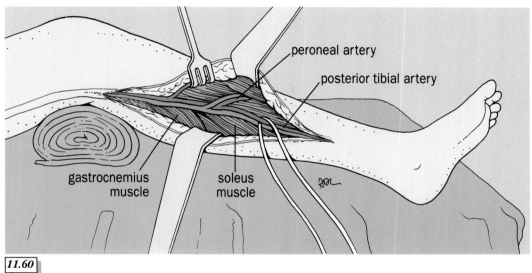

11.60

peroneal artery

posterior tibial artery

gastrocnemius muscle

soleus muscle

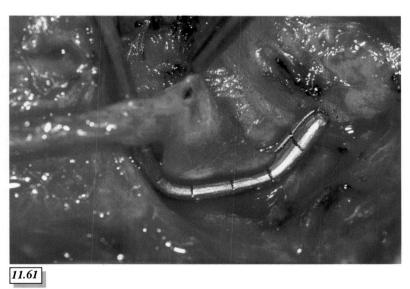

11.61

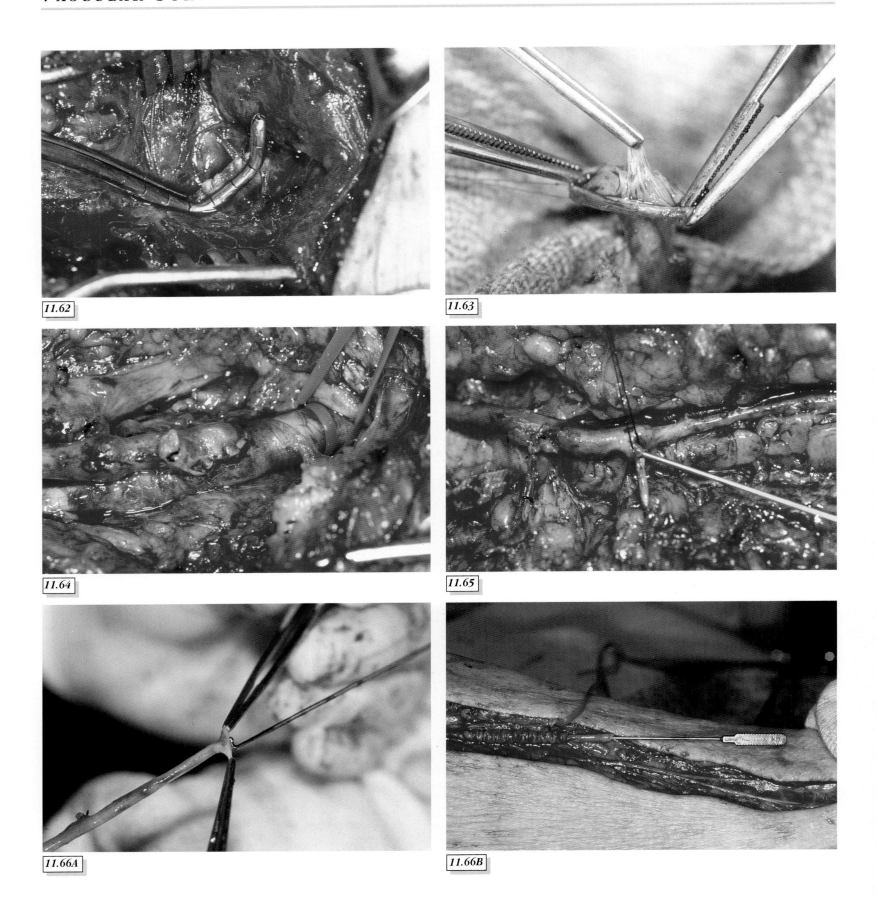

11.62

11.63

11.64

11.65

11.66A

11.66B

11.24

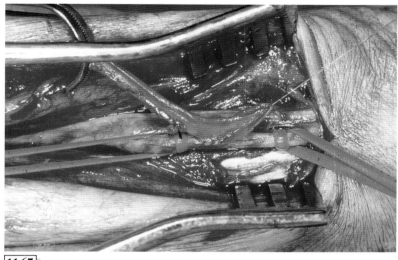

11.67

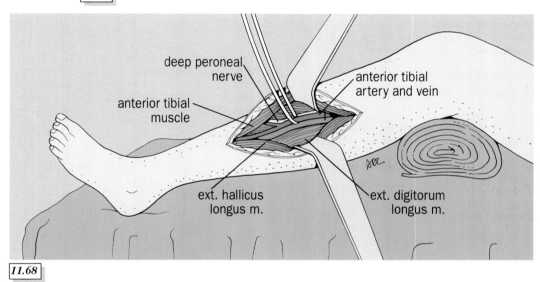

deep peroneal
nerve

anterior tibial
muscle

anterior tibial
artery and vein

ext. hallicus
longus m.

ext. digitorum
longus m.

11.68

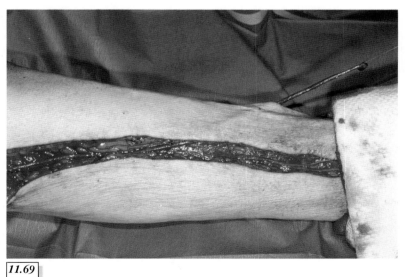

11.69

CAROTID ENDARTERECTOMY

Noninvasive carotid artery evaluation is performed preoperatively, along with CT scan of the head and arteriogram, usually intra-arterial digital subtraction arteriogram by brachial or femoral route.

CAROTID ENDARTERECTOMY	
INDICATIONS	• diameter stenosis greater than 80% in patients having hemispheric transient ischemic attacks (TIAs) or amaurosis fugax
	• lesions less than 80% with hemispheric TIAs or amaurosis fugax despite antiplatelet therapy
	• ulcerated lesions without demonstrated stenosis in patients having hemispheric TIAs or amaurosis fugax unresponsive to antiplatelet therapy
	• previous ipsilateral cerebrovascular accident with high-grade stenosis
	• asymptomatic high-grade stenosis greater than 80% of diameter in good-risk patients
CONTRA-INDICATIONS	• acute profound stroke
	• stroke in progressive evolution
ANESTHESIA	• radial artery line
	• regional cervical block or general endotracheal anesthesia, depending on surgeon's preference
POSITIONING	• supine, with head turned to opposite side and neck gently extended
	• Foley catheter
PREP	• Betadine skin prep

PROCEDURE

A decision must be made regarding the use of indwelling shunts during the carotid cross-clamp period. The options are no shunting, routinely shunting all patients, or the use of selective shunts. The use of shunts introduces the inherent risk of embolization. Selective shunting decisions can be made on the basis of the patient's response to carotid cross-clamp while awake under a regional block. If the patient is asleep, then a stump pressure in the carotid artery of less than 50 mmHg suggests the need for an indwelling shunt. Electroencephalographic (EEG) monitoring has also been used. Irrespective of the presence of a shunt, the technique of meticulous dissection and gentle handling of tissue is never more important than in carotid surgery.

A modified vertical incision is made in a conveniently marked skin crease along the anterior border of the sternocleidomastoid muscle (Fig. 11.70). This incision gives excellent exposure and an acceptable cosmetic result. Care should be taken to avoid the great auricular nerve at the superior portion of the neck incision, since its division will cause numbness of the ear. Inevitably, branches of the cervical plexus will be divided with the skin incision and will cause numbness in the anterior portion of the neck. It is useful to have both unipolar and bipolar cauteries available to control bleeding about the cranial nerves. The superior limit of the dissection is the posterior belly of the digastric muscle. The inferior limit is usu-

ally the omohyoid muscle. Lymph nodes are occasionally present over the lower carotid area and are usually encountered in great proliferation in the upper part of the incision.

As the dissection deepens, knowledge of the location of the major cranial nerves encountered in carotid surgery will help avoid postoperative morbidity from cranial nerve dysfunction (Fig. 11.71). The plane of dissection should be governed by the location of the carotid artery. Once the carotid sheath has been entered, the anterior facial vein should be identified and traced posteriorly to the internal jugular vein (Fig. 11.72). The facial vein is ligated and divided. Frequently there are branches in the inferior part of the dissection near the omohyoid muscle, which should be dissected and ligated. Branches of the ansa hypoglossal nerve will be seen and should be preserved at this juncture. The common carotid will usually be seen first and dissection should be carried out posteriorly to identify the vagus nerve and to protect it. Dissection can then be carried superiorly, but the dissection about the carotid bifurcation should not be vigorous, exposing only sufficient artery to allow dissection distally in the carotid branches. Multiple small branches are seen coming from the external carotid to the sternocleidomastoid muscle and these should be carefully divided. The plane of dissection of the lymph nodes is determined by the position of the carotid artery, and the lymph nodes may be swept anteriorly or posteriorly. In the superior part of the incision, a branch of the occipital artery crosses the hypoglossal nerve (Fig. 11.73). Several small veins will be present in the same region. These are ligated with fine sutures to allow the hypoglossal to swing anteriorly. This will free several centimeters of internal carotid. The vagus nerve will be seen laterally and posteriorly, and may be in close proximity to the internal carotid in this region. At this level, the internal carotid can be visualized to be free of atherosclerotic plaque, which is frequently noted inferiorly and medially. The area that appears to be free of disease can be gently dissected and encircled with a vessel loop without disturbing the artery.

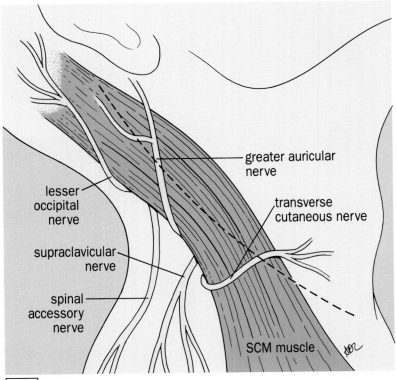

greater auricular nerve

transverse cutaneous nerve

lesser occipital nerve

supraclavicular nerve

spinal accessory nerve

SCM muscle

11.70

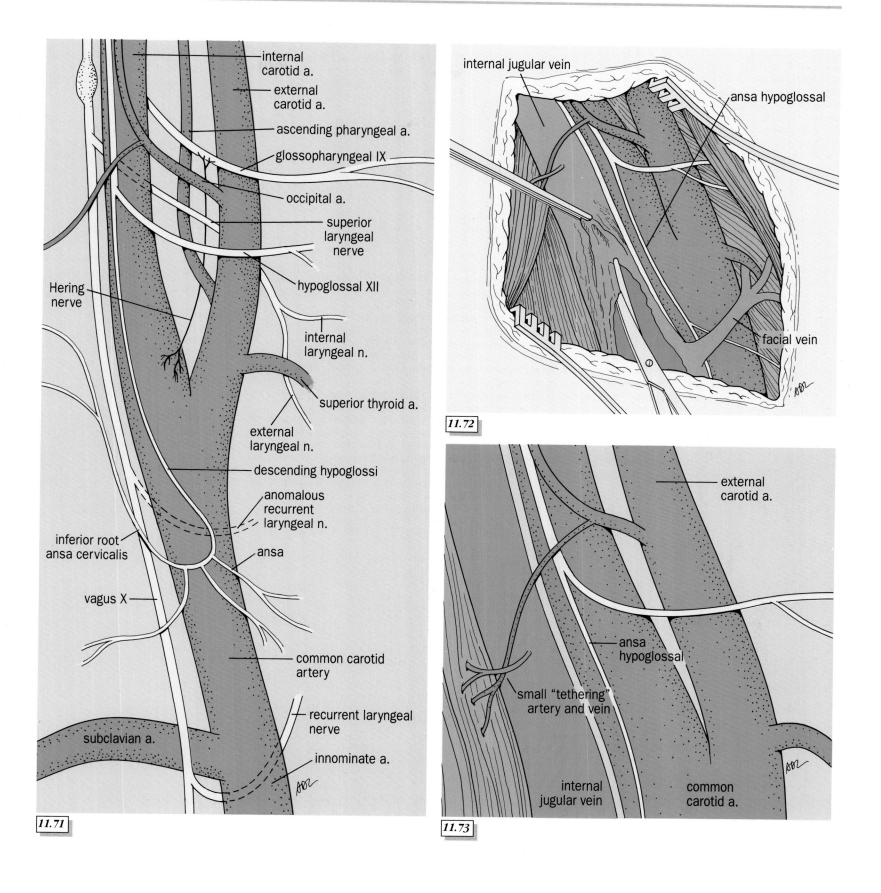

11.71

internal carotid a.

external carotid a.

ascending pharyngeal a.

glossopharyngeal IX

occipital a.

superior laryngeal nerve

hypoglossal XII

Hering nerve

internal laryngeal n.

superior thyroid a.

external laryngeal n.

descending hypoglossi

anomalous recurrent laryngeal n.

inferior root ansa cervicalis

ansa

vagus X

common carotid artery

recurrent laryngeal nerve

subclavian a.

innominate a.

11.72

internal jugular vein

ansa hypoglossal

facial vein

11.73

external carotid a.

ansa hypoglossal

small "tethering" artery and vein

internal jugular vein

common carotid a.

Attention is then focused on the external carotid artery, where the superior thyroid artery is mobilized anteriorly and laterally but not posteriorly, thus avoiding injury to the superior laryngeal nerve. The external carotid is freed above the superior thyroid, and by general dissection, staying close to the vessel, it can be encircled without disturbance of the carotid sinus nerve or the area of the carotid bifurcation and maximum plaque formation (Fig. 11.74). Branches of the ansa hypoglossal may be divided during this course of dissection, but they should be traced prior to division to make certain that they are not branches of the vagus nerve, and represent a nonrecurrent recurrent nerve, an occasional anomaly seen in the neck. The common carotid is likewise encircled, with care taken to identify the vagus nerve.

The patient is systemically heparinized (1 mg/kg). The vessels are occluded in a sequential fashion starting with the internal carotid, followed by the common carotid and then the external carotid to avoid embolization of material into the cerebral circulation. At this juncture, if a shunt is to be employed routinely, the vessel is opened and the shunt inserted. If selective shunting is to be performed, the EEG should be observed carefully for the ensuing 3 minutes to see if any abnormalities occur, although most such abnormalities tend to occur in the first 30 seconds. Stump pressures may be taken by removal of the clamp on the internal carotid and placement of a 20-gauge needle, attached to a strain gauge. Pressures above 50 mmHg suggest that a shunt is not required, and the needle is removed and the clamp replaced on the internal carotid artery. During placement of the clamps, it is important to avoid injury to the cranial nerves. It is during common carotid clamp placement that injury to the vagus nerve most often occurs.

The arteriotomy is usually begun in the common carotid artery. The plaque may then be cut and the arteriotomy extended into the internal carotid artery. It is important to make this incision laterally to avoid separation of the internal from the external carotid (Fig. 11.75). In addition, a laterally placed arteriotomy will tend to straighten out a small coil in the vessel. The arteriotomy is extended beyond the visible plaque. Proximally it extends in the common carotid artery to a point where a natural change in the thickened plaque is seen.

The endarterectomy is begun in the bifurcation area. The plane of dissection for the endarterectomy is important and it is best to place this in a plane in the midportion of the media. It is usual to have the deeper plane of the dissection in the midportion of the vessel where the plaque is thickest, and frequently it will extend into the deeper layers of the media (Fig. 11.76). One should advance to a more superficial plane in the proximal part of the dissection in the common carotid, and in the distal portion in the internal carotid. One attempts to dissect into the subintimal plane distally so that a "feathering" of the intima is present. Once the plaque has been separated distally, the plaque in the common carotid artery is transected by cutting obliquely so that a rough transition or a shelf of plaque is avoided. The operation is completed by an eversion endarterectomy of the external carotid (Fig. 11.77). This is best accomplished in a more superficial plane directly below the plaque to establish a good endpoint. It is useful to evert the plaque first from the superior thyroid and then from the external carotid separately. If a satisfactory endpoint is not achieved in this manner, a separate arteriotomy may be made in the external carotid artery to retrieve the endpoint. Tags of tissue are removed to leave as smooth a surface as possible.

After the endarterectomy has been completed, the interior of the vessel is washed with heparinized saline to remove any loose debris and also to assess any additional tags as well as the endpoint. The arteriotomy closure is begun at the internal carotid artery. Six–0 Prolene suture is used, with very small bites of tissue taken. Near the completion of the arteriotomy, the vessel is flushed in all directions and the interior of the vessel is washed with heparinized saline. The arteriotomy is completed; the clamp is momentarily released from the internal carotid and then reapplied. Forceps are applied to the proximal internal carotid to prevent flow of blood or air in this region. The clamp is removed from the external carotid, the common carotid, and after several heartbeats the internal carotid.

Protamine sulfate is used to reverse the heparin to the point of cessation of bleeding. Routine patching of the closure with saphenous vein or ePTFE is advocated by some surgeons to prevent recurrence (Fig. 11.78). Women with internal carotid arteries less than 4 mm in diameter are particularly susceptible to intimal hyperplasia. The wound is irrigated with antibiotic-containing solution, and a closed drain is inserted. The platysma is closed with a running suture of 3–0 Vicryl; 5–0 Vicryl is used for the subcuticular closure.

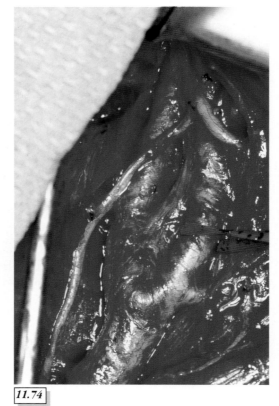

11.74

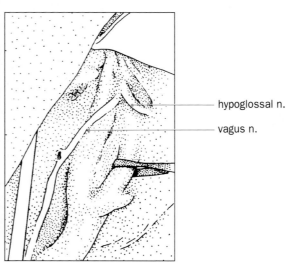

hypoglossal n.

vagus n.

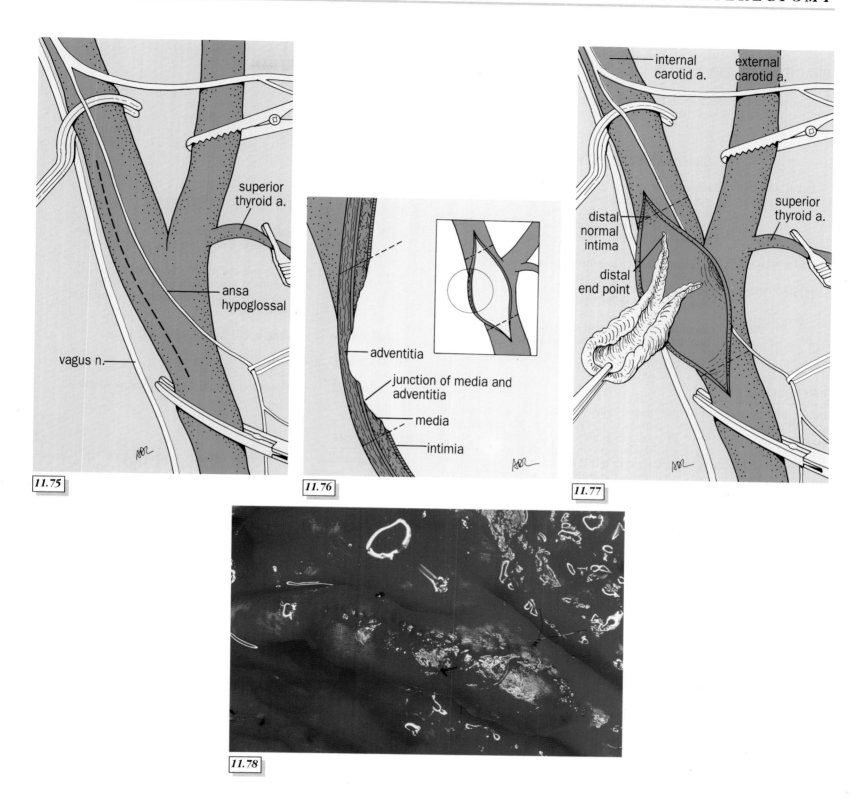

superior
thyroid a.

ansa
hypoglossal

vagus n.

11.75

adventitia

junction of media and
adventitia

media

intimia

11.76

internal
carotid a.

external
carotid a.

distal
normal
intima

distal
end point

superior
thyroid a.

11.77

11.78

BRACHIAL ARTERY REPAIR

Noninvasive vascular tests should be performed prior to surgery. Arteriography also may be helpful. Prophylactic antibiotics are recommended.

BRACHIAL ARTERY REPAIR

INDICATIONS	•injury from arterial catheterization or trauma that may produce pseudoaneurysm formation or hand ischemia from vessel thrombosis •alteration or loss of distal pulses after catheterization, even in the absence of limb-threatening ischemia
ANESTHESIA	•local anesthesia, for most patients
POSITIONING	•supine, with arm 90° from the body and the hand in supination (Fig. 11.79)
PREP	•shoulder and entire arm painted with iodine solution; hand covered with a stockinette

PROCEDURE

An incision is made along the medial border of the biceps tendon just above the elbow. Should mobilization of the radial and ulnar arteries be necessary, the incision may be extended in an S-shaped fashion across the antecubital fossa, and the bicipital aponeurosis may be divided (Fig. 11.80). The median and medial cutaneous nerves of the forearm are carefully identified while the area is mobilized about the injured vessel (Fig. 11.81). For catheter trauma, simple repair with interrupted sutures after thrombectomy will suffice. For more extensive injury involving one-half or less the circumference of the vessel, simple debridement and vein patch angioplasty are necessary. A portion of basilic or cephalic vein of sufficient length to bridge the defect is opened longitudinally and sutured with a continuous 6–0 polypropylene stitch. Less frequently, intimal damage from trauma is extensive requiring either an interposition vein graft or proximal and distal vessel reapproximation. For bypass repair the artery and vein are opened obliquely and sutured with continuous 6–0 polypropylene suture to produce a spatulated anastomosis (Fig. 11.82). A completion arteriogram and assessment of distal pulses and Doppler pressure provide objective evidence of a satisfactory repair.

EXTREMITY EMBOLECTOMY

Anticoagulation with heparin (1 mg/kg) is begun preoperatively, in the absence of absolute contraindications. Noninvasive vascular tests are rapidly performed, and arteriography, while not always necessary, may be helpful. Fluid and electrolyte administration, along with cardiac and urine output monitoring, is begun at the time of diagnosis. Prophylactic antibiotics are administered.

EXTREMITY EMBOLECTOMY

INDICATIONS	•acute ischemia accompanied by pain, pallor, poikilothermy, pulselessness, paresthesia, and paresis •cardiac sources in 90% of emboli •if symptoms are present for 6 to 8 hours, ischemic side effects may produce significant tissue damage
ANESTHESIA	•general endotracheal, epidural, or local
POSITIONING	•supine
PREP	•entire extremity painted with iodine solution

PROCEDURE

Details of approach to the brachial, femoral, popliteal, and tibial vessels are described elsewhere (see Figs. 11.36, 11.55, 11.58, 11.81). Exposure necessitates mobilization of the vessel just proximal to its bifurcation. A transverse arteriotomy incision allows primary closure without suture stenosis of the vessel (Fig. 11.83). With distal vessels occluded, the embolectomy catheter is first passed proximally. The balloon is slowly inflated so that the catheter is withdrawn without significant traction, thus avoiding intimal injury. Multiple passes are attempted until good flow is achieved and no clot is obtained on the final two passes (Fig. 11.84). The distal embolectomy is accomplished in a similar fashion. The artery is repaired with 6–0 polypropylene sutures. For an aortic saddle embolus we use 5F Fogarty catheters and bilateral groin incisions. Intraoperative arteriography and assessment of the pulses and Doppler pressures complete the procedure.

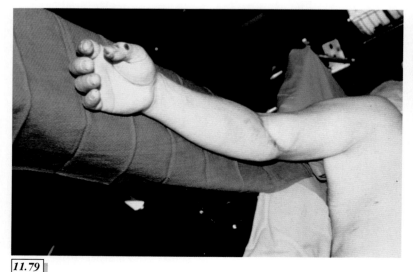

11.79

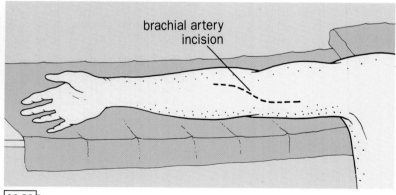

brachial artery incision

11.80

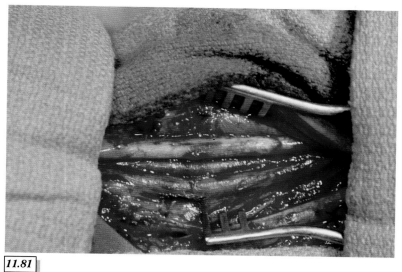

11.81

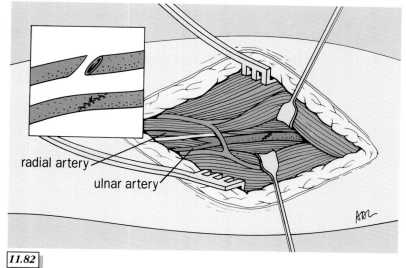

radial artery

ulnar artery

11.82

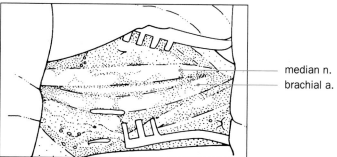

median n.

brachial a.

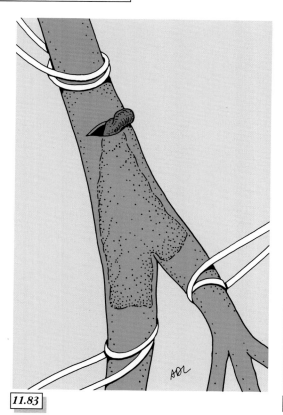

11.83

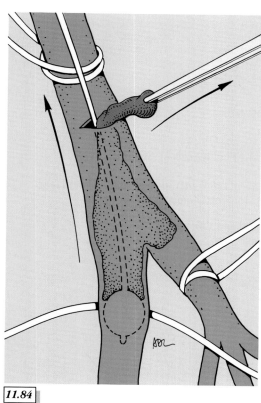

11.84

SURGERY FOR VENOUS DISEASE

PORTAL HYPERTENSION DECOMPRESSION PROCEDURES

An attempt should be made to correct the coagulopathy prior to surgery. Also prior to surgery, an attempt should be made to improve the patient's liver function and nutrition (Child's classification), if time permits. Control of ascites and cleansing of old blood from the intestines decreases postoperative morbidity. Preoperative endoscopy should confirm the presence of bleeding varices. Splenoportography is achieved by venous phase studies of celiac and superior mesenteric artery contrast injections (Fig. 11.85). Visualization of the left renal vein is necessary for the distal splenorenal bypass. Anatomic and hemodynamic studies can be obtained at that time. The blood bank should have an adequate amount of blood components available. Autotransfusion scavengers are valuable. Prophylactic antibiotics should also be administered.

Shunting procedures are an extremely effective means of controlling gastrointestinal hemorrhage from variceal bleeding.

They do not improve longevity, which is directly related to the severity of the liver disease. Selective shunts (distal splenorenal) decompress gastroesophageal varices to prevent recurrent bleeding, but maintain hepatopetal blood flow thus providing hepatotrophic substances and clearing toxic metabolic by-products (Fig. 11.86). The incidence of postoperative encephalopathy is somewhat diminished. A distal splenorenal shunt is not appropriate for patients with exsanguinating hemorrhage who require immediate reduction in portal pressure to survive.

Systemic or nonselective shunts (mesocaval and portacaval) decompress the entire portal system, preventing recurrent hemorrhage (Fig. 11.87). In producing hepatofugal portal flow, they may worsen the hepatic encephalopathy. These shunts are used mainly for patients with exsanguinating hemorrhage. Previous right upper quadrant surgery is a contraindication to the use of portacaval shunts.

Surgical mortality in these high-risk patients is related to their preoperative Child's classification and to the urgency of their procedure. Elective Child's A and B patients have an operative mortality rate of 10% to 15% for all procedures, while the operative risks are doubled for Child's C patients. Emergency surgery doubles the elective mortality rate for all patient groups.

DISTAL SPLENORENAL SHUNT

DISTAL SPLENORENAL SHUNT	
INDICATIONS	•failure of sclerotherapy and medical management to control bleeding from varices
ANESTHESIA	•general endotracheal
POSITIONING	•supine
PREP	•entire abdomen painted with iodine solution

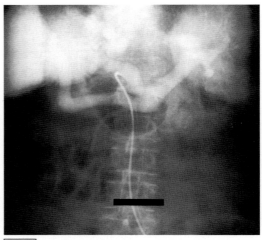

11.85

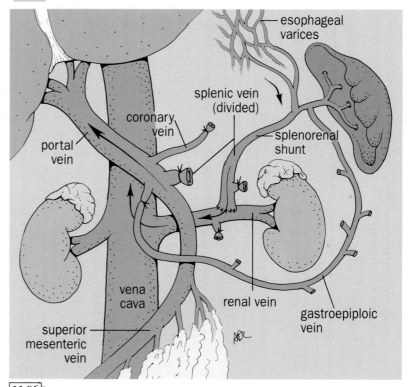

11.86

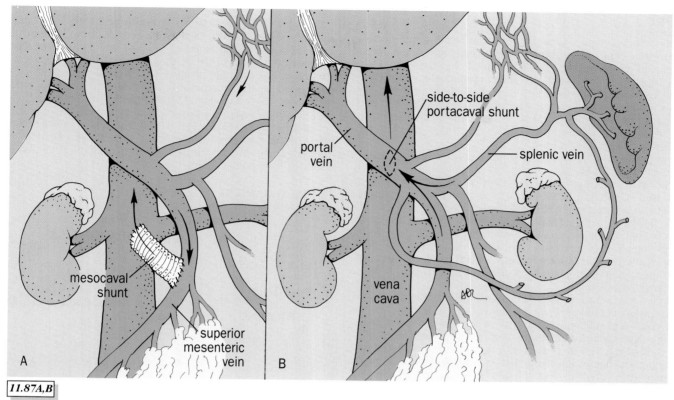

11.87A,B

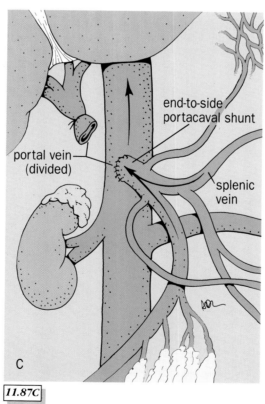

11.87C

PROCEDURE

A long midline incision is made, avoiding tributaries of the caput medusae (see Fig. 11.1). After exploration, the transverse colon and omentum are mobilized cephalad while the small bowel is retracted to the right side of the abdomen. Treitz's ligament is divided, allowing retraction of the bowel to the patient's right side. More extensive dissection of the preaortic lymphatic tissue at this level will expose the renal vein (Fig. 11.88). The renal vein should be mobilized from the vena cava to the renal hilum. The gonadal and, if necessary, the adrenal veins are divided to allow free movement of the renal vein (Fig. 11.89).

The splenic vein can now be mobilized without dissection of the gastrocolic ligament. In dividing and following the inferior mesenteric vein centrally, the peritoneum covering the inferior border of the pancreas is identified and incised. Cephalad retraction of the pancreas exposes the engorged splenic vein (see Fig. 11.88), and gentle dissection frees it from the pancreatic bed (Fig. 11.90). Small tributaries are sequentially ligated until the vein is fully mobilized from the pancreas (Fig. 11.91). Prior to division of the splenic vein at its junction with the superior mesenteric vein (SMV), a plastic catheter is introduced to obtain preshunt pressures. After division, the splenic vein is approximated to the renal vein to begin a tension-free anastomosis.

A plastic catheter is introduced into the renal vein at the site of the planned venotomy to obtain preshunt pressures. After clamping, a small portion of the renal vein wall is excised to allow for a widely patent anastomosis. A 6–0 polypropylene continuous suture approximates the posterior wall from within (Fig. 11.92). The anterior wall can be completed with multiple continuous or simple interrupted 6–0 polypropylene sutures to prevent pursestringing. After flushing, the anastomosis is completed (Fig. 11.93; see also Fig. 11.85). The coronary and right gastroepiploic veins are then ligated to complete the selective shunt. Pressures are again taken through the splenic vein.

The peritoneum is approximated with interrupted absorbable sutures to prevent hematoma formation from compressing the shunt. Abdominal wall closure is performed as described for aortic aneurysm surgery. Postoperative fluid restriction reduces the development of ascites.

MESOCAVAL SHUNT

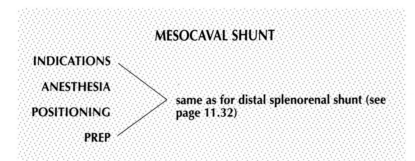

MESOCAVAL SHUNT

INDICATIONS

ANESTHESIA

POSITIONING

PREP

same as for distal splenorenal shunt (see page 11.32)

PROCEDURE

A long midline or bilateral subcostal incision is necessary for adequate exposure (see Fig. 11.1). After exploration, the transverse colon and omentum are retracted cephalad. The peritoneum is incised just to the right of Treitz's ligament, over the mesenteric vascular pedicle, revealing the SMV at the base of the transverse mesocolon (Figs. 11.94, 11.95). Further dissection centrally exposes the right and middle colic veins. The SMV is mobilized up to the uncinate process of the pancreas.

The vena cava is identified by dissection in the retroperitoneum to the right side of the patient's SMV. The duodenum is retracted cephalad after fully mobilizing the second, third, and proximal fourth portions (Fig. 11.96). A sufficient portion of the anterior and lateral walls of the cava can easily be cleaned to allow placement of a large Satinsky clamp. A prosthetic graft is chosen for the bypass (16- to 20-mm diameter).

The vena caval anastomosis is performed with 5–0 continuous suture after an ellipse of caval wall is excised. A clamp is then placed on the graft just above the anastomosis to allow flow in the cava. Portal pressures are measured in the SMV at the site of planned venotomy. Clamps are applied so that the right posterolateral wall of the mesenteric vein is rotated upward for the anastomosis. The venotomy excises a small amount of mesenteric vein wall (Fig. 11.97). Appropriate graft length is chosen to prevent either tension or bowing. The anastomosis is performed with 6–0 continuous suture (Figs. 11.98, 11.99). Flushing is performed prior to tightening of the sutures. Mesenteric vein pressure can now be repeated with the graft clamped and released. Closure is identical to that described for the distal splenorenal shunt.

PORTACAVAL SHUNT

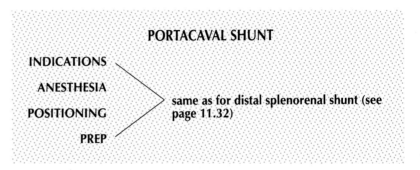

PORTACAVAL SHUNT

INDICATIONS

ANESTHESIA

POSITIONING

PREP

same as for distal splenorenal shunt (see page 11.32)

PROCEDURE

A long, right subcostal incision is made, extending laterally well into the flank. After exploration, the portal vein is exposed by incising the peritoneum over the portal triad (Fig. 11.100). The common duct is retracted cephalad to expose the dilated portal vein. Complete encirclement of the portal vein proximally and distally by division of small tributaries is necessary for full mobilization (Fig. 11.101). Portal pressure may be measured through a small vein in the omentum.

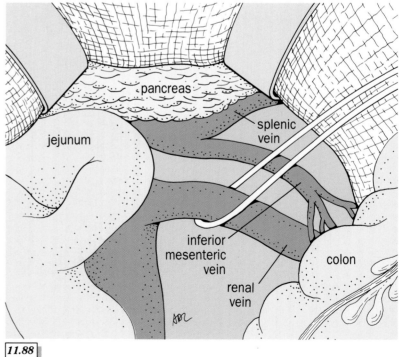

pancreas

jejunum

splenic vein

inferior mesenteric vein

renal vein

colon

11.88

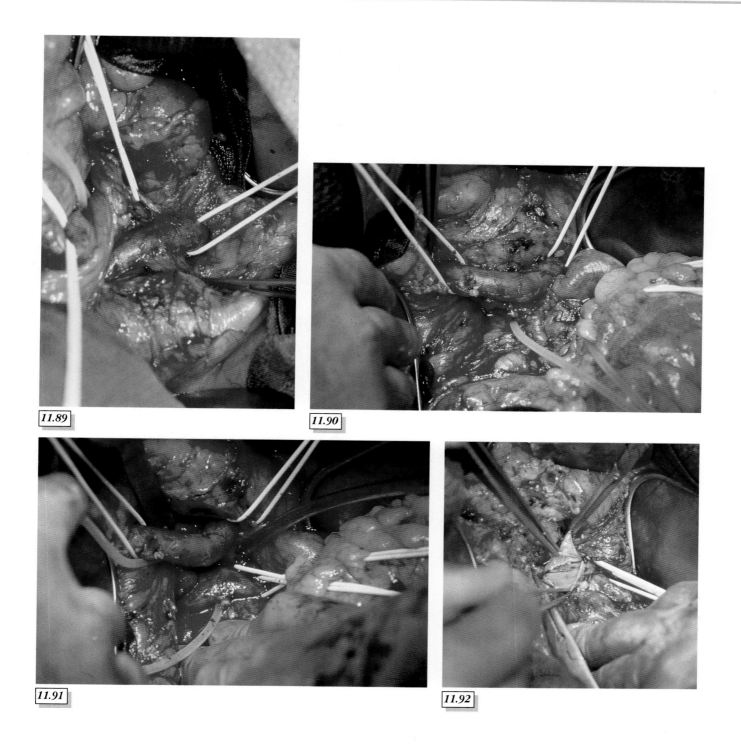

11.89

11.90

11.91

11.92

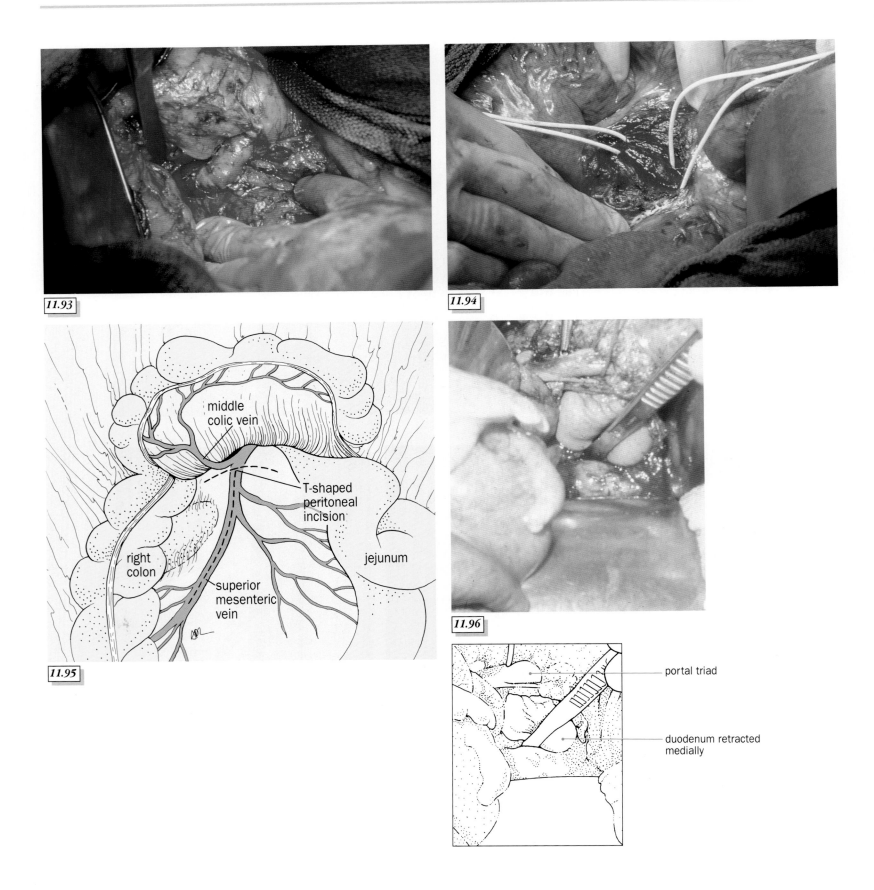

11.93

11.94

middle
colic vein

T-shaped
peritoneal
incision

right
colon

superior
mesenteric
vein

jejunum

11.95

11.96

portal triad

duodenum retracted
medially

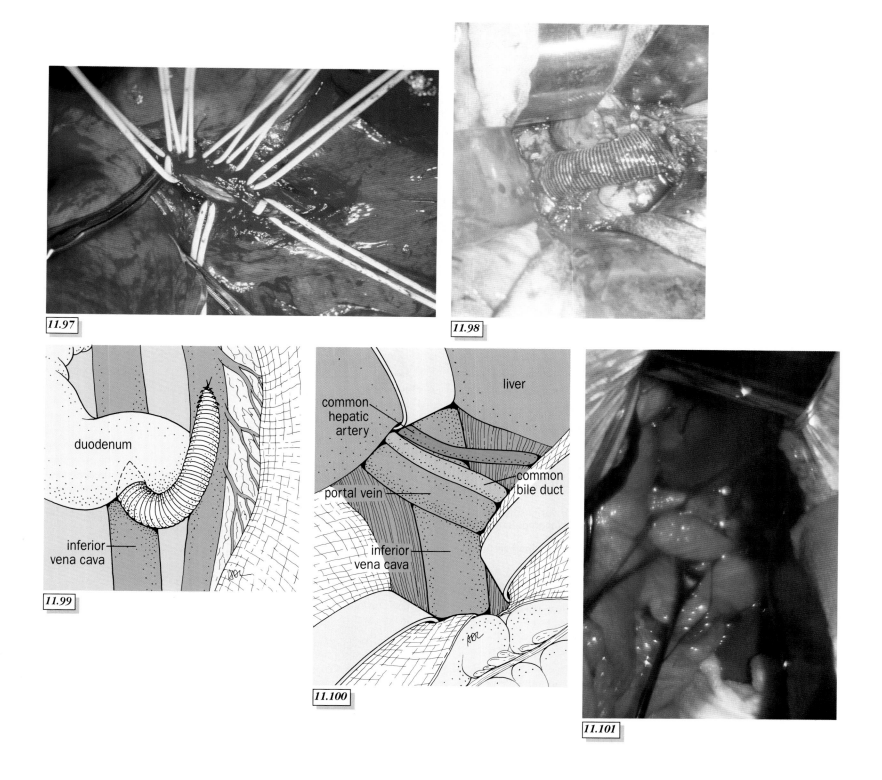

11.97

11.98

11.99

duodenum

inferior
vena cava

11.100

common
hepatic
artery

liver

portal vein

common
bile duct

inferior
vena cava

11.101

The vena cava is exposed posterior to the portal triad after incision and ligation of the peritoneum (Fig. 11.102). Kocherization of the duodenum is often necessary to obtain adequate exposure for the shunt (for Kocher maneuver, see Fig. 8.41). Large retroduodenal collaterals are divided when encountered. Further exposure can be obtained by removal of a portion of the caudate lobe of the liver with cautery. Absorbable mattress sutures are often necessary for hemostasis.

For an end-to-side portacaval shunt, the portal vein is divided high in the hilum after obtaining portal venous pressures. The remaining end is oversewn with 5–0 polypropylene suture. The vena cava is occluded with a Satinsky clamp and an ellipse of caval wall is removed. The anastomosis is performed with 6–0 polypropylene continuous suture taking care to avoid pursestringing (Fig. 11.103; see also Fig. 11.87C).

For a side-to-side anastomosis, sufficient length of the portal vein must be mobilized to reach the vena cava. After placement of a Satinsky clamp on the cava, a small ellipse of vein wall is removed. Clamps are placed horizontally on the portal vein and are rotated upward to expose its posterior surface. An oblique ellipse of vein wall is removed to correspond with the axis of the caval venotomy (Fig. 11.104; see also Fig. 11.87B). Continuous 6–0 polypropylene suture is used to repair the posterior wall from within the lumen as the first step of the anastomosis. Finally, the anterior wall is closed with a continuous suture technique.

Appropriate flushing should be performed with either procedure. Portal pressure once again may be measured through the omental vein with the shunt functioning. Multiple-layer closure of the incision completes the operation.

VENOUS STRIPPING AND LIGATION

Whether the patient has primary or secondary varicosities can most often be discerned by a simple history and physical examination. Noninvasive venous tests should also be performed.

VENOUS STRIPPING AND LIGATION

INDICATIONS	• symptomatic larger superficial varicosities related to valvular insufficiency or incompetent perforators • sclerotherapy candidates with proximal greater or lesser saphenous varicosities
CONTRA-INDICATIONS	• previous history of deep venous thrombosis, open sores, or acute cellulitis a relative contraindication to superficial venous stripping
ANESTHESIA	• general endotracheal or epidural
POSITIONING	• supine
PREP	• limb shaved and marked with an indelible pen (Fig. 11.105), and circumferentially painted with iodine • entire limb painted with iodine solution

PROCEDURE

To strip the greater or lesser saphenous varicosities, a small transverse incision is made over the appropriate vein at the ankle (Fig. 11.106). A transverse venotomy is made with a #11 scalpel blade. The stripper is introduced into the vein at the ankle level and advanced toward the groin (Fig. 11.107). If it can be guided to the groin, a small cutdown is made over the fossa ovalis at the now palpable saphenofemoral junction (Fig. 11.108). Occasionally, due to the many tortuous and widened venous channels, the stripper cannot be advanced to the groin. In that case, a cutdown is made over the vein at the level of blockage and a new stripper is inserted proximally.

Prior to placement of traction on the stripper, the accompanying nerve (saphenous or sural) should be dissected free for a distance of 4 to 5 cm. The vein is divided, oversewing the end with 3–0 silk suture ligatures. The bulbous tip is attached to the stripper as it is withdrawn subcutaneously for a distance of 5 cm from the incision site (Fig. 11.109). Subcuticular 5–0 absorbable suture is used to close the ankle incision.

Identifiable incompetent perforators away from the path of the stripper should then be ligated while dilated tributaries are stripped through small (1 cm) stab wounds (Fig. 11.110). A nerve hook or a crochet hook ensures rapid encirclement of the varicosity. For extensive tributaries, multiple stab wounds at 6-cm intervals are necessary for local stripping of the varicosities with a hemostat.

In each case, a single inverted 5–0 absorbable subcuticular suture suffices to approximate the skin. When all incisions in the leg below the groin are repaired, the stripper is slowly withdrawn (Fig. 11.111). The leg is sequentially ace wrapped using sterile technique during the stripping to assure hemostasis (Fig. 11.112). The groin incision is closed with 4–0 absorbable subcuticular sutures and the legs are elevated 20° overnight. The following morning the ace wraps are removed and reapplied prior to ambulation and discharge. They are kept in place for 3 days, after which time showering and elastic compression stocking use is permitted.

AMPUTATIONS IN THE ISCHEMIC EXTREMITY

Success in amputation surgery requires meticulous technique and decision making regarding level of amputation, based on sound clinical judgment and objective testing. Early involvement of rehabilitation specialists will encourage the patient and speed functional recovery. Indications for amputation include chronic ischemia with dry gangrene, nonhealing and painful ulcer, or severe and unremitting rest pain. Certainly all attempts at revascularization should have been exhausted. Other indications include acute ischemia where systemic toxicity, including myoglobinemia, threatens the patient's life, and gangrene complicated by infection, so called "wet gangrene," particularly in the diabetic.

Clinical criteria for determining amputation level are helpful, but not absolute, particularly if revascularization with development of collateral flow has occurred. They include the following:

1. Digit or transmetatarsal amputation requires at least one palpable pedal pulse
2. Healing will not occur in skin that shows dependent rubor
3. Venous filling time should be less than 20 to 25 seconds for toe or transmetatarsal healing
4. Healing will not occur if infection, ulceration, or gangrenous skin changes are present at the amputation level
5. A below-knee amputation will usually heal if there is a palpable femoral pulse.

Many techniques have been developed for evaluating objective criteria for amputation level. Doppler segmental and photoplethysmographic pressures are the easiest to obtain and are noninvasive. Objective criteria include the following:

1. Doppler ankle systolic pressure of 70 mmHg required for forefoot amputation, and a pressure of 35 mmHg for digit amputation
2. Doppler-detected flow in popliteal artery necessary for below-knee healing
3. Doppler systolic calf pressure of 70 mmHg or calf pressure of 50 mmHg with thigh pressure of 80 mmHg required for below-knee amputation healing
4. Photoplethysmographic digit or transmetatarsal pressure of 20 mmHg or greater necessary for healing of digit amputation.

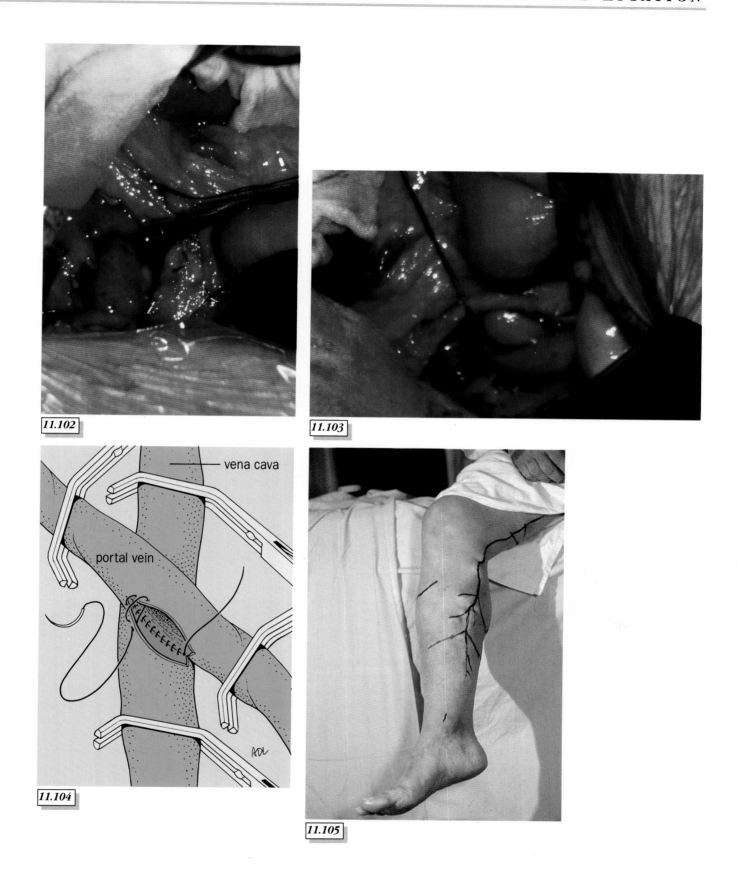

11.102

11.103

vena cava

portal vein

11.104

11.105

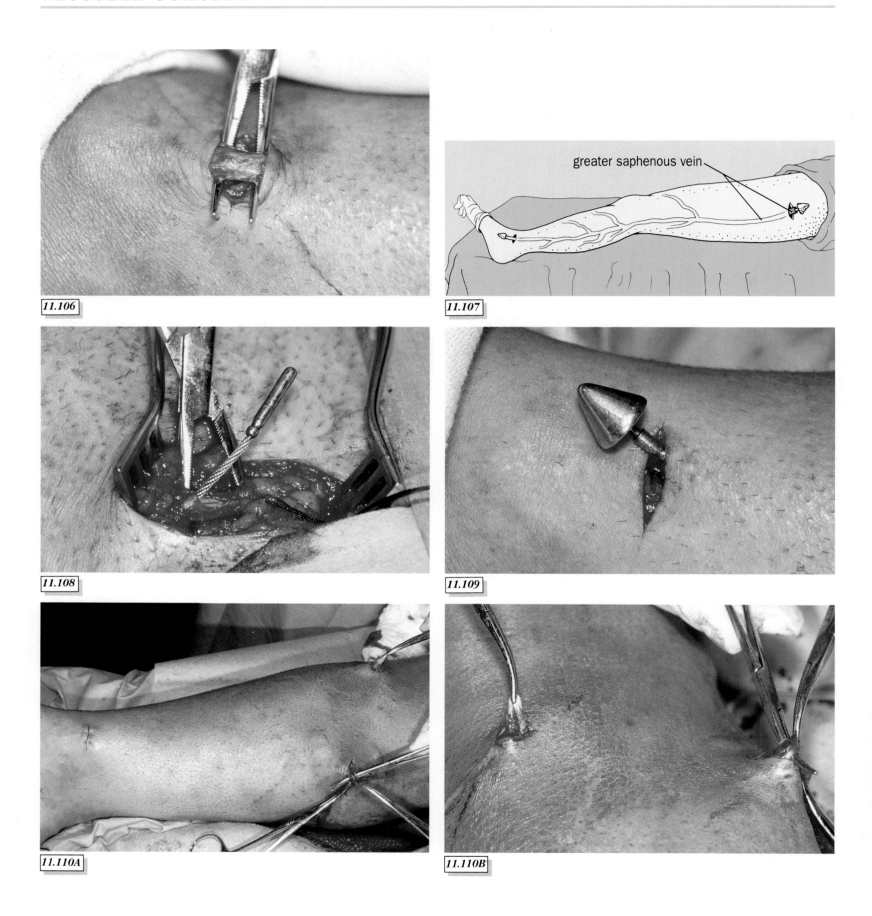

11.106

11.107

greater saphenous vein

11.108

11.109

11.110A

11.110B

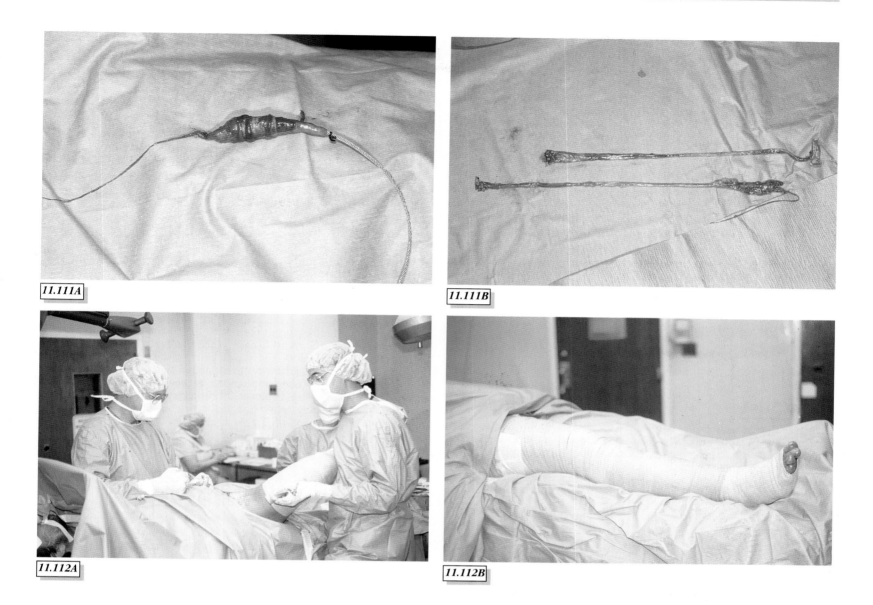

11.111A

11.111B

11.112A

11.112B

Gentle handling of tissue, careful hemostasis, and approximation of skin without tension are hallmarks of amputation surgery. The classical admonition is that only the knife and the needle are permitted to touch the skin, and that incisions are made cleanly without undermining. In the face of infection or acute ischemia, delay to preserve length of the limb is balanced against systemic toxicity. Skin may be left open for delayed secondary healing if infection is part of the process. Skin sutures usually remain in place for 3 weeks, and ambulation is not permitted for the first 7 to 10 days.

TRANSPHALANGEAL AMPUTATION

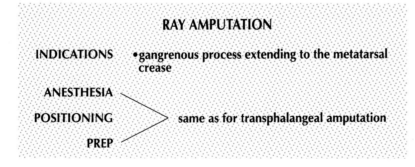

TRANSPHALANGEAL AMPUTATION

INDICATIONS	•locally infected gangrene or severe ischemic pain limited to single digit
ANESTHESIA	•ankle block, spinal, or general endotracheal
POSITIONING	•supine
PREP	•Betadine skin prep

PROCEDURE

A circular skin incision at the base of the toe, at the level of the proximal phalanx, is most commonly used (Fig. 11.113). Other incisions are acceptable as long as closure is without tension. The bone is transected at the level of the proximal phalanx. The skin is closed with nonabsorbable sutures or may be left open with the skin loosely approximated.

RAY AMPUTATION

RAY AMPUTATION

INDICATIONS	•gangrenous process extending to the metatarsal crease
ANESTHESIA	
POSITIONING	same as for transphalangeal amputation
PREP	

PROCEDURE

A circular skin incision at the base of the toe is again used, but a dorsal, vertically placed skin incision is extended over the metatarsal head. The metatarsal head is divided at its neck, with care taken to avoid injury to the digital vessels. The gangrenous toe is removed with the metaphalangeal joint and divided metatarsal bone. If possible, the dead space is closed with absorbable sutures and the skin is closed with interrupted nonabsorbable material.

TRANSMETATARSAL AMPUTATION

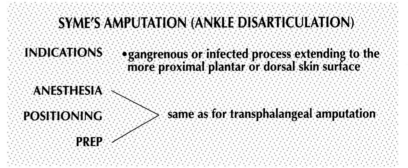

TRANSMETATARSAL AMPUTATION

INDICATIONS	•gangrene involving multiple toes, particularly extending to the metatarsophalangeal crease •same as for transphalangeal amputation
ANESTHESIA	
POSITIONING	same as for transphalangeal amputation
PREP	

PROCEDURE

The operation is based on a long plantar flap, which has a better blood supply than the thinner dorsal skin (Fig. 11.114). The dorsal incision is placed 0.5 to 1 cm distal to the planned line of bone resection in the midmetatarsal area. The incision extends from the first to the fifth metatarsal. The plantar incision is more distally placed at the metatarsophalangeal crease. The two incisions are joined by a gentle distal curve from the dorsal incision. This incision is taken to the metatarsal bones, which are divided with an air-driven saw. Bone and tendon are removed, but muscle is left attached to the plantar flap. After careful hemostasis, the wound is irrigated with antibiotic-containing solution, and the plantar flap judged for looseness of approximation and fit (Fig. 11.115). Absorbable sutures are used to close the fascia, and carefully placed monofilament skin sutures are used. A rigid plaster dressing is advised unless there is concern about infection.

SYME'S AMPUTATION (ANKLE DISARTICULATION)

Syme's amputation is increasingly performed because of the ease of prosthetic use. The amputation is based on using a well-vascularized posterior heel pad to cover the disarticulated ankle.

SYME'S AMPUTATION (ANKLE DISARTICULATION)

INDICATIONS	•gangrenous or infected process extending to the more proximal plantar or dorsal skin surface
ANESTHESIA	
POSITIONING	same as for transphalangeal amputation
PREP	

PROCEDURE

A dorsal skin incision extends across the ankle from the medial to the lateral malleolus. The plantar incision is constructed distal to the heel pad and connects the two malleoli (Fig. 11.116). All of the extensor tendons are divided anteriorly, and the incision is deepened to open the talotibial

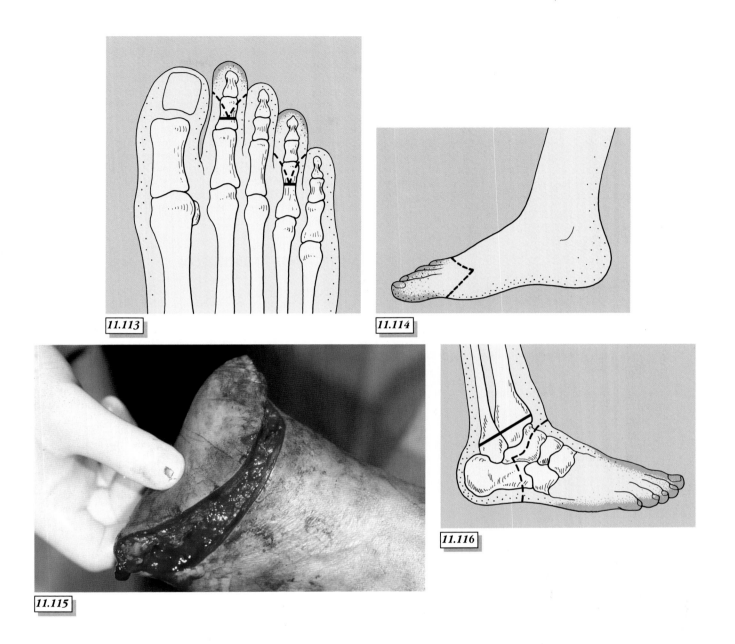

11.113

11.114

11.115

11.116

joint. Medially, the posterior tibialis tendon is divided, as are the posterior tibial vessels. The joint is opened by plantar flexing of the foot, thereby gaining access laterally to the peroneus tendons, which are now divided. The plantar incision is deepened to the calcaneus. A careful dissection is begun directly on the bone in order to excise the calcaneus from the heel pad without injury to the skin of the heel or to its blood supply. The Achilles tendon is the last attachment to be divided. The distal tibia and fibula are divided directly at the malleoli, making certain that all of the articular cartilage is removed. After careful hemostasis, the heel pad is brought anteriorly and carefully sutured to the dorsal skin with atraumatic technique. It is important to maintain the positioning of the heel pad, and an immediately placed rigid cast dressing will work well for this. The final result allows easier rehabilitation and ease of prosthetic use (Fig. 11.117).

BELOW-KNEE AMPUTATION

BELOW-KNEE AMPUTATION

INDICATIONS	•gangrene or infection extending above the ankle, but not involving the proximal calf anteriorly or posteriorly, to within 3 cm of the tibial tubercle •inadequate blood supply to heal a more distal amputation
ANESTHESIA	•spinal or general endotracheal
POSITIONING	•supine
PREP	•Betadine skin prep, with gangrenous or infected tissue covered with a sterile dressing

PROCEDURE

As with the transmetatarsal amputation, the long posterior flap is used because of its superior blood supply. The anterior skin flap is made 1 cm distal to the intended level of bone division, which as a general rule is four to five fingerbreadths distal to the tibial tuberosity. A transverse incision, equal to the anterior half of the calf circumference, is made. Medially and laterally oriented longitudinal incisions are placed at the midcalf plane. They are equal in length, plus 1 cm, to the diameter of the calf at the level of bone transection. The posterior skin flap is completed by joining these incisions in a gentle curve (Fig. 11.118). The skin incisions are completed prior to muscle transection.

The anterior compartment muscles are divided sharply at the level of bone transection. The anterior tibial vessels are secured with nonabsorbable sutures. The tibia is divided at the predetermined level using an air-driven saw, without stripping of the periosteum. The fibula is divided at a convenient location and will be shortened after the limb is removed. By distally distracting the tibia, a view of the posterior tibial and peroneal vessels and nerves can be obtained. These vessels are carefully tied, frequently requiring suture ligatures. The posterior tibial nerve is pulled down, ligated, and divided, allowing it to retract into the soft tissue. The posterior muscles are sharply divided at the posterior skin incision using the amputation knife.

After the specimen has been removed, the fibula is shortened 1 cm proximal to the tibial division using a rongeur. The anterior lip of the tibia is cut in a 30° angle, encompassing the anterior one-third of the bone. Sharp edges are filed. Frequently, a portion of the gastrocnemius and soleus muscles is trimmed to allow approximation of the flaps. Hemostasis using fine absorbable ties is completed. The wound is irrigated with antibiotic-containing solution. Interrupted 3-0 Dexon is used to close the fascia over the tibia. Careful skin apposition using simple or vertical mattress sutures of 5-0 monofilament suture completes the closure (Fig. 11.119).

A rigid plaster dressing has its best application in this amputation level, and should be applied unless infection is a serious concern. Early rehabilitation can begin.

ABOVE-KNEE AMPUTATION

Conservation of length increases the likelihood of successful rehabilitation, but must be balanced against the need for primary healing.

ABOVE-KNEE AMPUTATION

INDICATIONS	•gangrene or infection involving knee •inadequate blood supply to heal at a lower level •contracture of knee, particularly in a patient with ipsilateral stroke
ANESTHESIA	•spinal or general endotracheal
POSITIONING	•supine
PREP	•Betadine skin prep, with infected or gangrenous tissue covered with sterile dressing

PROCEDURE

A slightly "fish-mouthed" or circular incision is made 2 to 3 cm distal to the planned level of bone division (Fig. 11.120). The muscles of the anterior, medial, and lateral compartments are divided in a plane resembling a funnel. The femur is divided without removing the periosteum. The femoral vessels are individually suture ligated. The sciatic nerve is also ligated after it is placed on stretch, and allowed to retract to prevent its adherence to the edge of the skin closure and the development of a painful neuroma. The posterior muscles are also cut in the same plane as the anterior group of muscles. Careful hemostasis and irrigation with antibiotic-containing solution is standard. A small anterior lip of the femur is removed, and the edges of the bone are filed. The fascia is closed over the end of the femur with 3-0 Dexon. The skin is carefully closed with 5-0 monofilament suture (Fig. 11.121). Although a rigid dressing may be used, its usefulness in this setting is limited by its bulk and weight.

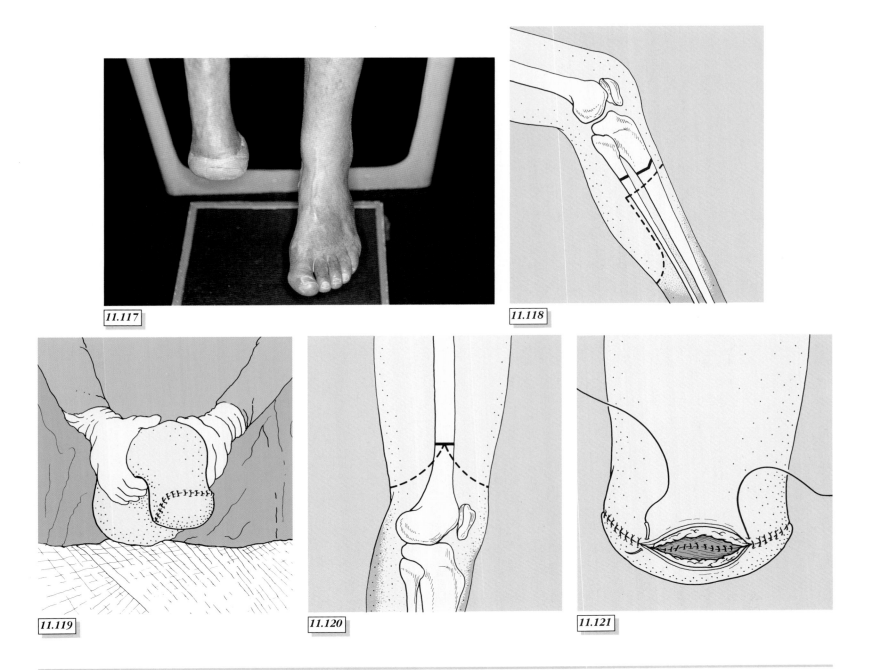

11.117

11.118

11.119

11.120

11.121

BIBLIOGRAPHY

Bergan J, Yao J, eds. *Techniques in Arterial Surgery*. Philadelphia, Pa: WB Saunders Co; 1990.

DeWeese JA. *Rob & Smith's Operative Vascular Surgery*. 4th ed. St Louis, Mo: CV Mosby Co; 1985.

Greenhalgh RM. *Vascular Surgical Techniques: An Atlas*. Philadelphia, Pa: WB Saunders Co; 1989.

Shah D, Chang B, Leopold P, Cosen J, Leather R, Karmody A. The anatomy of the greater saphenous venous system. *J Vasc Surg* 1986;3:273–283.

Taylor L, Edwards J, Porter J. Present status of reversed vein bypass grafting: five-year results in a modern series. *J Vasc Surg* 1990;11:193–206.

Veith F. Special vascular exposures. In: Veith F, ed. *Semin Vasc Surg* 1990;2:214–235.

Wylie EJ, Stoney RJ, Ehrenfeld WC. *Manual of Vascular Surgery I*. New York, NY: Springer-Verlag; 1980.

Wylie EJ, Stoney RJ, Ehrenfeld WC. *Manual of Vascular Surgery II*. New York, NY: Springer-Verlag; 1986.

12

Renal and Hepatic Transplantation Surgery

Michael J. Moritz • John S. Radomski • R. Anthony Carabasi • Bruce E. Jarrell

The technical problems associated with renal and hepatic failure are not markedly different from those of vascular and general surgery. However, several points deserve special attention. The debility, poor nutrition, and catabolic state common in patients with renal and hepatic failure impair wound healing. In addition, these patients, immunocompromised by their disease states and then therapeutically immunosuppressed after transplantation, are more susceptible to infectious complications. Lastly, both diseases have a bleeding tendency—the uremic platelet defect of renal failure and the deficient synthesis of clotting factors in hepatic failure. The uremic platelet defect is estimated by a "bleeding time," and is reversible with cryoprecipitate transfusion or DDAVP (desmopressin) administration.

All of these factors reduce the surgical margin of safety and mandate close attention to basics. Strict observance of aseptic technique is critical. Meticulous hemostasis is crucial to avoid hematoma formation, with increased risk of wound breakdown and/or infection. As vascular suture lines may ooze, use of a topical hemostatic agent, particularly Oxycel cotton, to fill the interstices can speed hemostasis and avoid further suturing.

HEMODIALYSIS ACCESS

Familiarity with the venous anatomy of the arm is useful (Fig. 12.1). The nondominant arm is preferentially used, unless the vessels in the dominant arm are much more suitable—especially for a wrist fistula. In general, prosthetic grafts are made of expanded polytetrafluoroethylene (ePTFE). "Thin-walled" grafts are not suitable. The loop graft requires a prosthesis that will not kink (eg, ringed graft), generally 6 mm in diameter. For the upper arm graft, either a 4- to 7-mm tapered graft or a 6-mm straight graft is used. If no contraindications exist, systemic heparin may be given before artery clamping. However, with the uremic platelet defect, only one fifth of the usual dosage is needed (1000 units for the average adult). Either polypropylene or Goretex suture can be used. (Note that only the sizes for polypropylene are given in the text.) Dressings are wrapped around the extremity loosely. Tape on the skin should be avoided.

Table 12.1 summarizes the advantages and disadvantages of the three most common techniques of hemodialysis access.

WRIST FISTULA

Radiocephalic Arteriovenous Fistula

WRIST FISTULA	
INDICATIONS	• chronic renal failure • hemodialysis chosen over peritoneal dialysis
ANESTHESIA	• local infiltration
POSITIONING	• supine, arm on an arm board
PREP	• radial artery, cephalic vein, and incision marked preoperatively (Fig. 12.2) • Betadine prep to entire hand and forearm with stockinette

PROCEDURE

After infiltration of local anesthesia, a longitudinal incision is made between the radial artery and the cephalic vein into the subcutaneous tissue. First, the vein is dissected in the subcutaneous plane. Once an adequate vein has been identified, the artery is dissected after the fascial plane has been opened over it. By sharp dissection, each of these vessels is controlled, and the side branches are divided between fine silk ties. An adequate length of both vessels is mobilized so that they can be brought together side to side *without tension* for 15 mm. The radial artery is controlled with yellow vessel loops and the cephalic vein with blue loops. The dorsal sensory branch of the radial nerve should be preserved and is controlled with a white vessel loop (Fig. 12.3). The vessels are controlled by doubly looping the arterial (yellow) loops about the artery proximally and distally. One end of the loop is also passed around the vein and slight tension is applied (Fig. 12.4). The vessels are thereby controlled and brought into juxtaposition for anastomosis. Clamps are not necessary for control. The arteriotomy and venotomy are made and a stay suture is placed in both artery and vein (Fig. 12.4). A side-to-side anastomosis 10 to 12 mm in length is constructed with running 7–0 polypropylene suture.

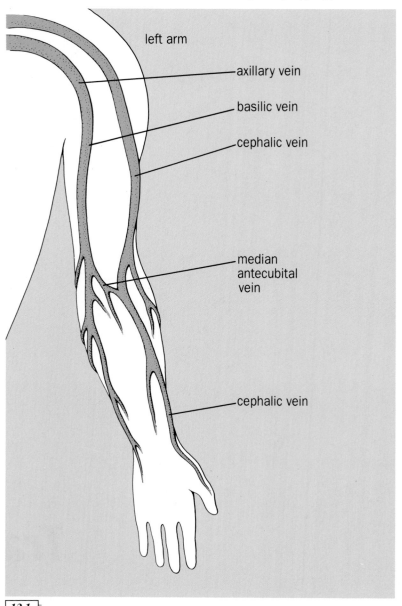

left arm

axillary vein

basilic vein

cephalic vein

median antecubital vein

cephalic vein

12.1

TABLE 12.1 HEMODIALYSIS ACCESS: THE THREE MOST COMMON TECHNIQUES

TECHNIQUE	ADVANTAGES	DISADVANTAGES
WRIST FISTULA	• no prosthetic material • lowest risk of infection • lasts longest	• must have patent radial artery and suitable cephalic vein patent from wrist to antecubitus • few patients with suitable vessels • requires at least 6 weeks to "mature" before use
FOREARM LOOP GRAFT	• can be used 10 days postop • may cause dilation of cephalic vein for future access procedures • easy to declot (when needed) • if graft fails, other procedures can be done in same arm	• prosthetic graft with risk of infection • requires adequate antecubital veins • slightly lower success rate than upper arm graft • shorter life span
UPPER ARM GRAFT	• can be used 10 days postop • highest early success rate • suitable vessels almost always available	• prosthetic graft with risk of infection • if graft fails, other procedures usually cannot be done in the same arm

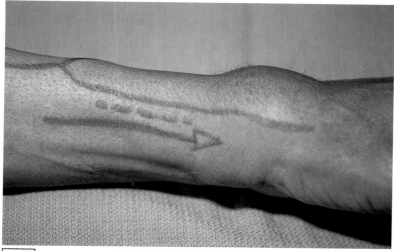

12.2

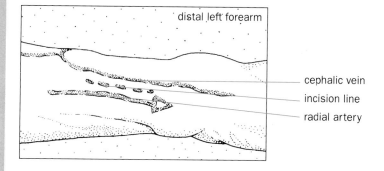

distal left forearm

cephalic vein
incision line
radial artery

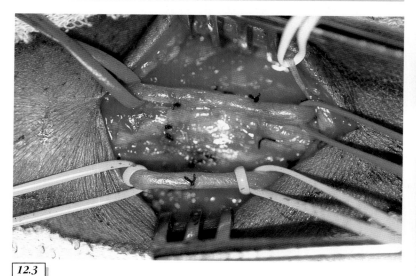

12.3

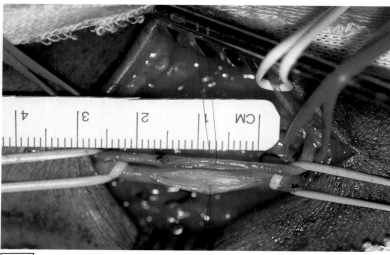

12.4

The back wall is done first from "inside," then the front wall. The vessels are flushed by sequentially releasing tension on the loops. The knot is tied and the loops are released. A thrill should be palpable in the vein and the vein becomes distended—both proximally and distally (Fig. 12.5).

If the vein cannot reach the artery side to side without tension, an end-to-side (vein-to-artery) anastomosis is constructed. The cephalic vein is ligated distally and divided. The end of the vein is brought to the side of the artery for anastomosis, which is performed as previously indicated. The final result shows the vessel loops held loosely about the artery and the comparatively large cephalic vein headed proximally (Fig. 12.6).

After hemostasis is secured, the wound is closed in two layers with interrupted 3–0 absorbable sutures in the subcutaneous tissue and loosely tied interrupted or running simple sutures of 4–0 nylon in the skin.

FOREARM LOOP GRAFT

Brachial Artery to Antecubital Vein Loop Arteriovenous Dialysis Graft

FOREARM LOOP GRAFT	
INDICATIONS	• same as for wrist fistula (see page 12.2)
ANESTHESIA	• regional block or local
POSITIONING	• same as for wrist fistula (see page 12.2)
PREP	• Betadine prep to entire arm with stockinette • perioperative prophylactic antibiotics as for insertion of any intravascular prosthesis • incision and course of subcutaneous tunnel marked preoperatively (Fig. 12.7)

PROCEDURE

After the patient's arm is marked with the incision and the course of the subcutaneous tunnel, a transverse incision is made one fingerbreadth below the antecubital crease over the brachial artery and the cephalic, basilic, or other suitably sized antecubital vein. The vein is freed by sharp dissection for an adequate length. If there is no adequate superficial vein, a deep vein accompanying the brachial artery (the basilic vein) may be of sufficient caliber.

The bicipital aponeurosis is opened to expose the brachial artery, which is freed by sharp dissection for an adequate length. Preferentially, the dissection is carried onto the ulnar and radial arteries. The radial artery can be used for the anastomosis if it is accessible and of sufficient caliber. This will reduce the risk of a steal phenomenon. The artery and vein are controlled with vessel loops (Fig. 12.8).

A longitudinal counterincision is made at the apex of the tunnel distal to the point at which the graft will lie. Subcutaneous tunnels are created with a tunneler and the graft is pulled through the tunnels (Fig. 12.9). The graft must not lie beneath the counterincision, but proximal to it. The graft is trimmed to an appropriate length and beveled.

The artery is controlled proximally and distally with vascular clamps. A Fogarty soft jaw clamp can be used proximally and a bulldog (Vascu-Statt II) distally. An arteriotomy is performed and the end-of-graft to side-of-artery anastomosis is carried out with running 6–0 polypropylene suture. An anastomosis usually begins at the heel and the corner stitch is tied or "parachuted" (see Figs. 11.7 and 11.8 in Chapter 11). The artery is flushed proximally and distally through the graft. A vascular clamp is then placed on the graft adjacent to the arterial anastomosis and the clamps are released, restoring arterial flow. The vein is controlled with vessel loops, a venotomy is made, and an end-of-graft to side-of-vein anastomosis is

performed with running 6–0 polypropylene suture. Before the knot is tied, the graft is filled with blood from the arterial end and is allowed to bleed through the venous anastomosis. Flow is then established to the graft (Fig. 12.10). Minor oozing from the anastomoses is controlled with Oxycel cotton. A thrill should be palpable in the graft and the vein.

After hemostasis is secured, the wounds are closed with interrupted 3–0 absorbable sutures in the subcutaneous tissue, and with running subcuticular sutures or interrupted nylon sutures in the skin. A minimum of 10 days should be allowed for graft incorporation prior to any graft puncture for dialysis; this minimizes the incidence of perigraft hematoma.

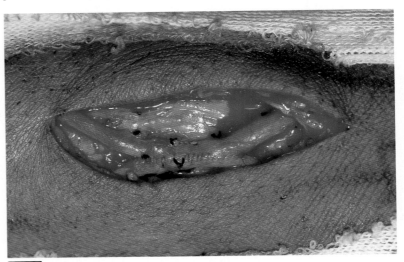

12.5

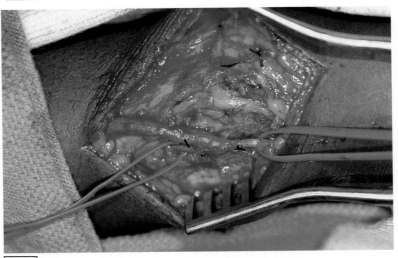

12.6

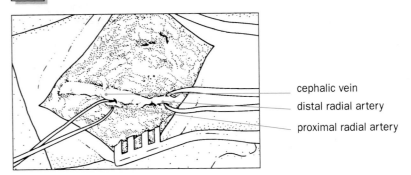

cephalic vein

distal radial artery

proximal radial artery

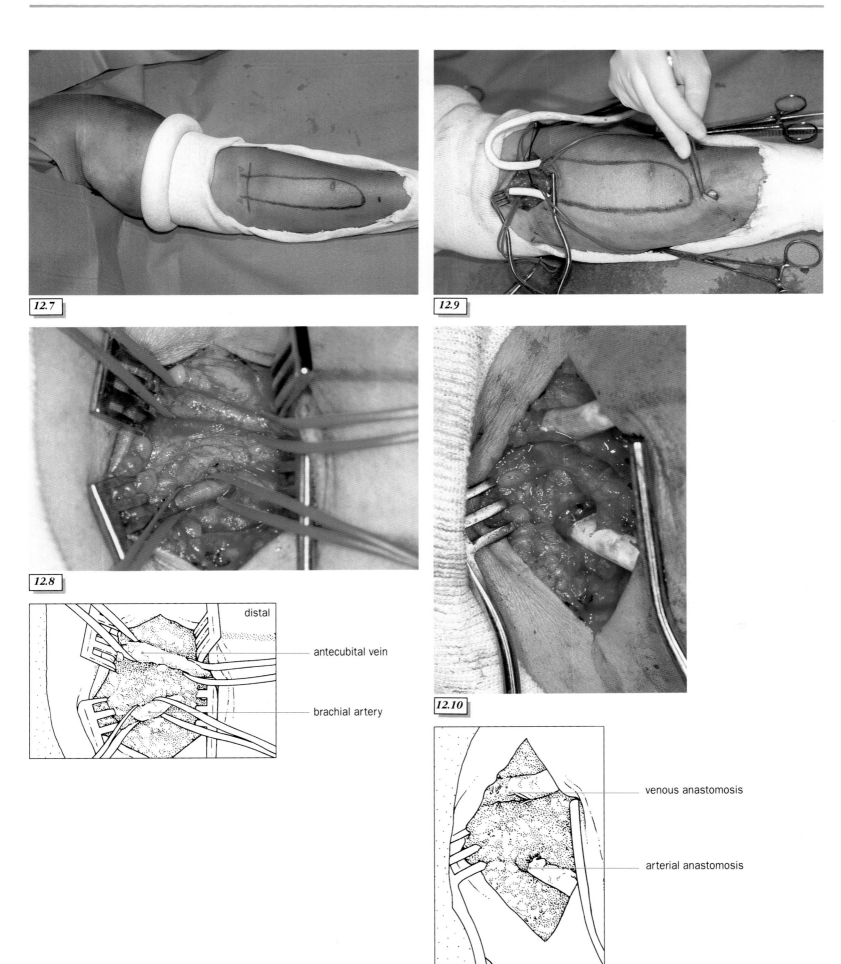

12.7

12.9

12.8

distal

antecubital vein

brachial artery

12.10

venous anastomosis

arterial anastomosis

UPPER ARM GRAFT

Brachial Artery to Axillary Vein Arteriovenous Dialysis Graft

UPPER ARM GRAFT	
INDICATIONS	• same as for wrist fistula (see page 12.2)
ANESTHESIA	• in decreasing order of preference: regional interscalene block, general endotracheal, or local
POSITIONING	• same as for wrist fistula and forearm loop graft (see page 12.2)
PREP	• axilla and upper chest shaved • Betadine prep to entire arm, axilla, and upper chest, with stockinette for arm (Fig. 12.11) • perioperative prophylactic antibiotics

PROCEDURE

The brachial artery is exposed through a longitudinal incision over the arterial pulse and proximal to the elbow crease (see Fig. 12.11). After dissection is carried through the deep fascia, the brachial artery is identified and encircled with a vessel loop. With careful sharp dissection, the brachial artery is freed from the surrounding venae comitantes for a sufficient length. Care is taken to avoid the median nerve, which crosses from lateral to medial over the artery in this portion of the arm (Fig. 12.12).

A transverse incision is made 2 to 3 cm inferior to the deltopectoral groove (see Fig. 12.11) and is carried down through skin and subcutaneous tissue. The pectoralis major muscle is split in the direction of its fibers and a self-retaining retractor is placed. The pectoralis minor muscle is identified and transected, partially or completely; although the anastomosis can be performed with this muscle retracted medially, it is easier if it is transected near its insertion on the coracoid (Fig. 12.13). The axillary vein is identified by palpation, inferior to the axillary artery pulse, and is freed for a sufficient length (Fig. 12.14) so that a side-biting vascular clamp can be applied.

A gentle curve for the tunnel connecting the two incisions is marked (Fig. 12.15). A tunneler is passed from the arm incision proximally. A tapered 4- to 7-mm graft (4 mm at the arterial end, 7 mm at the venous end) is tied to the tunneler and drawn through the tunnel, with care taken to avoid twisting the graft (Fig. 12.16).

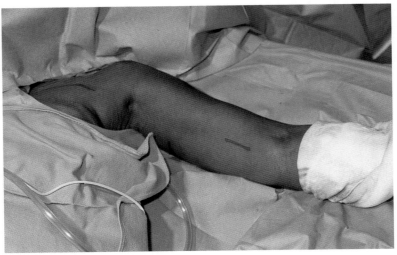

12.11

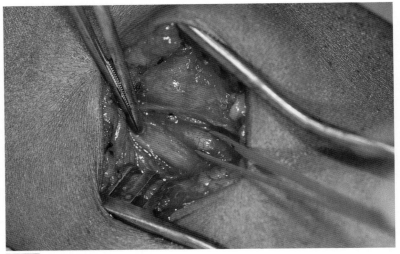

12.12

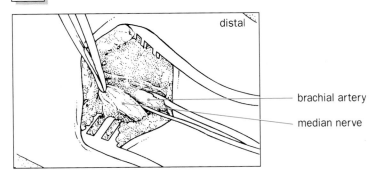

distal

brachial artery

median nerve

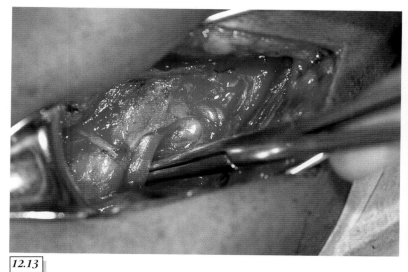

12.13

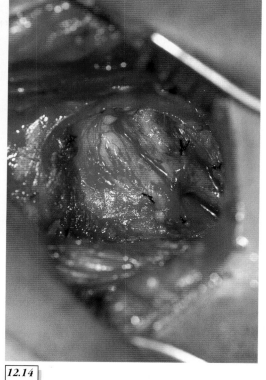

12.14

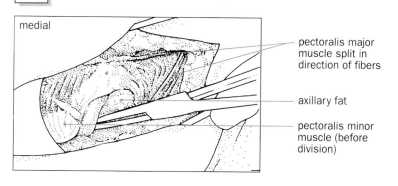

medial

pectoralis major
muscle split in
direction of fibers

axillary fat

pectoralis minor
muscle (before
division)

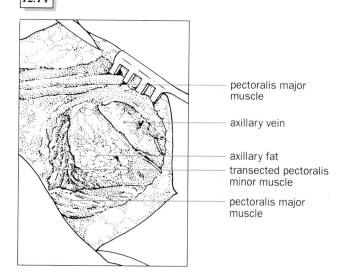

pectoralis major
muscle

axillary vein

axillary fat
transected pectoralis
minor muscle

pectoralis major
muscle

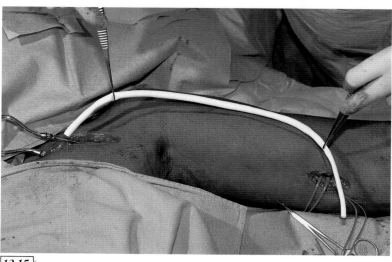

12.15

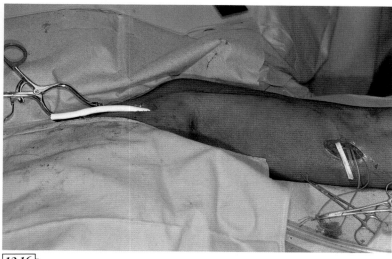

12.16

The venous anastomosis is usually performed first. The axillary vein is elevated and a side-biting clamp (eg, large Derra) is applied with the handle medially (Fig. 12.17). The graft is trimmed to an appropriate length and beveled. A venotomy is made and an end-of-graft to side-of-vein anastomosis is constructed with running 5–0 polypropylene suture (Figs. 12.17, 12.18). After the anastomosis is completed, the side-biting clamp is released briefly to check hemostasis.

The brachial artery is occluded with vascular clamps as in the previous procedure. The graft is trimmed to the appropriate length and an arteriotomy is performed. The anastomosis is constructed with running 6–0 polypropylene suture (Fig. 12.19). Prior to tying of the suture, the graft is filled from the venous end and allowed to bleed through the anastomosis. The graft is then occluded and the brachial artery flushed distally and proximally. The suture is tied and the clamps are removed, with blood flowing first to the graft and then to the forearm. Hemostasis is obtained with Oxycel cotton. A thrill should be palpable in the graft.

Both wounds are irrigated, hemostasis is obtained, and the wounds are closed with interrupted 3–0 absorbable sutures in the subcutaneous tissue and, usually, running subcuticular sutures in the skin. A minimum of 10 days should be allowed for graft incorporation prior to any graft puncture for dialysis.

ORGAN RETRIEVAL SURGERY
LIVING-RELATED RENAL DONOR

The donor workup includes at least a complete history and physical examination, routine blood tests, 24-hour urine collection for creatinine clearance and protein, and arteriography. Although either kidney can be removed, the following principles apply in order of priority:

1. If one kidney is suspect (eg, slightly smaller than normal), that kidney should be donated because the donor's renal function must be compromised as little as possible.
2. The kidney with the fewest arteries (preferably one) is donated.
3. The right kidney is easier to remove, as dissection of the vein is more straightforward.
4. The left kidney has more complex venous anatomy, but the longer vein facilitates transplantation.

It is important to remember that normal renal size is both age- and gender-dependent. The range of normal for adults is about 11 to 15 cm in length, with the right side 0.5 cm shorter than the left side (as measured by nephrogram phase of arteriogram).

LIVING-RELATED RENAL DONOR

INDICATIONS	•altruism and an appropriate recipient
ANESTHESIA	•general endotracheal
POSITIONING	•lateral decubitus, table flexed and kidney rest raised (Fig. 12.20)
PREP	•brisk diuresis initiated with fluids and diuretics and maintained throughout the procedure •subcutaneous heparin 2 hours preoperatively (deep venous thrombosis prophylaxis) •calf compression boots and bladder catheter placed •flank and lower chest prepped with Betadine and sterilely draped

PROCEDURE

A flank incision parallel to the ribs is made from the edge of the paraspinal muscles to the lateral border of the rectus. The incision level depends on the position of the kidney; the incision may be made at the eleventh rib or interspace, the twelfth rib (Fig. 12.21), or subcostally.

The muscle layers are opened. If needed, the pleura is reflected superiorly and the rib resected subperiosteally. The peritoneum is reflected anteriorly. Gerota's fascia is opened longitudinally. The kidney is sharply dissected free of perinephric fat (Fig. 12.22). The kidney is reflected posteriorly and the renal vein (Fig. 12.23) is dissected free circumferentially to the vena cava. The kidney is then reflected anteriorly and the artery is fully dissected. All venous and arterial branches except those to the kidney are divided between silk ties. Lastly, the ureter is dissected free with its accompanying soft tissues down to the iliac vessels. The fatty tissue between the lower pole and the ureter is protected. The dissection is thus completed (Fig. 12.24).

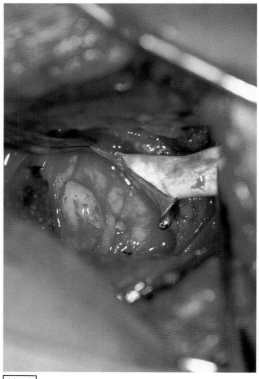

12.17

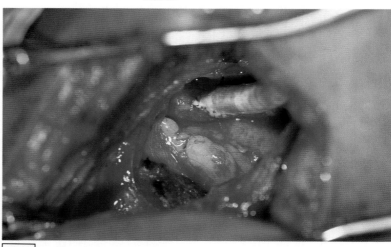

12.18

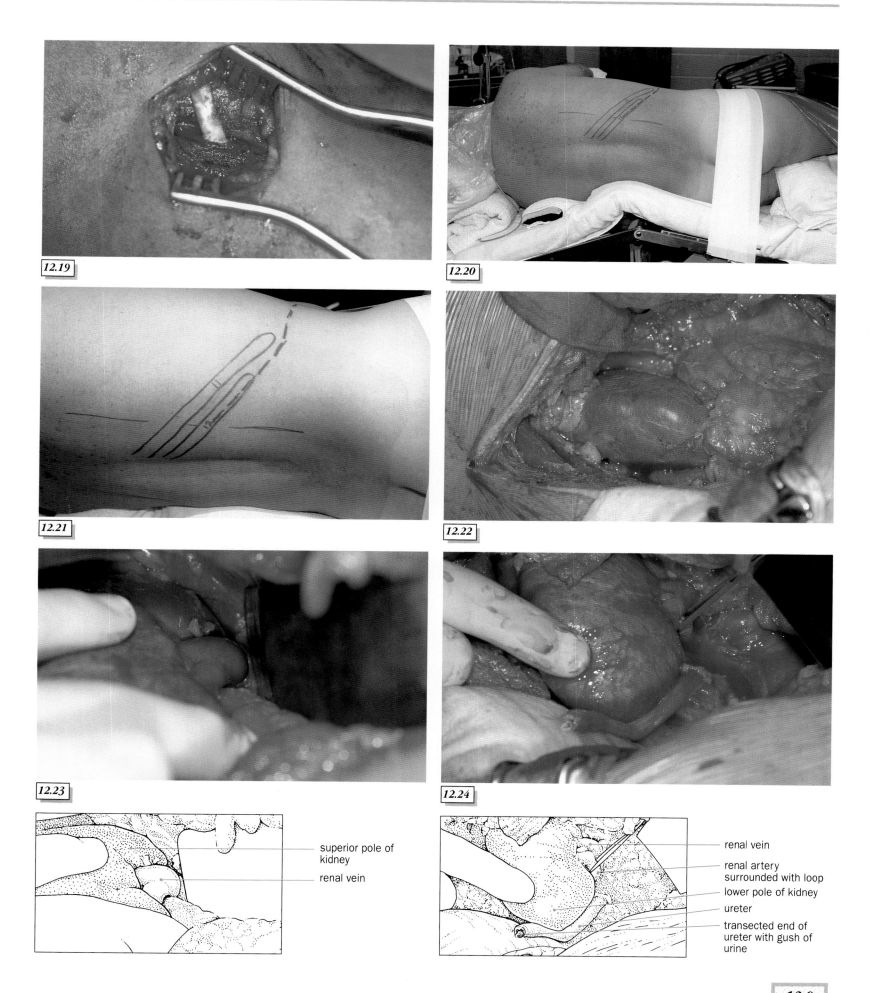

12.19

12.20

12.21

12.22

12.23

12.24

superior pole of
kidney

renal vein

renal vein

renal artery
surrounded with loop

lower pole of kidney

ureter

transected end of
ureter with gush of
urine

The patient is anticoagulated with heparin. The ureter is clamped, divided, and ligated distally with a chromic tie. Vascular clamps are placed on the proximal renal artery and the vena cava. The vessels are transected close to the clamps and the kidney is removed.

The kidney is taken to the recipient's operating room and its artery perfused with cold lactated Ringer's solution with the following additives (per 400 mL): 100 mL of 25% albumin, 2000 units of heparin, and 2.5 mg of phentolamine. The flushed kidney is uniformly pale (Fig. 12.25).

The heparin is reversed with protamine and the vessels are controlled. The artery is doubly ligated with silk, or is ligated with silk and suture-ligated with polypropylene. The vena cava is closed with running 5–0 polypropylene (Fig. 12.26). Hemostasis is checked and the incision is then closed with #1 PDS pericostal sutures (if necessary), two layers of running #1 PDS sutures in the muscle layers, and staples for the skin.

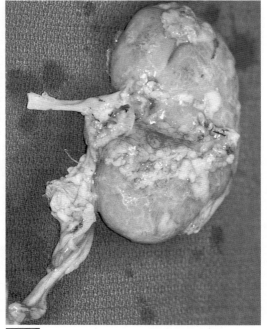

12.25

CADAVER RENAL DONOR

CADAVER RENAL DONOR

INDICATIONS	• brain death (most heart-beating cadaver donors provide several vascularized organs; kidneys alone are retrieved when family refuses other organs or when other organs are not usable)
POSITIONING	• supine
PREP	• Betadine prep from chin to pubis and to table on each side

PROCEDURE

A midline incision is made from xyphoid to pubis. The right colon is mobilized medially. The right kidney is sharply freed from within Gerota's space and the ureter dissected inferior to the iliac vessels. The same dissection is performed for the left kidney, ending with the creation of a window in the left colonic mesentery. No attempt is made to identify the renal arteries or veins.

The midgut is mobilized superiorly until it is attached only by the superior mesenteric vessels. Next the great vessel dissection is begun. During this dissection, the anomalies to watch for include (1) iliac artery branches to the lower poles, (2) precaval branches to the right lower pole, and (3) postaortic left renal vein. The aorta is dissected anteriorly from its bifurcation proximally, dividing the inferior mesenteric artery. The left renal vein is identified. The superior mesenteric artery (SMA) is divided between silk ties or umbilical tapes. The lymphatic vessels about the stump of the SMA are divided so that a vascular clamp can be placed 1 cm superior to its origin (Figs. 12.27, 12.28).

The inferior vena cava bifurcation is dissected free. Two umbilical tapes are passed about both the aorta and the vena cava. The donor is heparinized. The ureters are divided distally, close to the bladder, and a culture of each is taken. The aorta and the vena cava are ligated distally and cannulated proximally with a flanged aortic cannula and a medium chest tube, respectively (Figs. 12.29, 12.30). The aorta proximal to the SMA is crossclamped with a vascular clamp as the aortic flush is begun and the caval cannula is allowed to drain, exsanguinating the donor and cooling the kidneys. Currently, cold flush (2 to 4 liters) is used for an adult donor.

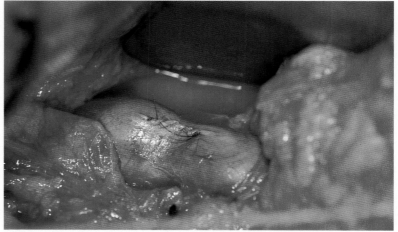

12.26

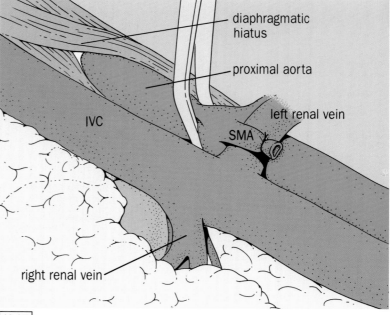

diaphragmatic hiatus

proximal aorta

left renal vein

IVC

SMA

right renal vein

12.27

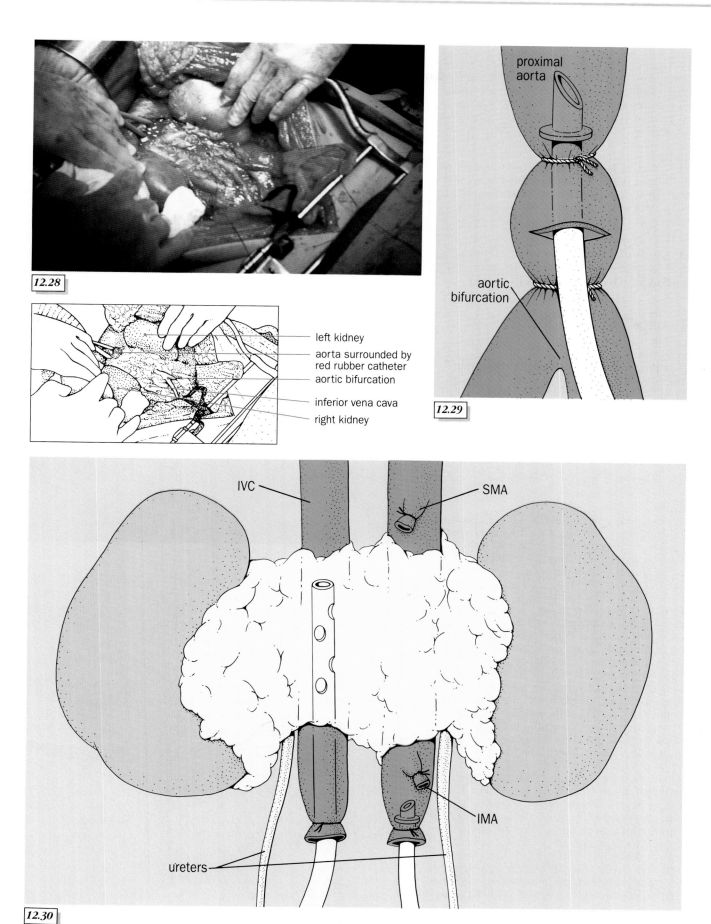

12.28

left kidney
aorta surrounded by red rubber catheter
aortic bifurcation
inferior vena cava
right kidney

proximal aorta

aortic bifurcation

12.29

IVC

SMA

IMA

ureters

12.30

The entire block of aorta and inferior vena cava with attached kidneys and ureters is removed as follows. The aorta and the vena cava are transected distal to the cannulas and are elevated. The lumbar vessels are sequentially divided, staying directly on (or in) the anterior spinal ligament and, superiorly, the diaphragmatic crura. Note that the renal arteries and a retroaortic left renal vein are *very* posterior. The dissection is continued superiorly to the level of the crossclamp, where the aorta and the vena cava are transected, and the entire block is removed (Fig. 12.31).

On the back table the block is split. Multiple renal arteries are more easily and safely identified from within the aorta. The posterior midline of the aorta is opened and the lumen examined for multiple arteries (Fig. 12.32). The anterior midline of the aorta is then opened, protecting the left renal vein. The inferior vena cava is opened in a similar fashion, or preferably the left renal vein is taken off with a small cuff of vena cava. The kidneys are sterilely packaged.

CADAVER MULTIPLE-ORGAN DONOR—HEPATECTOMY

CADAVER MULTIPLE-ORGAN DONOR—HEPATECTOMY

INDICATIONS
- brain death
- heart-beating cadaver with adequate renal and hepatic function
- appropriate liver recipient (size- and blood group-compatible)

POSITIONING
- supine

PREP
- Betadine prep from chin to pubis and to table on both sides

PROCEDURE

The much larger exposure in this procedure makes the kidney dissection easier. The technique for liver retrieval involves four stages: (1) initial essential steps; (2) optional steps, postponed until after the cold flush if the donor is not stable (rapid flush technique); (3) cannulation and cold flush; and (4) completion of dissection and removal of the organs.

INITIAL STEPS

A midline incision from the suprasternal notch to the pubis is made and the sternum is split. The pericardium is opened down to the diaphragm and the diaphragm is divided for 1 to 2 cm. A sternal retractor and a large Balfour retractor are placed. The falciform ligament is ligated and divided.

The left triangular ligament is divided to the midline with the cautery. Then the arterial supply to the liver is assessed with the following maneuvers. The lesser omentum is opened, and a left hepatic artery from the left gastric artery, which runs across the lesser omentum with the hepatic vagal fibers (Fig. 12.33), is searched for (Fig. 12.34). If the artery is present, it is carefully preserved, dissecting it back to the left gastric artery and celiac axis. The porta hepatis is then palpated between two fingers, feeling for the "normal" proper hepatic artery and for a branch from the SMA. When an SMA branch is present, it is posterior and medial to the common bile duct and lateral to the portal vein (see Fig. 12.33, inset). A branch from the SMA will be in this location regardless of its size; that is, whether it is an accessory right, replaced right, or replaced proper hepatic artery.

The supraceliac aorta is then controlled. In the stable donor, the common hepatic artery is identified at the medial edge of the porta hepatis, and its anterior surface is traced to the celiac axis and aorta with the cautery and sharp dissection. In the unstable donor, the diaphragmatic crura over the aorta are directly opened with the cautery and the aorta is thus exposed. Exposure must be adequate to place a crossclamp, but the aorta need not be circumferentially dissected free.

OPTIONAL STEPS

Such steps make the "cold" dissection easier and quicker, but are not essential. The first option is the dissection of the anterior aspect of the arteries described previously.

Next, freeing the retroperitoneal attachments of the midgut by dividing the right line of Toldt and the line of insertion of the small bowel mesentery allows the bowel to be reflected superiorly. This provides complete exposure of the inferior vena cava and the aorta. The renal veins are identified where they enter the inferior vena cava. The SMA is isolated and encircled more than 3 cm from the aorta. Because a hepatic artery from the SMA is its first branch, located within 2 cm of its origin, this is a safe place to control and later ligate the SMA.

CANNULATION AND FLUSH

Except in pediatric donors (less than 25 kg), a portal cannula is placed via the inferior mesenteric vein at the ligament of Treitz. The largest cannula that the inferior mesenteric vein can accommodate is inserted. (Sizes range from IV extension tubing to a 14-French flanged aortic cannula.) The aortic and caval bifurcations are dissected free. The patient is heparinized and aortic and caval cannulas are placed as described earlier for cadaver renal harvest (see Figs. 12.29, 12.30). Note that if there is no heart retrieval or if the cardiac surgeon agrees, the inferior vena cava can be vented into the pericardium instead of placing a caval cannula.

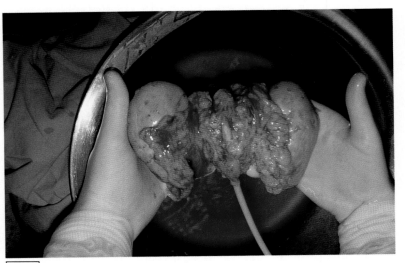

12.31

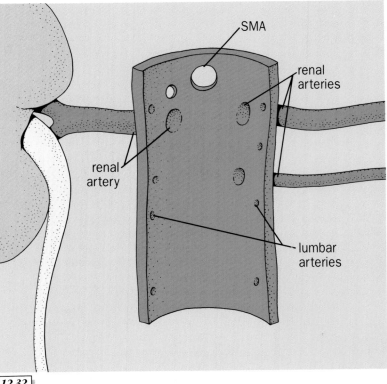

12.32

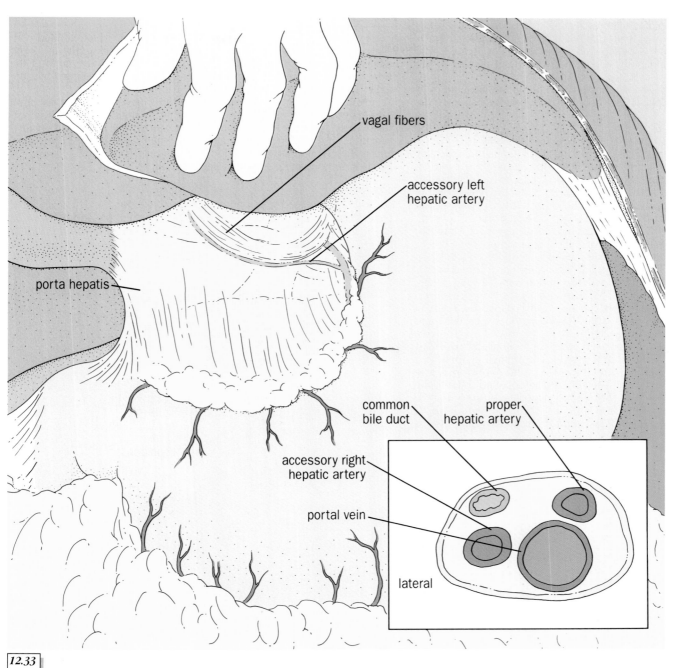

vagal fibers

accessory left
hepatic artery

porta hepatis

common
bile duct

proper
hepatic artery

accessory right
hepatic artery

portal vein

lateral

12.33

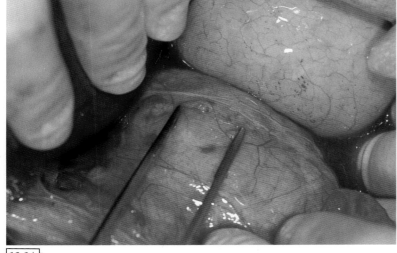

12.34

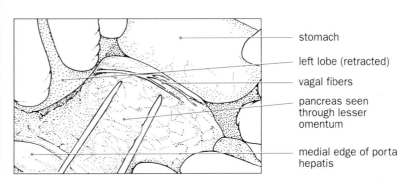

stomach

left lobe (retracted)

vagal fibers

pancreas seen
through lesser
omentum

medial edge of porta
hepatis

At the chosen time, the supraceliac aorta is cross-clamped and the flushes are begun (Fig. 12.35). If no caval cannula is used, the right atrium is opened widely to vent the vena cava. The distal SMA is ligated. The viscera are topically cooled with several liters of slush placed in the peritoneum.

Because composition of flush solutions is in evolution, no prescription is given. However, the principle of rapid cooling and exsanguination of the organs is constant.

COMPLETION OF DISSECTION AND REMOVAL OF ORGANS

The principle is to remove the liver quickly and with minimal trauma. Any fine surgery is best delayed and done on the back table with perfect lighting and exposure. Arterial and portal tributaries may be ligated if desired, but they may simply be cut long and ligated on the back table.

The cold dissection is begun after the heart (if donated) is excised. The common hepatic artery and the celiac axis are dissected free. The porta hepatis is dissected along the duodenum—never superiorly toward the liver. The gastroduodenal artery is divided. The common bile duct is divided distally. The gallbladder is opened and irrigated with cold solution until the effluent from the bile duct is clear. An SMA branch to the liver is searched for between the bile duct and the portal vein (see Fig. 12.33, inset). If none is found, the portal vein is dissected to its origin and transected. The aorta is opened distal to the celiac axis, and a segment that includes the celiac axis and extends proximally is dissected and transected, completing the hilar dissection.

If an SMA branch is found, it is traced inferiorly behind the pancreas. The SMA is dissected from its origin distally, the branch is identified (always the first on the right side of the SMA), and the branch and proximal SMA are freed completely. The aorta is then opened distal to the SMA, taking only a Carrel patch of SMA and celiac axis and protecting the very close orifices of the renal arteries.

Using heavy scissors, the pericardium around the inferior vena cava is divided. The diaphragm is divided, leaving diaphragm on the "bare area" (Fig. 12.36). The inferior vena cava is transected just above the insertions of the renal veins (taking half of the right adrenal gland). The retroportal lymphatic vessels are divided and the liver is removed. On the back table, the biliary tree and vessels are reflushed if desired, and the organ is sterilely packaged for transport. The iliac vessels also are removed for use as conduits, if needed. Then the kidneys are removed.

In the recipient operating room, the diaphragm is removed, the vessels are dissected free, and all branches are tied (Fig. 12.37). The common bile duct is never dissected.

RENAL TRANSPLANTATION

RENAL TRANSPLANTATION	
INDICATIONS	• chronic renal failure in a patient sufficiently healthy for surgery and immunosuppression
ANESTHESIA	• general endotracheal
POSITIONING	• supine
PREP	• abdominal skin prepped and draped with towels • for recipients of living-related kidneys, ipsilateral proximal thigh is prepped and draped into the field so that the saphenous vein is available to augment short vessels, if necessary

PROCEDURE

A Foley catheter is sterilely inserted into the bladder, which is filled with approximately 200 mL of saline containing neomycin (2 g/300 mL). The catheter is clamped, connected to long tubing with a Kelly clamp at the end, and then unclamped. The long tubing and clamp are draped into the sterile field (Fig. 12.38).

The most common procedure is described, namely, that for an adult recipient of a first or second cadaver donor kidney transplant. Special circumstances (such as living-related donor, pediatric recipient, retransplantation, and ileal loop) are mentioned where appropriate. The procedure is divided into four segments: (1) exposure, (2) back-table work, (3) revascularization, and (4) ureteral implantation.

EXPOSURE

The kidney is placed extraperitoneally into the right or left iliac fossa. (Exceptions to this occur in small children, when the ureter is to be placed into an ileal loop, or for other special cases in which the kidney may be placed intraperitoneally.) The right side is slightly preferred, as the iliac vein is deeper on the left. Either kidney (right or left) may be placed on either side.

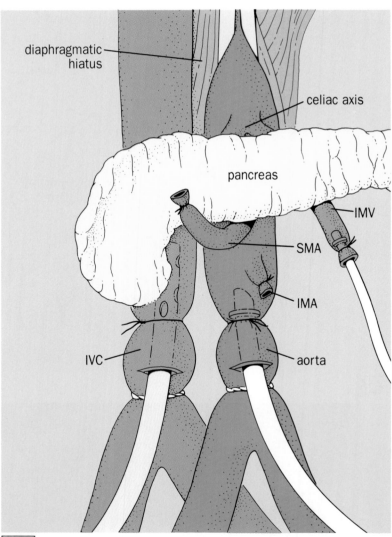

12.35

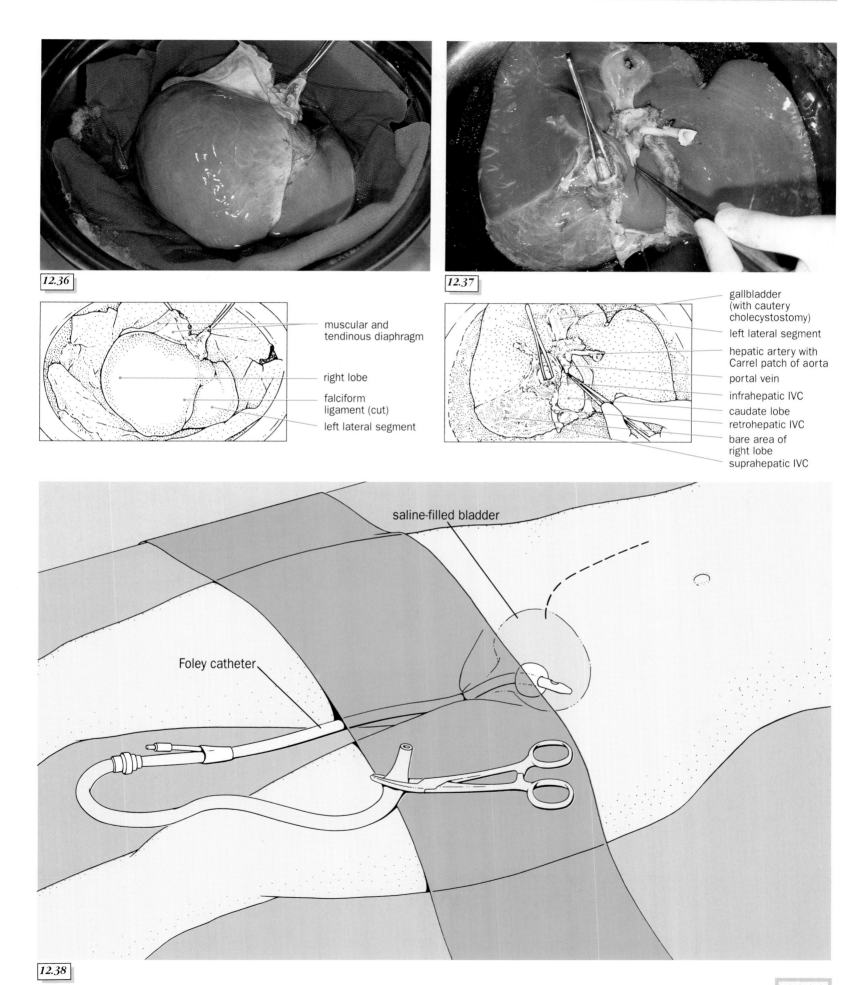

12.36

muscular and
tendinous diaphragm

right lobe

falciform
ligament (cut)

left lateral segment

12.37

gallbladder
(with cautery
cholecystostomy)

left lateral segment

hepatic artery with
Carrel patch of aorta

portal vein

infrahepatic IVC

caudate lobe

retrohepatic IVC

bare area of
right lobe

suprahepatic IVC

saline-filled bladder

Foley catheter

12.38

For optimal exposure, a J-shaped incision is used, which begins 1 cm above the symphysis pubis and extends obliquely to the linea semilunaris and then vertically (Fig. 12.39). The advantages of the J incision are discussed later. The linea semilunaris is palpable as the lateral edge of the rectus muscle. The direction of the linea is variable, more medial and vertical in men, more lateral and oblique in parous women, and intermediate in nulliparous women.

The incision is carried to the fascia and hemostasis is obtained with the cautery. The anterior rectus sheath is opened and the rectus muscle divided with the cautery to the midline. The linea semilunaris is then identified and opened as follows. Both above and below the linea semicircularis, the linea semilunaris includes the aponeuroses of three muscles (the external and internal obliques and the transversus abdominus) plus the transversalis fascia. As the muscles are aponeurotic, no further muscle need be divided (Fig. 12.40).

Beginning at the point where the lateral edge of the rectus is exposed, the posterior leaf of the internal oblique aponeurosis, the transversus abdominus aponeurosis, and the transversalis fascia are successfully opened for entrance into the preperitoneal space. Gentle blunt dissection is used to reflect the peritoneum medially, and the entire incision is opened.

The retroperitoneal space is opened and deepened down to the psoas muscle using gentle blunt and sharp dissection to reflect the peritoneum medially. The spermatic cord is always preserved in men. In women, the round ligament is divided. The epigastric vessels should be preserved, if possible. The surgeon's hands point directly posteriorly to develop the retroperitoneal plane (Fig. 12.41). The fat lateral to the psoas muscle, which is quite bulky in obese patients, can be left in place with correspondingly less bleeding. If the blunt dissection is done carefully, the bridging vessels can be cauterized as they are stretched, avoiding any oozing. For reoperations, this plane must be developed solely with sharp dissection. The entire incision is deepened to the level of the psoas and then self-retaining retractors are placed (Fig. 12.42). An upper-hand retractor is used superiorly, usually with the malleable blade, and a large aneurysm-type Balfour retractor with interchangeable blades is used below. A shallow blade is used laterally against the ileum (a deep blade slides out) and a deep blade medially for the peritoneum. Minimal dissection is required to create a pocket for the kidney.

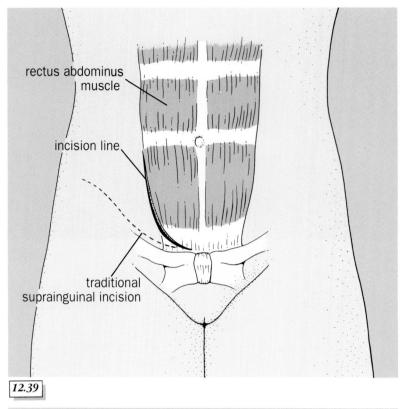

12.39

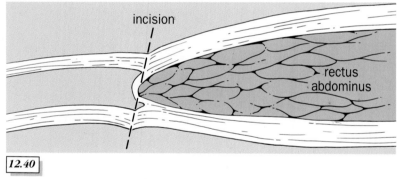

12.40

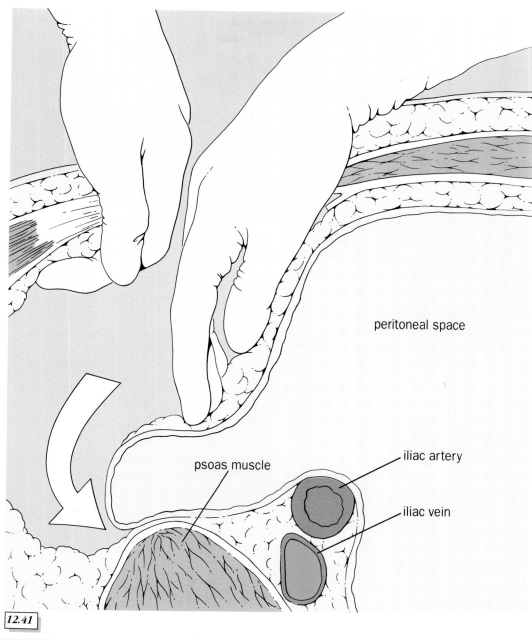

peritoneal space

psoas muscle

iliac artery

iliac vein

12.41

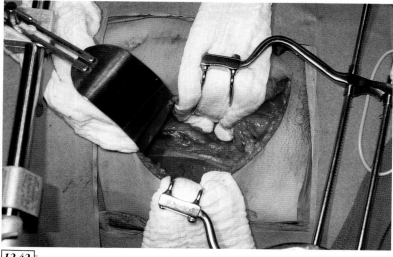

12.42

The iliac vessels (Fig. 12.43) are dissected free of surrounding lymphatics. The genitofemoral nerve runs with the lymphatics between the medial edge of the psoas and the right common iliac artery, and must be preserved (Fig. 12.44). The lymphatic vessels are preferentially reflected rather than divided, though the remaining tissue is divided between silk ties to avoid lymphatic leaks and collections. As only end-to-side anastomoses are used, the internal iliac artery is not dissected. The optimal position on the iliac vessels is chosen, and the minimal length of vessels needed is exposed. The artery is freed circumferentially and reflected medially, whereas the vein is dissected only on its anterior two thirds. The internal iliac vein usually is not dissected. Infrequently, a short renal vein (usually from a living-related donor) will require division of the internal iliac veins to elevate the external iliac vein from the depths of the pelvis. This technique (Fig. 12.45) requires careful isolation of the one to three posterior venous branches in the depths of the pelvis. As these branches are very short, only one tie is placed on each. The iliac vein is clamped proximal and distal to the branches. The branches are then cut on the iliac side, the iliac vein is elevated and rotated, and the posterior holes are sewn under direct vision. This completes the exposure.

This exposure has two advantages over the traditional suprainguinal incision. First, much less muscle is transected, with less time and effort spent to control bleeding. Second, this exposure allows the surgeon to choose any location for the vascular anastomoses, from the bifurcation of the vena cava and the aorta above, to the inguinal ligament below. In general, the anastomoses are placed higher (on the common iliac vessels) in a narrower pelvis and lower (on the external iliac vessels) in a wider pelvis. The location is adjustable to compensate for atherosclerotic plaques, short vessel or ureteral length, scarring from prior transplantation, or other anatomic variations.

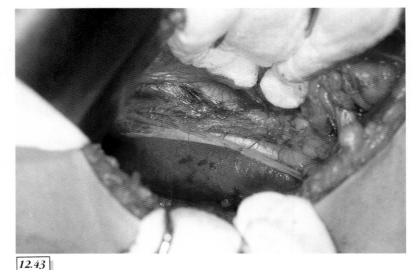

12.43

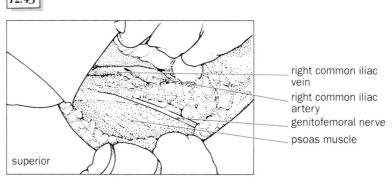

right common iliac vein
right common iliac artery
genitofemoral nerve
psoas muscle

superior

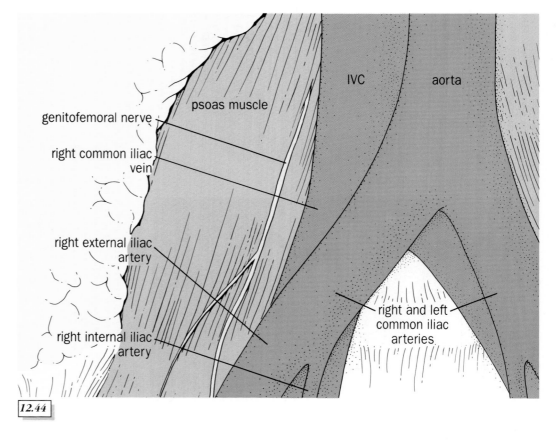

genitofemoral nerve
right common iliac vein
right external iliac artery
right internal iliac artery

psoas muscle
IVC
aorta
right and left common iliac arteries

12.44

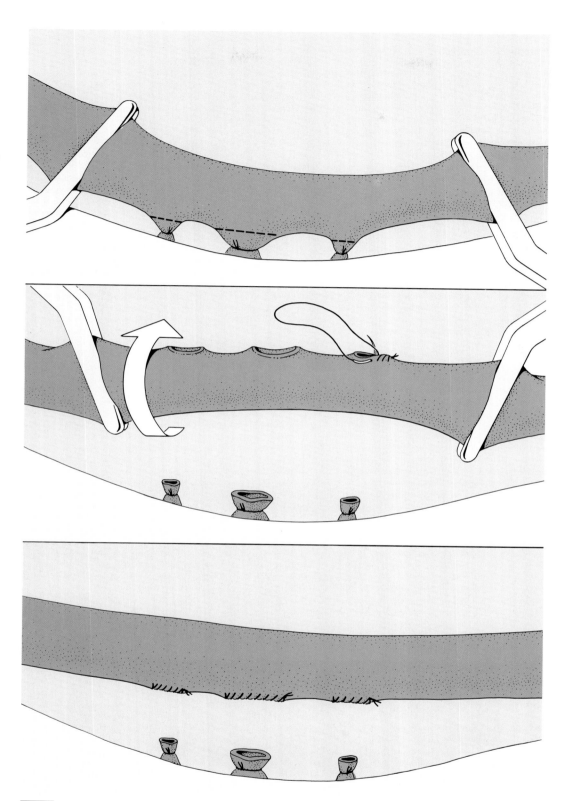

12.45

RENAL TRANSPLANTATION

12.19

BACK TABLE

The kidney is sterilely removed from storage and the perfusion solution is cultured. The vein and then the artery are dissected from the great vessel toward the hilum, ligating all branches with silk. Great care is taken to preserve the ureteral blood supply. On the artery, no branch is ligated until there is certainty that it supplies no renal parenchyma or the ureter. If there are multiple veins, the smaller one(s) can be ligated. For living-related donor kidneys, the vein can be lengthened, if necessary, with autogenous saphenous vein. One of two variations, a longitudinal sleeve technique (Fig. 12.46) or a transverse cuff technique (Fig. 12.47) can be used.

If there are multiple renal arteries, they are joined so that only one arterial anastomosis is made to the recipient. Several techniques to reconstruct the arterial supply may be used. Multiple adjacent arteries can be included on a single large Carrel patch (Fig. 12.48). If two arteries are too far apart, "excess" aorta can be removed and a single patch recreated (Fig. 12.49). A transected polar artery, usually having length enough only to reach the main renal artery, may be implanted therein (Fig. 12.50). Finally, two arteries (without patches) can be joined by slitting their nearest sides to create a large "pair-of-pants" anastomosis (Fig. 12.51), a reconstruction generally used for living-related kidneys.

REVASCULARIZATION

The kidney is placed in the pocket on a cardiac insulating pad cut to size (Fig. 12.52). Stay sutures are generally avoided. The kidney is not "flopped" from side to side, avoiding both the time lost in changing exposure and the chance of entangling sutures.

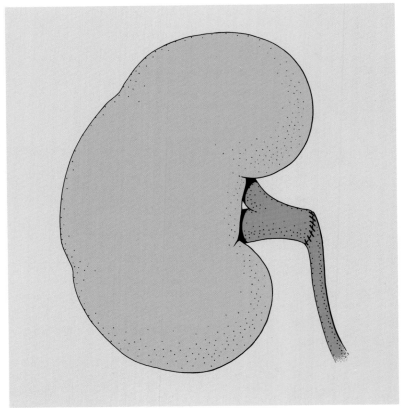

12.46

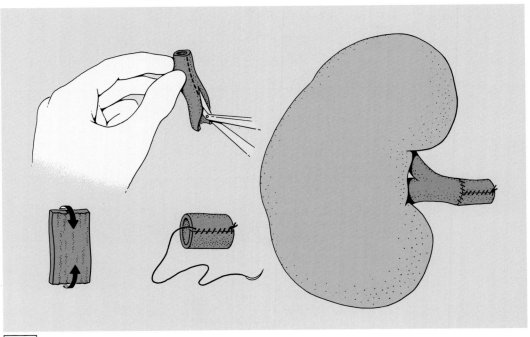

12.47

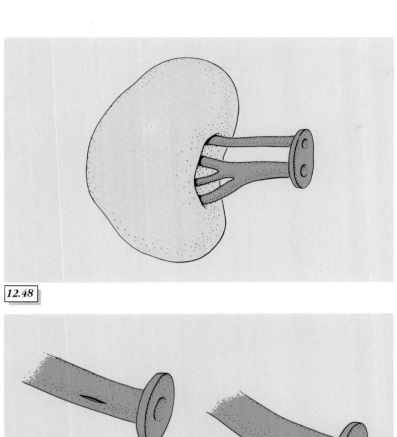

12.48

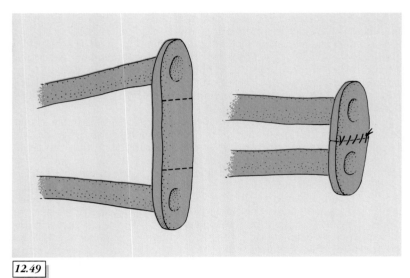

12.49

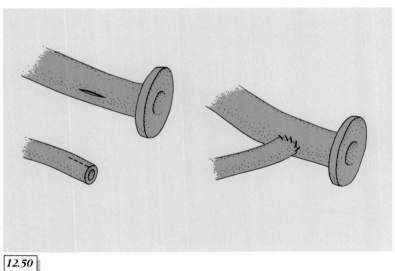

12.50

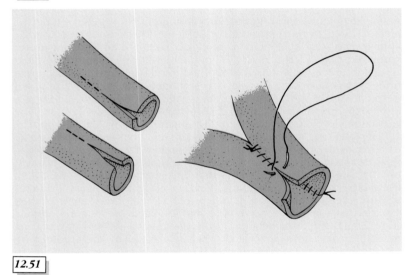

12.51

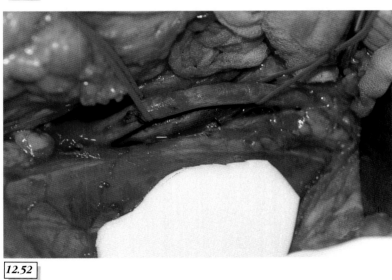

12.52

The venous anastomosis is always done first. The artery is retracted medially, a side-biting clamp is placed on the iliac vein (usually a Kay or Kay–Lembert clamp), and a longitudinal venotomy is made (Fig. 12.53A). The vein is carefully aligned to avoid any twist (and trimmed if necessary, although this is rare), and the cephalad corner stitch is placed (Fig. 12.53B). The back wall is then sewn from within with a single running stitch of 5–0 or 6–0 polypropylene suture (Fig. 12.53C), which is continued onto the front wall (Fig. 12.53D).

A Henle clamp is placed across the renal vein, the side-biting clamp removed, and the anastomosis checked for hemostasis (Fig. 12.54). Usually, the patient is then given systemic heparin (one fifth the usual dosage). The chosen segment of iliac artery is occluded above and below with vascular clamps. The arterial anastomosis is then performed in an identical manner to that described earlier (see Fig. 12.53E). Prior to tying, the clamps are released briefly to flush out any debris, while the renal artery is occluded gently with forceps. After tying, the arterial clamps are released, again occluding the renal artery briefly. The artery and vein are then opened simultaneously. With this technique, residents and fellows can perform this operation with adequate exposure and with warm ischemia times that average less than 40 minutes.

URETERAL IMPLANTATION

A simplified extravesical ureteroneocystostomy is used. After a tunnel is created deep to the epigastric vessels, the ureter is trimmed to the appropriate length; its accompanying vessel is tied and the ureter spatulated (Fig. 12.55A, inset). Bluntly and with the cautery, the fat is cleared from the superolateral area of the bladder and a stab cystotomy is made with a hemostat. The mucosa is grasped with an Allis clamp and elevated (Fig. 12.55A). A small feeding tube (5- or 8-French) is used as a temporary stent and is placed into the ureter and bladder. The anastomosis is performed with 4–0 PDS suture in a triangular fashion. The two running legs are begun with two sutures, both at the apex of the ureteral spatulation, and each runs one third of the way around, taking small bites on the ureter and large full-thickness bites on the bladder; each is then tied (Fig. 12.55B,C). The remaining one third is done with interrupted sutures, all placed and held untied. It is vital that all sutures include ureteral and bladder mucosa. The temporary stent is then extracted with an Adson nerve hook and the interrupted sutures are tied (Fig. 12.55D). The watertightness of the anastomosis is tested by retrieving the tubing attached to the bladder catheter and filling the bladder with saline colored with indigo carmine. (Note that if there is initial difficulty in identifying the bladder, further filling of the bladder via this tubing will make it easier to find and to perform the stab cystotomy.) A urometer is attached to the tubing.

Meticulous hemostasis is obtained, with careful checking of the pocket and both sides of the renal hilum. A closed suction drain is brought through a separate stab incision and placed posterior to the kidney down to the bladder. The wound is closed with a single layer of running #1 PDS suture in fascia, running 3–0 absorbable suture in Scarpa's fascia, and staples for the skin.

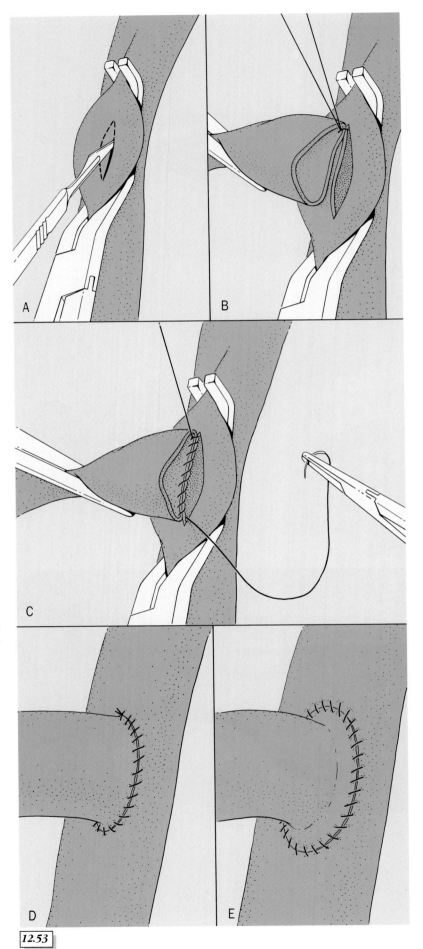

12.53

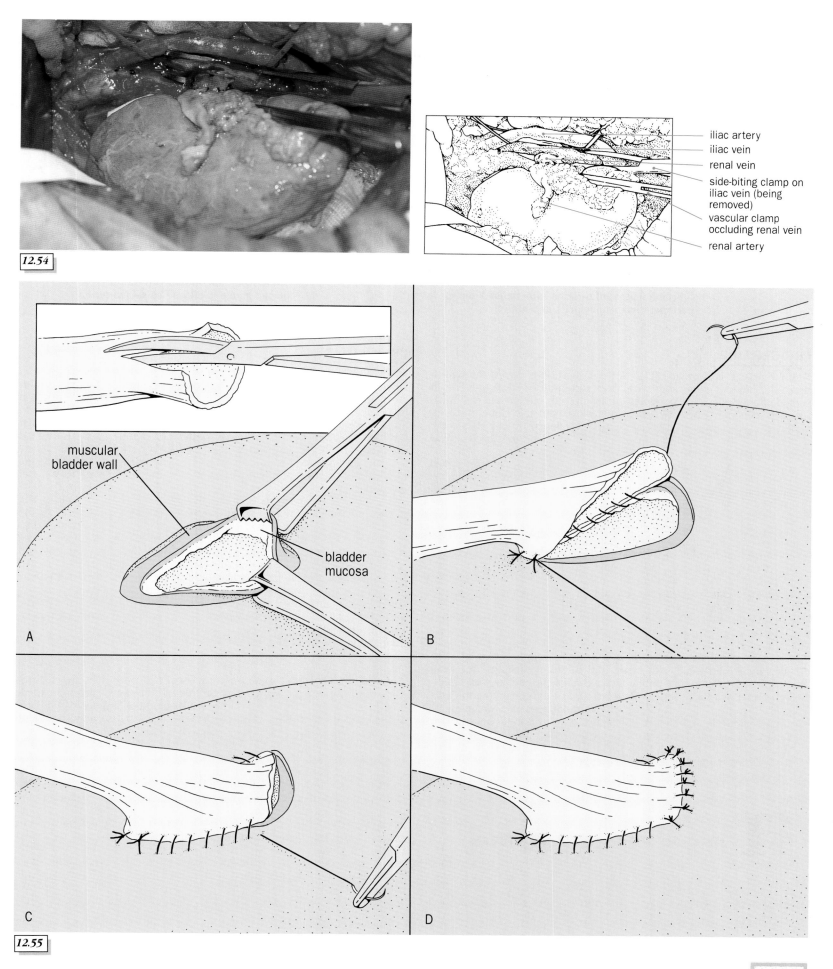

iliac artery
iliac vein
renal vein
side-biting clamp on
iliac vein (being
removed)
vascular clamp
occluding renal vein
renal artery

12.54

muscular
bladder wall

bladder
mucosa

A

B

C

D

12.55

TRANSPLANT NEPHRECTOMY

TRANSPLANT NEPHRECTOMY

INDICATIONS	•acute rejection unresponsive to antirejection therapy •symptomatic chronic rejection (pain, infection, hematuria, fever) •primary graft nonfunction
ANESTHESIA	•general endotracheal
POSITIONING	•supine
PREP	•Betadine prep to abdomen •Foley catheter inserted only if patient makes substantial amount of urine from native kidneys •perioperative prophylactic antibiotics

PROCEDURE

The old incision is reopened (Fig. 12.56). Dissection is carried through the skin, subcutaneous tissue, and fascia. Great care must be taken to reflect the peritoneum medially, as it is densely adherent to the abdominal wall in this area. Dissection is carried sharply downward onto the kidney (see Fig. 12.56). The subcapsular plane can then be developed by blunt dissection. The kidney is freed gently throughout, until it can be mobilized upward (delivered) into the wound.

Care is taken to avoid any manipulation of the hilum. No attempt is made to isolate the iliac vessels or the anastomoses, as troublesome and dangerous bleeding may ensue. The renal and iliac vessels are generally very soft and friable, and demand great respect. A large Crafoord clamp is placed across the renal parenchyma adjacent to the hilum of the kidney. A second Crafoord clamp is carefully positioned below the first one. The kidney is then transected and removed from the field. Cultures of the kidney should be obtained at this time. The superficial Crafoord clamp is then removed. To obtain control more proximally, the clamp can be placed deep to the other Crafoord clamp, and the more superficial of the two removed. With careful sharp dissection, the remaining renal parenchyma is removed. The branches of the renal artery and vein are identified and oversewn with 4–0 or 5–0 polypropylene sutures or tied with silk. Again, no attempt is made to visualize or to remove the main renal vessels. Leaving this small portion of grafted tissue does not cause problems. The ureter is then identified, traced distally as far as possible, ligated, divided, and removed.

The wound is irrigated with saline and carefully examined for hemostasis. Small bleeding points on the retained renal capsule are cauterized. A closed suction drain is placed in the renal space and brought out through a lateral stab wound. The fascia is closed with running #1 PDS suture and the skin with staples. A baseline ultrasound is obtained on the third postoperative day and the drain is removed after this time if there is minimal drainage. The patient is observed closely for signs of sepsis or bleeding during the first 48 hours postoperatively.

HEPATIC TRANSPLANTATION

Orthotopic liver transplantation has become more common due to recent improvements in technique and to the introduction of cyclosporine as an immunosuppressant. This procedure is a technical tour de force, requiring from 6 to 12 hours. The success of the procedure is strongly dependent on the proper execution of each step. Failure to perform each step correctly may result in loss of the patient. Therefore, attention to every detail is critical.

HEPATIC TRANSPLANTATION

INDICATIONS	•fulminant liver failure •chronic liver failure (eg, cirrhosis, biliary atresia)
CONTRA-INDICATIONS	•thrombosis of portal and superior mesenteric veins •sepsis, malignancy
ANESTHESIA	•general endotracheal
POSITIONING	•supine
PREP	•entire abdomen, both groins, and left axilla prepped and draped into field •Thompson table-mounted retractor placed above to elevate costal margins (Fig. 12.57)

PROCEDURE

RECIPIENT HEPATECTOMY

Two arterial lines, at least four venous lines, and a Foley catheter are inserted. A hypothermic patient is more prone to cardiac arrest and to other complications during this prolonged procedure. Therefore, all intravenous products administered during the procedure must be warmed. Moreover, the room is kept much warmer than usual, and the patient's legs, arms, and head are wrapped in foil insulators to maintain core temperature above 34°C. The patient is moved to the right side of the operating room table. The arms are extended to 90°, but no further.

The bilateral subcostal incision extends from the right midaxillary line to the left midclavicular line, and also is extended superiorly in the midline to the xyphoid (Fig. 12.58). In making the incision, many collaterals in the subcutaneous tissue must be controlled. The xyphoid may be removed. Once the abdomen is open, the falciform ligament and associated collaterals are ligated and divided. The abdomen is explored briefly, but since many patients have vascular adhesions, exploration may not be safe to perform. While subsequent steps are present here in a certain order, in general the easier steps are performed earlier and the more difficult ones performed later. The order varies from patient to patient, depending on previous surgery, degree of adhesions, and other intra-abdominal findings. Hemostasis is crucial, and the cautery is used liberally.

PORTA HEPATIS DISSECTION. If the patient has not had prior right upper quadrant surgery, the porta hepatis may be free of adhesions, allowing expedient dissection. The first step is to place a hand in the foramen of Winslow and obtain digital control of the portal structures. Dissection should be carried out away from the duodenum and toward the liver to avoid the small vessels along the duodenum. The dissection is initiated on the common bile duct, at or above the level of the cystic duct entrance. The common duct is ligated and divided high, preserving length caudally. The dissection proceeds to the left side of the porta hepatis, where the hepatic artery is dissected and divided, leaving a stump for revascularization of the graft. The hepatic artery is ligated and divided with a long silk tie on the stump (Figs. 12.59, 12.60; note that in the case shown the patient's proper hepatic artery arose from the SMA and thus it is to the right of the portal vein). The portal vein is dissected, but not ligated. Tissue posterior to the portal vein should be divided to skeletonize the portal vein. Small branches on the anterior surface of the portal vein draining the pancreas may be present, and are ligated to avoid tearing during later clamp placement.

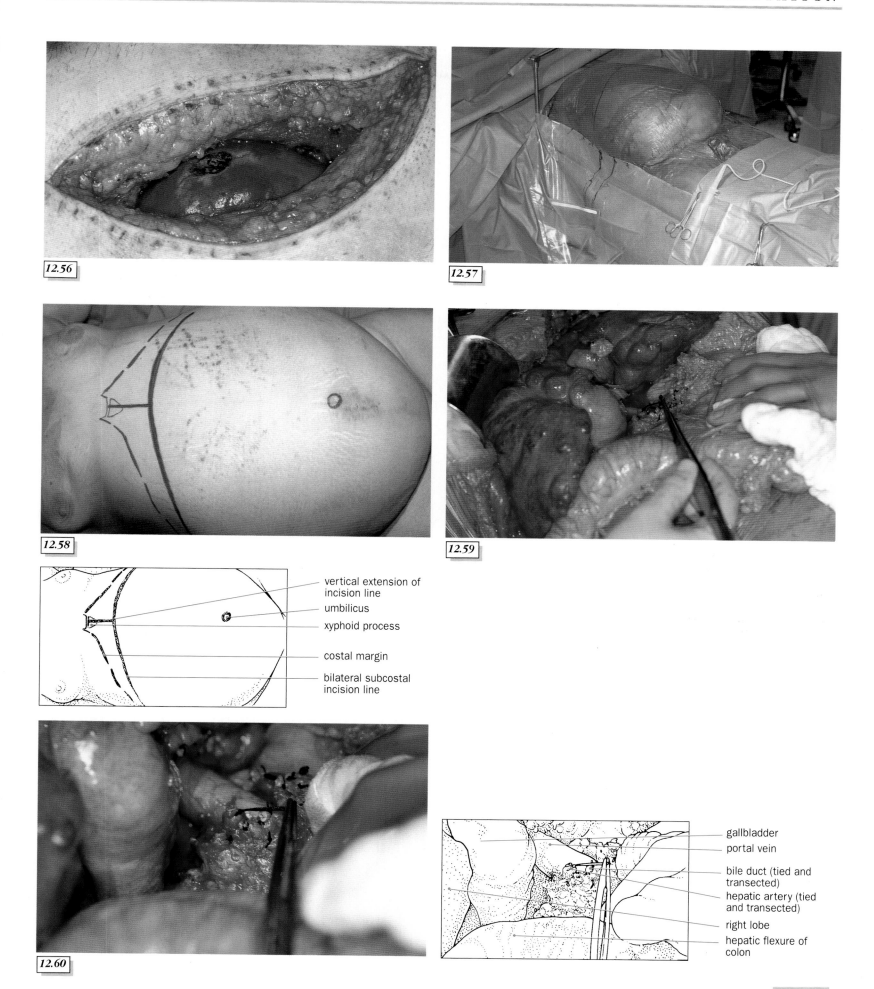

12.56

12.57

12.58

vertical extension of
incision line

umbilicus

xyphoid process

costal margin

bilateral subcostal
incision line

12.59

12.60

gallbladder

portal vein

bile duct (tied and
transected)

hepatic artery (tied
and transected)

right lobe

hepatic flexure of
colon

SUPRAHEPATIC DISSECTION. The next area for dissection is the suprahepatic portion of the liver. The left triangular ligament attachments to the diaphragm are divided. Dissection then proceeds anterior to the suprahepatic inferior vena cava down to the ligamentous portion of the diaphragm enveloping the vena cava. This ligament is left attached, allowing a firmer grip for the vena cava clamp when it is applied later. The right triangular ligament is divided, exposing the bare area of the liver. Full mobilization of the right lobe of the liver allows better exposure of the retrohepatic inferior vena cava, making its dissection safer.

INFRAHEPATIC INFERIOR VENA CAVA EXPOSURE. Once the liver is mobile, exposure of the infrahepatic inferior vena cava becomes easier but should be performed with caution. In patients with severe portal hypertension or previous surgery, this area may be treacherous. Also, mobilization and displacement of the liver from its fossa distorts the vena cava, impairs venous return, and may cause hypotension. Minimal dissection is performed to avoid the many varices present. Posterior to the portal vein, the peritoneum over the vena cava is opened. The anterior surface of the infrahepatic vena cava is identified. Dissection proceeds anteriorly and cephalad until either the liver or the small hepatic veins are encountered. Dissection proceeds on the right side of the vena cava, staying high to avoid injury to the right renal vein. Once the lateral vena cava has been cleared, the vena cava may be encircled with a finger and its left side identified. The inferior vena cava is then surrounded with a Penrose drain (Fig. 12.61). Many lymph nodes may be present in this area. The left renal vein is below the dissection and does not come into view.

POSTERIOR RETROHEPATIC INFERIOR VENA CAVA EXPOSURE. Exposure of this portion of the abdomen may be difficult in the patient with a large liver, a narrow rib cage, or multiple adhesions, who (rarely) requires a right thoracotomy for exposure. In general, a broad approach to the inferior vena cava from the right side of the liver is advocated to minimize the risk of uncontrollable bleeding due to poor exposure. The goal is to identify the right adrenal vein, which may enter the vena cava at any level between the right renal vein and the diaphragm. This vein is carefully ligated and divided. Then, the posterior vena cava can easily be swept free of tissue under direct vision. This allows the surgeon to encircle the suprahepatic vena cava, while visualizing the entire area. Occasionally, this step is extremely treacherous because of previous surgery or multiple varices in the area. The liver is mobilized at this stage (Fig. 12.62).

If the posterior hepatic areas cannot be safely dissected, both the suprahepatic and the infrahepatic inferior vena cava must be controlled before one can proceed. However, the dissection of the entire area does not have to be performed at this time. Rather, the liver can be removed and then access to and hemostasis of the area obtained. At this point, the donor liver should be ready for implantation.

SHUNTING. Crossclamping the inferior vena cava is essential to removal of the liver. This prevents venous return from the lower body to the heart, producing profound effects on hemodynamics. The issue of whether a venous bypass is necessary to return blood to the heart during clamping has been approached in several ways. One approach, advocated by Starzl and Shaw, has been to bypass routinely. A second approach is that of selective shunting, in which the suprahepatic vena cava is clamped and the patient is monitored to determine the effects of clamping. If no hypotension occurs, the patient may undergo transplantation without shunting. If significant hypotension occurs, shunting is utilized. A third approach is that of no shunting, which has been used by a number of centers also with excellent results.

For bypass, the left axillary and femoral veins are dissected free and cannulated with a closed loop of tubing, which passes from the femoral vein through a bypass pump to the left axillary vein (Fig. 12.63). A Y connector is present near the femoral end of the shunt for cannulation of the portal vein, if desired. Thus, blood from both the femoral and portal systems is shunted to the right atrium. Portal venous decompression is

usually not necessary when portal hypertension is chronic. No anticoagulation is used during this procedure. Technically, the veins should be dissected carefully because of their proximity to vital structures, and because of the importance of hemostasis for the 1 to 2 hours of shunting, at which time these incisions are hidden from the surgeon's view. Secondly, the cannulas should not be inserted until bypass is ready to be instituted. These cannulas can initiate thrombosis and/or produce pulmonary embolus.

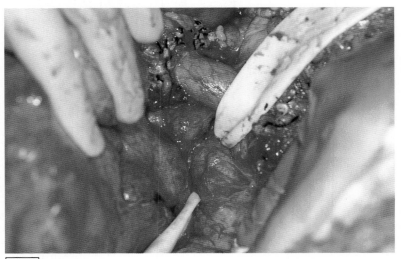

12.61

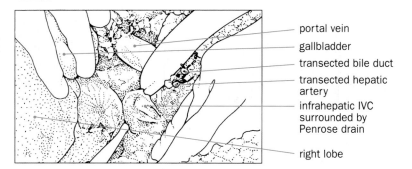

- portal vein
- gallbladder
- transected bile duct
- transected hepatic artery
- infrahepatic IVC surrounded by Penrose drain
- right lobe

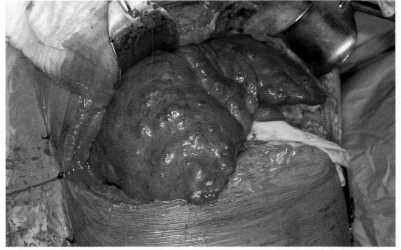

12.62

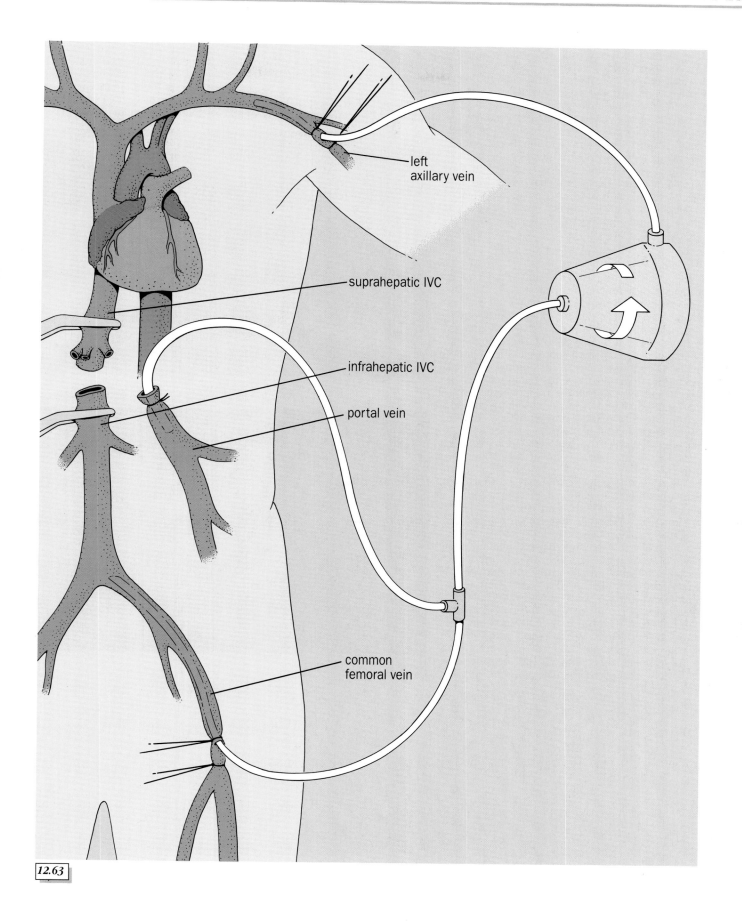

left
axillary vein

suprahepatic IVC

infrahepatic IVC

portal vein

common
femoral vein

12.63

LIVER REMOVAL. Once the liver is ready for removal, a vascular clamp is applied to the portal vein. A large Crafoord clamp is placed on the infrahepatic inferior vena cava and a large, very secure clamp (Pott's gastrointestinal forceps) is placed on the upper vena cava. It is important to place this clamp parallel to the operating table (Fig. 12.64). The liver is then excised using a knife on the upper vena caval area. An incision is made into the liver substance rather than into the vessel and a large margin of tissue is left with the clamp. The portal and infrahepatic vena cava are then transected, leaving a long length of vessel past the clamp. The liver is removed (see Fig. 12.64). Hemostasis is obtained in the retrohepatic area using 2–0 silk sutures. The suprahepatic vena cava is then prepared for suturing. A right-angle clamp is used to open each hepatic vein. This allows transection of their common septa, creating a wide cuff (Fig. 12.65). It is critical that no phrenic veins are left unattended.

LIVER REIMPLANTATION
The liver is brought into the field and the suprahepatic vena cava is sutured using 3–0 polypropylene in a running fashion (Fig. 12.66). On completion of the suprahepatic anastomosis, the liver is retracted superiorly and the infrahepatic vena cava is sutured in a similar fashion. Prior to completion of this anastomosis, 0.5 to 1 L of cold lactated Ringer's solution is infused into the portal vein and allowed to flush through the infrahepatic vena cava. The infrahepatic vena cava sutures are tied following completion of the flush. The portal venous anastomosis is then approached. First, several sponges are placed above the right dome of the liver to push the liver inferiorly and approximate the portal venous ends. The portal bypass (if used) is discontinued. The portal venous anastomosis is performed using running 5–0 or 6–0 polypropylene. Before completion, the sutures are not tied but, instead, are held under enough tension to approximate the edges loosely. The portal clamp is released briefly to vent stagnant blood from the portal vein. At this point, the clamps are ready for removal.

Advance notice must be given to the anesthesiologists so that they have the patient in optimal physiologic condition for clamp removal. This includes maintenance of blood pressure and pretreatment of the patient with calcium, bicarbonate, and other drugs in preparation for the release of potassium, acid ions, and other adverse materials by the liver. The clamps on the portal vein and the suprahepatic inferior vena cava are removed first. When the patient is stable, the infrahepatic vena caval clamp is removed. The three anastomoses are checked for major sites of hemorrhage and are controlled if necessary. The pack is removed from above the liver and the liver is warmed with warm saline to raise the core temperature. Hemostasis is rechecked. The portal venous anastomosis is inspected and allowed to dilate to its full diameter. The suture is then tied. At this point, the liver is usually pink and firm, with minimal edema. After the patient is stable and hemostasis present, the bypass (if used) is ended, the cannulas are removed, and the veins are repaired. Then, the hepatic artery is approached. The recipient hepatic

artery stump is isolated and sutured to the donor hepatic artery (with its aortic Carrel patch) using 6–0 polypropylene with magnification. The clamps are removed and the vessel is checked for pulse and thrill. If, on occasion, the hepatic artery of the recipient is either inadequate or thrombosed, a segment of vessel (iliac artery) from the donor should be used to create an anastomosis to the recipient's aorta or iliac artery.

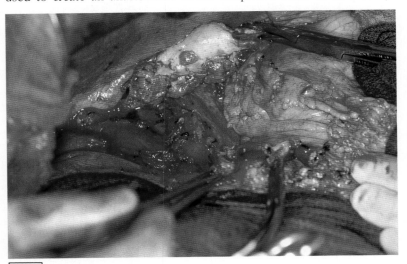

12.64

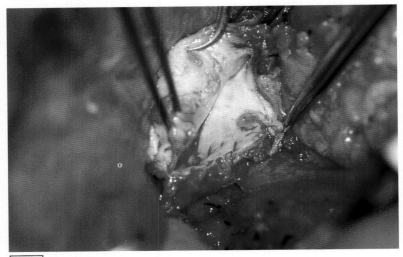

12.65

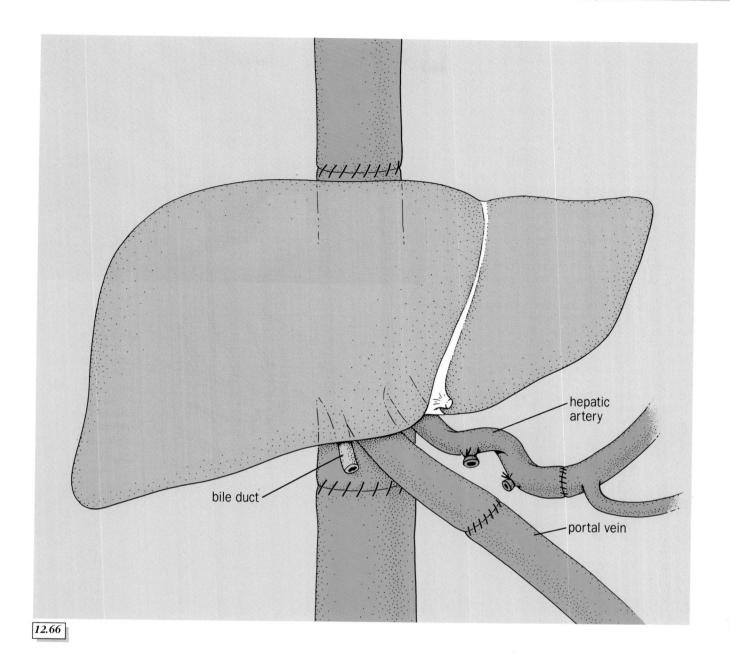

bile duct

hepatic
artery

portal vein

12.66

It is critical to have a technically excellent hepatic artery anastomosis, because thrombosis will result in graft failure. The portal vein and hepatic artery anastomoses are thus completed (Fig. 12.67; note the position of the hepatic artery medial to the portal vein; this is a different recipient from the previous photographs).

After hemostasis has again been obtained, the gallbladder is removed using the cautery. Dissection is performed to within 1 cm of the common duct—but no closer—to preserve its blood supply. In patients with no bile duct disease, the ducts may be sewn end to end (choledochocholedochostomy) (Fig. 12.68). The donor bile duct is transected flush with the surrounding tissues and is not dissected to avoid devascularization. A 5-French T-tube is inserted through the recipient bile duct, 1 to 2 cm distal to the anastomosis. This is done by placing a 2–0 silk suture through the long limb of the T-tube and inserting the needle from within the lumen of the bile duct directly through the wall. The suture is pulled through, dragging the T-tube with it (see Fig. 12.68, inset). The bile duct is sewn end to end using interrupted 5–0 polypropylene (some centers use absorbable sutures). The anastomosis is tested for watertightness by filling the duct with indigo carmine dye. A cholangiogram is performed to document patency of the anastomosis and biliary tree.

If the patient's bile duct is unacceptable, a choledochojejunostomy is performed (Fig. 12.69). A Roux-en-Y segment of bowel is created and anastomosis is created from the end of the bile duct to the side of the bowel. A short 5-French stent is placed through the anastomosis and sutured into place with a fine absorbable suture. This stent does not drain externally. The anastomosis may be performed with polypropylene or absorbable suture. The abdomen is then inspected for hemostasis. A biopsy of the liver is performed using a Tru-cut needle. Two large drains are placed above the right and left lobes of the liver in the area of the posterior hepatic dissection. A third drain is placed near the bile duct anastomosis. After hemostasis is attained, the wound is closed with running #1 PDS suture in the fascia and staples in the skin.

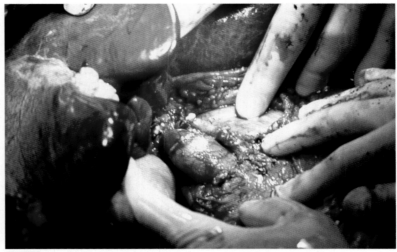

12.67

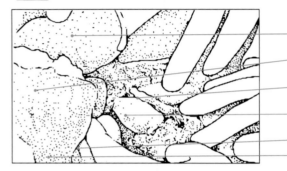

lateral segment of left lobe

median segment of left lobe

hepatic artery after anastomosis

portal vein after anastomosis

gallbladder

right lobe

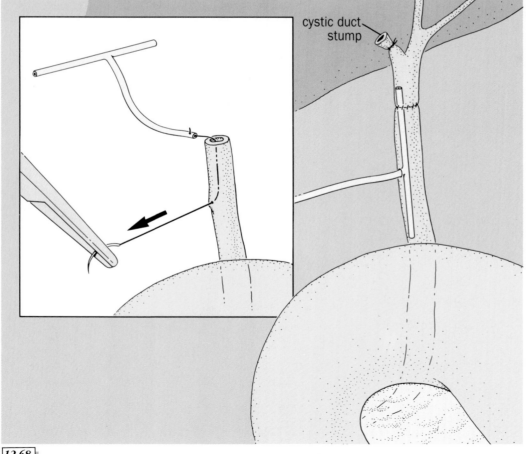

12.68

cystic duct stump

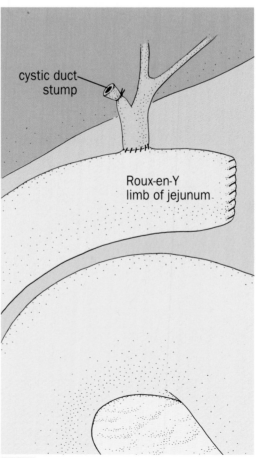

cystic duct stump

Roux-en-Y limb of jejunum

12.69

BIBLIOGRAPHY

Bay WH, Hebert LA. The living donor in kidney transplantation. In: Cerilli GJ, ed. *Organ Transplantation and Replacement*. Philadelphia, Pa: Lippincott; 1988:272–283.

Chapman JR, Allen RD. Dialysis and transplantation. In: Morris PJ, ed. *Kidney Transplantation*. 3rd ed. Philadelphia, Pa: Saunders; 1988:37–58.

Cosimi AB. The donor and donor nephrectomy. In: Morris PJ, ed. *Kidney Transplantation*. 3rd ed. Philadelphia, Pa: Saunders; 1988:93–103.

Lempert N. Cadaver kidney organ procurement. In: Cerilli GJ, ed. *Organ Transplantation and Replacement*. Philadelphia, Pa: Lippincott; 1988:287–295.

Maddrey WC, ed. *Transplantation of the Liver.* New York: Elsevier; 1988.

Ney C, Friedenberg RM, eds. *Radiographic Atlas of the Genitourinary System.* Philadelphia, Pa: Lippincott; 1981.

Waltzer WC, Rapaport FT, eds. *Angioaccess.* New York: Grune and Stratton; 1984.

Wood RP, Shaw BW. Multiple organ procurement. In: Cerilli GJ, ed. *Organ Transplantation and Replacement.* Philadelphia, Pa: Lippincott; 1988:322–336.

index